Ingeborg Stadelmann

A Consultation with a Midwife

*I would like to dedicate this book
to all the children who are being born
this very moment,
and all parents
who receive their child
in its own
way of being.*

Ingeborg Stadelmann

A Consultation with a Midwife

Sensitive, natural guidance
through pregnancy, childbirth,
the postnatal period and breastfeeding
with
herbal medicine,
homoeopathy and
aroma therapy

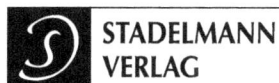

STADELMANN VERLAG

Nota bene

This book serves the purposes of elucidation, information and self-help. Every reader is called upon to decide on her own whether – and to what extent – she should follow the suggestions for action and make use of the naturopathic applications. This book is not intended, however, to replace professional advice. In cases of doubt or if an illness has already set in, a midwife or doctor must be consulted in order to determine the correct diagnosis and the corresponding treatment.

If used wrongly or in incorrect dosages, naturopathic substances can cause undesirable side effects. It is essential to pay close attention to the pointers and read the book carefully. Remember: "All things are poison and nothing is without poison; only the dosage keeps a thing from being poisonous!" (Paracelsus, alchemist and physician, 1493 – 1541)

ISBN 13: 978-3-943793-00-0
© 1994, 2005, 2013 Ingeborg Stadelmann

𝒟 Stadelmann Verlag, Nesso 8, 87487 Wiggensbaach
Fax +49 (0)8370/8896
www.stadelmann-verlag.de
E-Mail: info@stadelmann-verlag.de

Translation of the third german printing of the thoroughly revised edition 2006
Illustrations: Torill Glimsdal-Eberspacher, Betzigau
Editing: Marina Burwitz, Munich

Translation by Judith Rosenthal
English German Language Service

Annotation:
Please do not hesitate to contact us for any improvements or interests for production or distribution. We are thankful to any ideas of improvement!

Contents

Foreword to the Newly Revised Edition

It's been a long time since I held the very first copy of my first book Die *Hebammen-Sprechstunde* in my hands. To this very day, I am very proud of the fact that the book was "born" in my own publishing company. Eleven years have passed since then, and a completely revised and updated new edition is now finally finished. This task became very urgent, because through the book I grew older and more experienced. A lot has happened in the meantime. In the first version I shared my professional everyday life as a free-lance midwife, and now I would like to tell you briefly all the things that were brought about by that book.

Contrary to the prophecies of experts in the field, the book became a bestseller: more than 500,000 copies have been sold, primarily in Germany, but the *Hebammen-Sprechstunde* can be found on every continent. I would like to take this opportunity to express my sincere thanks to all the readers who contributed to this vast circulation. To this day, I don't have time for marketing activities and advertising campaigns, but the book has nevertheless come to be widely known. "Good things spread of their own accord," as one old proverb tells us, and in this case it has proven true.

According to another saying, books change the world. That's something an elderly gentleman, himself an author, told me in 1993 when I was busy writing the book. He said: "You'll see: writing books is like having children. Books bring change too, not just children." I wanted to contradict him, but he just ignored me and grumbled: "I know, you midwives see it all differently, but just you wait!" And today I am that much the wiser, because he turned out to be right. The knowledge of experienced colleagues had always been very important to me, but I have also learned to pay more attention to what older folks have to say.

Today I can confirm that books really are like children – they are demanding, they are challenging, and they constantly present us with new tasks and new adventures. And I have learned that the written word, while it patiently waits to be corrected and supplemented, also carries a lot of weight when it comes to changing old habits or treading new paths. I am accordingly very proud of the fact that, with the help of the *Hebammen-Sprechstunde*, so many births have taken a positive direction for mother and child alike. What is more, through this book, there has been an increase in the number of midwives and doctors who have an open ear for natural childbirth and natural medicine. There are even hospitals which advertise that they conduct childbirth according to the "Stadelmann method." At midwife training institutions, my book is referred to as "the other textbook" and many an applicant uses it to prepare for a job interview. It sets a counterpoint to the traditional textbooks and also serves as an important guide for embarking on the venture of self-employment. I was especially delighted when a young doctor wrote to me: "Everything that's not in the manual can be found in your book."

It is therefore understandable, that the *Hebammen-Sprechstunde* or – to use the new English title – *Consultation with a Midwife* – represents a treasure trove of information especially for expectant parents, providing them the knowledge, support and confidence they need to get through the phases of pregnancy, birth and "childbed" – the weeks and months that follow. I am pleased to have succeeded in publishing a book in comprehensible "woman talk" which is considered both a bible by parents and an indispensable guide for the young midwife. That is exactly what I hoped for when I wrote the first manuscript. Now, in the context of the revision, I am sure that the book will continue to reach that goal. Midwives tell me: "Inge, it's just terrific – I quote your book during the antenatal class and every last doubt is dispelled." Or: "I suggest to the mother that she read about the topic in your book and then we can talk about it the next time I come to call." Expectant parents write me letters or send me E-Mails from every corner of the earth, recounting how they were able to help themselves during pregnancy, birth and the postnatal phase with the aid of information from the book. But I also receive inquiries as to where a midwife can be found who works and acts in the manner I have described. When I get these requests, or the more unpleasant reports about childbirth, I always hope that every woman will find a wise midwife sooner or later.

But not only the parents and the hospitals have changed. *The Consultation with a Midwife* can also be considered a pioneering work with regard to cooperation between midwives and pharmacists. My alliance with the pharmacist Dietmar Wolz of the Bahnhof-Apotheke in Kempten (Allgaeu, Germany) has been very fruitful: my *Original D® Aromamischungen* (the registered brand name for my aroma blends) have become as well known beyond the borders of Germany as "Stadelmann's tea blends from the pharmacy in Kempten." In many places, the book has led to pharmacies' stocking not only herbs and homoeopathic medicines but also aroma blends on a regular basis. A few have tried their hand at manufacturing the products themselves, but most of them are grateful to be able to offer my originals with the guaranteed highest natural quality. Throughout Germany, an increasing number of pharmacies cultivate an exchange with self-employed midwives, thus helping to ensure that expectant mothers receive not only the care of a midwife but also competent pharmaceutical advice, responding to their individual needs and thus allowing them to face motherhood with a sense of self-assurance.

My life and that of my family likewise changed; the old man was right on that count, too. In the meantime I no longer work in my beloved "Light of Earth" but carry my light – the message contained in the *Consultation* – out into the world. I used to have to tell women that I didn't have the capacity to take on another birth and now I'm booked out way in advance as a lecturer and further-training instructor. But I gladly pass on my knowledge in the hope that it will help to increase the number of midwives who provide expectant mothers with wise, clever, woman-oriented guidance throughout this wonderful and decisive phase of their lives.

With this newly revised edition I hope to provide you, dear readers, with answers to many of the questions that arise during this unique period in which a child comes to the world. I have updated the contents and, wherever I deemed it necessary, expanded it. I have added sections, for example on prenatal diagnostics and "elective caesareans" as well as death of the newborn and coping with the mourning that follows – an emotion which is unfortunately often repressed.

And I hope to change the world a little bit more with this new edition than I did with the first edition of the *Hebammen-Sprechstunde*. Above all, I hope that an increasing number of the standard examinations carried out during pregnancy will be carried out in midwives' practices and that the number of independent birth centres offering midwife accompanied birth will also grow, thus leading to a steady – if slow – increase in the number of extra-clinical births. As far as the hospitals are concerned, I hope that family-oriented births are not only offered in their advertising brochures but that professionally trained personnel is really available so that the offers on paper can become reality. In other words: that the birthing stool is fetched out of the corner or that the child actually does come into the world in a birthing pool – at the point of time that is appropriate for mother and child and without clinical intervention. It should be a matter of course that the parents are given all the time in the world to welcome the new member of their family. It is a further great hope of mine that more women will once again decide in favour of spending the postnatal phase at home, and that the newborns experience those so very important and unique first days of their lives in the shelter of the family.

For that to happen, however, society will have to change in such a way as to allow awareness, self-determination and security to accompany the beginning of life – and not a procedure pre-established by public institutions. To be sure, home births and giving birth in an independent birthing centre are associated with additional costs. But you are certainly willing to spend more for good quality when it comes to baby clothing and bedding and the pram. So don't be "penny-wise and pound-foolish": in the same way that children are always a rewarding investment, every investment you make for your child is also worthwhile. In many European countries, incidentally, parents have to co-finance births at home or in an independent birthing unit, and here in Germany patients will have to pay for an increasing proportion of their health care – whether in or out of hospital – out of their own pockets as time goes on. If you are guided less by financial considerations than a strong need for safety, remember that our grandparents were all still born at home and obviously all survived the experience well. Our great-grandparents surely wanted the greatest possible safety for mother and child back then as well, and placed their entire faith in the competence of a midwife.

The children who are born today and go out into the world are the adults of tomorrow and they need a good foundation. In my opinion, compromises in that foundation should not be made for reasons of cost. Rather, children should be provided with as much trust and love as possible. Whenever and wherever a birth takes place, it remains a decisive event in the shaping of that life. In the light of these considerations, I wish for more courage on behalf of the parents in taking responsibility for themselves, and for many children who have the courage to embark on life and enjoy the light of the earth their whole lives long.

Ermengerst 2005

Foreword to the First Edition

In the search for literature suitable for use as a reference for expectant parents it became clear to me that there was no book by midwives for parents. For years people have been asking me: "Where can we look up that information you gave us?" I therefore would like to respond to "my" women's request and gather all of my advice, tips and pointers between the covers of this book. It is to serve expectant parents as a reading and reference book throughout the period of pregnancy, childbirth and the postnatal period. I would like to grant my professional colleagues insight into the practice of midwifery on a self-employed basis and encourage them with my advice so they can accompany pregnant women with naturopathic methods and means.

Moreover, in this way I would also like to re-acquaint my readers with the midwife's profession. For it is our job to advise an expectant mother during pregnancy, prepare her for childbirth; accompany her while she is in labour, support her during the birth of her child, care for her during the postnatal period and, where necessary, call upon mother and child during the first eight weeks after childbirth. As you can see from this list, a midwife's working day is multi-faceted.

You should also be aware that in Germany health plans generally cover nearly all midwife services. For more information, see page 460.

A little bit about myself: I have been practising the midwife's profession since 1976. I was initially employed in a small maternity hospital where midwives customarily cared for the women and their newborns in the early postnatal phase. As early as 1977, I began offering antenatal classes on the side. In 1984 I embarked on self-employment. Now I cared for women at home following their stay at hospital. And I began to be approached by women who had given birth in the hospital as out-patients and wanted my help at home from the first day of the postnatal period. Soon there were the first requests for home births. A convinced obstetrician and some even more strongly convinced parents helped make this step into home obstetrics a lasting experience. My initial scepticism soon vanished. Intensive preparatory talks and getting to know the parents helped keep the risk as low as possible.

In 1986, along with a colleague, I founded a midwife's practice, which received a name "Erdenlicht" (Light of Earth) upon the proposal of a third midwife. There, we midwives aim to be a light on earth which helps children to lay their eyes on the light of the earth for the first time and offers parents a beacon in their process of becoming and being parents. Our services included antenatal classes, partner evenings, information on naturopathic methods, nappy-changing classes, postnatal exercise classes, the baby club, the baby massage course, the breastfeeding group, a nutrition circle on breastfeeding and what comes after it, seminars on the homoeopathic treatment of children's illnesses and lectures on aroma therapy and its use in the family. Since 1988 we have provided antenatal care on a regular basis as well.

I am myself the mother of three children. My two sons were both born in hospital; my daughter came into the world at home. Each of my children contributed enormously to my development as a midwife. During both pregnancy and childbirth, my first child acquainted me with medicalized childbirth – and all of the problems associated with it. Back then, programmed childbirth was customary. I had to learn from experience that an episiotomy can be really painful, as it caused an injury that still haunts me today.

My second pregnancy revealed to me that premature contractions, the same kind I had during the first pregnancy, can be quite normal. That tea can help. That the intake of foreign protein during pregnancy can cause the child extreme skin problems – problems which may be a burden to the child his whole life long. The birth led to the realization: no timing, no episiotomy, that's childbirth! I had the good fortune to experience what "childbearing" means, as opposed to "being delivered." To this day I am grateful to my colleague, and I would like to take this opportunity to mention that childbearing in hospital can also be a very wonderful and memorable experience for a family if the framework conditions are met. We love to remember the relaxing and rejuvenating postnatal period in the hospital. It was through my second pregnancy, the birth and the weeks that followed that I encountered homoeopathy and herbal medicine, the two forms of treatment I have called my own since then. I had the opportunity to learn that even extreme breastfeeding problems and sore nipples can be healed with naturopathic methods. Later, we learned as a family how to use natural medicine and the corresponding attitude to cope with skin problems in children.

My third pregnancy several years later allowed me to discover what it is like to bear a child in the family circle, what it means when the birth is accompanied by unprocessed psychological problems or changes. This child helped us to break out of a rigid structure: to experience a home birth as a midwife, to pursue full-time employment as a wife and mother, despite breastfeeding, to carry out an exchange of roles in the family in a small rural village! Since the birth of our daughter, my husband has been at home, takes care of the children, runs the household, supports me with my writing, encourages me and takes loads off of my back and my mind. Without my husband, I would never be able to work so comprehensively as a midwife. Because being a self-employed midwife means being on call for the next birth night and day, year in and year out as well as being available for women in pregnancy and the postnatal period to help them with all of their fears and acute problems.

It was thus that I discovered herbal medicine and homoeopathy for my profession. I encountered aroma therapy several years later. I also became aware of this method of healing in connection with the birth of a child. I was given the opportunity to accompany a woman who is very familiar with essential oils as she gave birth to her daughter. The experience was so memorable, that I have been intensively exploring the applications and effects of essential oils since that time.

I would like to dedicate this book explicitly to pregnant women, parents and children, for it was pregnant women, parents and children who helped me to attain my present state of knowledge.

In the following sections of the book – on pregnancy, childbirth and postnatal period – I will report alternately on my experience in the area of herbal medicine, homoeopathy and essential oils. I mean to provide pointers and advice – not compulsory prescriptions. Every pregnant woman will recognize for herself which form of therapy she feels drawn to. One will prefer tea blends, the other homoeopathic medicine; another will discover a liking for essential oils in the aroma lamp, massage oil or the bathtub.

I would like to remind the reader that all human beings – expectant parents included – are capable of making decisions and taking responsibility for themselves. Ultimately nobody can do this for us, our whole lives long.

In the appendix you will find chapters containing basic information on the use of medicinal herbs, homoeopathy and aroma therapy. The reader is advised to consult the respective chapter before applying those naturopathic methods.

This book should not be used to replace the advice of an experienced midwife, doctor or other therapist trained and certified in the care of pregnant women and mothers. Please remember that naturopathy is a form of treatment based on experience and is not free of side effects.

Ermengerst 1994

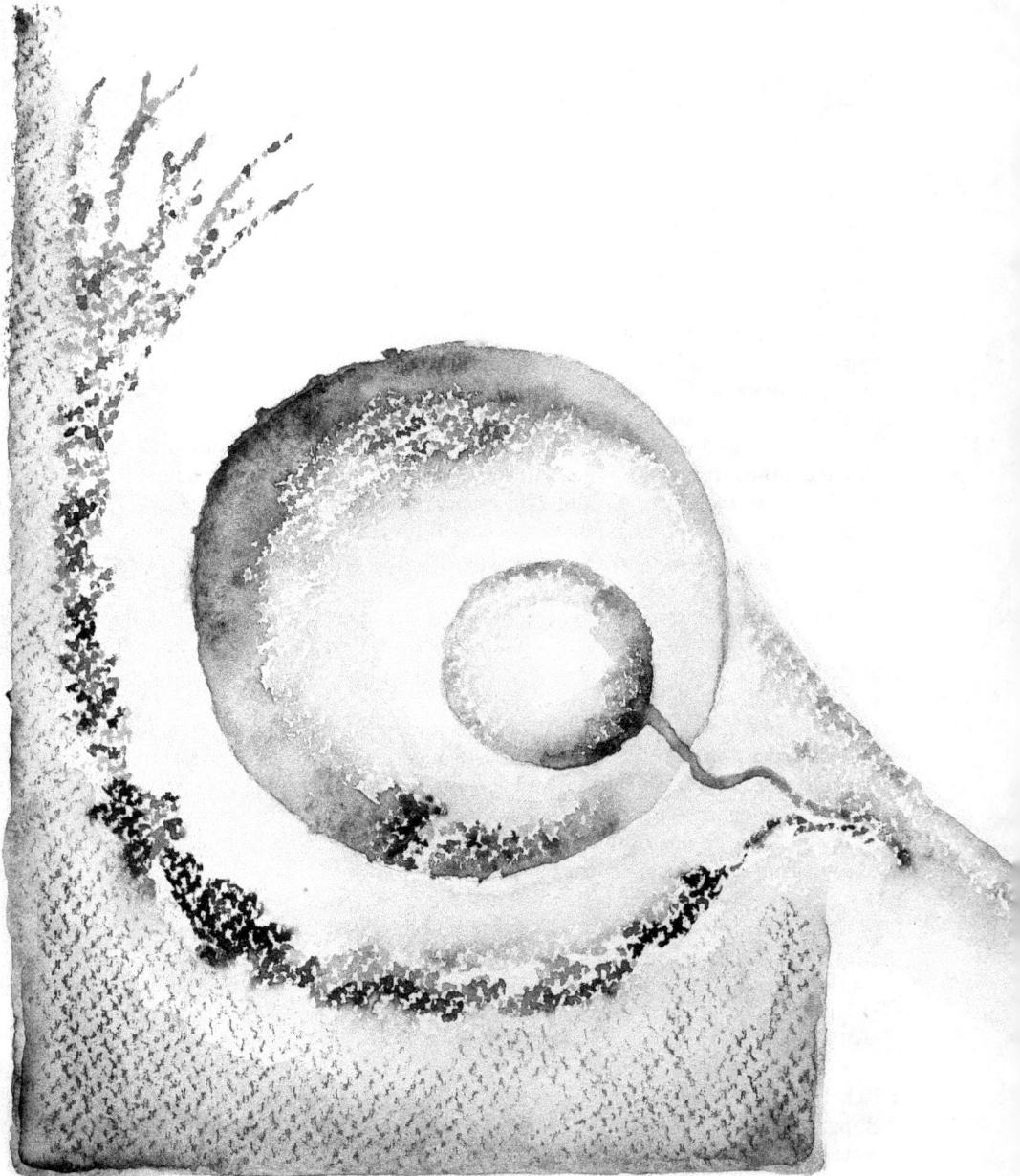

PREGNANCY

the two of us – three
warm
soft
incredible
you in me
we

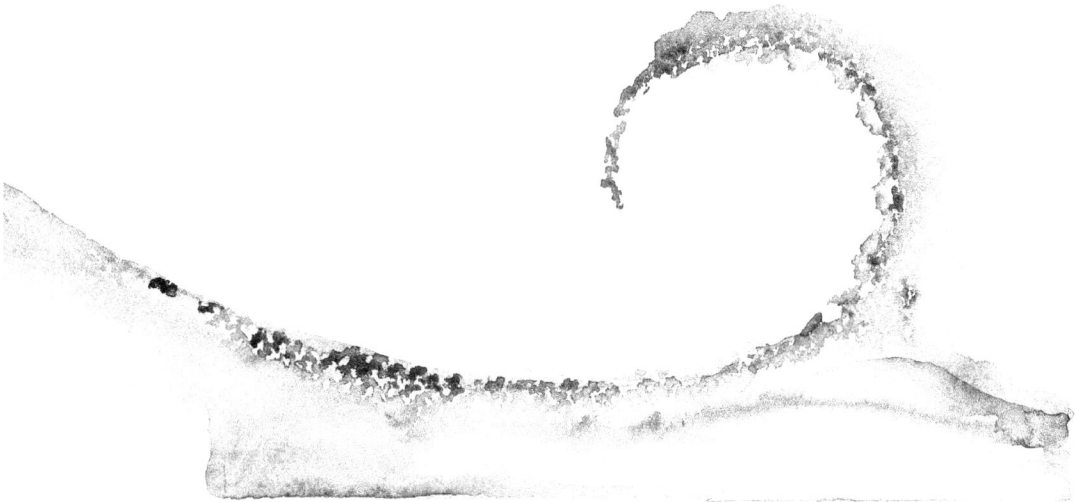

THE FIRST THREE MONTHS

We refer to the period from the first to the twelfth week of pregnancy, also called the first trimester, as a time of hormonal adjustment and new beginning.

These first three months are often marked by uncertainty and anxiety. Fatigue and sudden changes of mood can render them quite a challenge. The expectant mother is in two minds about whether she should tell people about her pregnancy and, if so, who – a pregnancy of which she herself perhaps has no more than a presentiment. Unfortunately, to an increasing degree, I have the impression that in this situation women have less and less a feeling of "anticipating a blessed event," but are burdened instead by a sense of helplessness and inner conflict. In our society, pregnancy is rarely still associated with hope and coming bliss, but with the "risk" involved. For in the age of the emancipated and successful woman, the pressure to bear a physically, mentally and socially healthy child has grown vastly. And whereas in former days people merely talked about happy anticipation, now the ins and outs of parentage and the ideal point in time at which to embark upon it are discussed in all thoroughness.

The first weeks of pregnancy are surely also influenced by the moment of the child's conception. A woman who has longed for a child for many years will indeed be imbued with a sense of hope. Yet the latter often goes hand in hand with worry, for the woman is usually well-informed about the possible risks during early pregnancy – the desire to become a mother has led her to many a doctor's office. This explains why such women often wait a while before consulting a midwife.

Particularly women who have enjoyed midwife accompaniment during previous pregnancies tend to seek contact to self-employed midwives at an early stage. In the past years, however, we have also noticed a slight increase in the number of women who come because they've heard from a friend that we offer assistance from the moment a pregnancy has been confirmed, or even before. This is why many women ring up for an appointment without wanting to tell us the reason for their interest. Then they come and say what Regina said to me those many years ago: "You know, I thought I'd just come and talk to you first. I think I'm pregnant. And if I am, I don't want to find out for sure with a strip of paper or an ultrasound that makes it so irreversibly visible. Because maybe I'm mistaken and then I would be really disappointed to find out that I'm not pregnant after all."

Such women are still a rarity in a midwife's practice, but that makes us all the happier when they do come. I can well understand a woman who wants to be alone with her uncertainty and dream the dream of motherhood for a little while yet, because the reality of a high-risk pregnancy or the knowledge of having a blighted ovum is often such a staggering disillusionment that nothing remains of that tiny moment of happiness.

But the fact of a real pregnancy can sometimes be just as staggering if the woman does not want to accept it and hopes that it is actually a case of blighted ovum. As a midwife and mother, I can sympathize with these feelings and I know that what the woman needs is someone who will listen to her and show her understanding for her current state. I know that it takes some time and a certain amount of self-reflection for the awareness of an initially unwanted pregnancy to ripen and for the woman to decide how she will react to a positive urine test or ultrasound result. By having themselves examined at an extremely early stage, many women learn a truth with which they are not quite ready to cope. As a consequence, they are hardly in a position to make the decision as to whether to keep the child or not. Talks with women in early pregnancy represent a very special challenge to us midwives, because in such cases we are required to remain totally objective and provide support to the woman in her momentary situation and her individual reaction for or against pregnancy. At the same time, it is important to explain to her that – if the suspicion of pregnancy is confirmed – she should realize that this child belongs to her and her biography, no matter how long she bears it within her, whether it decides to leave again of its own accord or whether she, as an expectant mother, makes the difficult decision to terminate the pregnancy. She will remain the mother of this child until her dying day and she should encompass it with her unending love. I explain to the woman that it will not be possible to erase this unborn child from her memory. Naturally, she doesn't have to tell everyone that she has made a conscious decision against her pregnancy, but it will be a part of her life from that time on. In situations of such difficult, momentous decisions, it is important not to disregard the child's father, but to try to understand him and his reactions. Again and again, men force women to decide against having the child. Demands such as these, for or against the child, are often made on an entirely rational basis. A man cannot decide with feminine emotions, for, after all, it is the woman who is pregnant. Conversely, we women should not react to a man with accusations, for a man can only react as a man and will quickly come to terms with the fact that he ultimately cannot make the decision. He is often not entirely conscious of his responsibility, or evades it, for a man's emotions are simply different. Women must be conscious of the fact that they will have to bear this decision alone for the rest of their lives, whereas men can easily ignore their paternal responsibility – particularly in view of the fact that their hormonal balance doesn't adjust to fatherly feelings very quickly.

When I conduct such difficult and at the same time such naturally human consultations, I find the most important thing is to react with a sense of calm and patience. I often have the impression that the woman has consciously chosen me as a neutral advisor – sometimes even an anonymous one if the consultation takes place by phone – and I am honoured by the trust she places in me. I advise her to make contact with a midwife near her, but also just to give herself a few days to decide what to do. I tell her that the conception already represents a piece of eternity in its own right, and that a few days won't make the slightest difference. We midwives always learn a lot from the women who later get back in touch with us to tell us their decisions. Particularly when we go on to accompany them during pregnancy, birth and the postnatal period, it is much easier for us to understand when this woman suddenly becomes pensive, or her partner quiet, or her cheeks are suddenly wet with seemingly inexplicable tears. Then we know that she is visiting the thoughts she confided in us way back in the beginning of pregnancy, before it was even clear whether the child was welcome or not. It is true: whether as midwives or as mothers, we women are bearers of secrets.

At the beginning of pregnancy, many women decide to hold onto their secret for a while – and later they often refer to this phase as one of the most wonderful periods of twosomeness with the child. Have you ever watched children exchanging secrets? Do you remember secrets you had as a child? Then maybe you can imagine why these young mothers with their radiant, transfigured smiles are suddenly so different as a friend or partner. They will only talk to others about their happy condition – the fact that a whole new little human being has settled in somewhere deep inside her – when they have digested it themselves. It is unfortunate that not many women experience such a phase of bliss these days, because many of them learn of what is actually still a very intangible and incomprehensible condition much too soon, due to the fact that health insurance companies cover the cost of control examinations from the very earliest possible date. As a midwife, I take the liberty of questioning the wisdom of this early detection system, because in my opinion women need a few weeks to absorb a reality that will have such a huge effect on their futures. I like to compare this situation with the pulse-quickening of couples in love, holding hands for the first time or exchanging their first kisses in a dark and secret place. In the urge to absorb and comprehend the experience, they, too, want to keep the wonderful state of falling in love to themselves for a little while.

Common Minor Problems during Early Pregnancy

After amenorrhoea – the absence of menstruation – the first symptoms that lead a woman to suspect she is pregnant are usually nausea, vomiting, abnormal cravings and swelling of the breasts.

Nausea/Vomiting

Within the context of my work, I have noticed that it is predominantly women who are not pregnant for the first time who come to midwives with complaints of nausea and vomiting. I don't know whether this is because they have only gotten to know the midwife in connection with the birth of their first child or in the postnatal period, or whether these symptoms actually increase with each pregnancy.

One thing I'm sure of, however, is that the child is already making itself "heard," saying: here I am, I need your time and attention and what is more, I am not my sister and I'm also not my brother. I'm me and I'm here!

This is easy for many women to understand, but it doesn't help much when she's at her job. During this phase, women unfortunately still can't count on much understanding from their co-workers, and even their partners have difficulty coming to terms with the new situation. The women who come for advice are happy that their complaints are taken seriously. "It's just part of being pregnant" – that's a sentence many women are literally sick of hearing.

The early phase of pregnancy – the beginning of a new life – is punctuated by lots of question marks. How will my life change? How will I cope? Will I manage everything? To be sure, there will have been other situations in life where these questions popped up, and in those situations, answers and help were found. For many women, these questions and problems were answered and solved by thinking things through, acting sensibly and receiving clear instructions from others, i.e. by rational means. Also, until now such decisions have only affected the woman herself. Now, however, with a baby inside, no matter how tiny, that's no longer the case. From start to finish, every decision is made for the child as well as the mother. "Responsibility" begins: "IT wants an answer I don't even know yet!" is how many women feel in this situation. A phase of life begins which is determined more strongly than ever before by "gut feeling" – the belly, which has been something of a stranger until now. Mothers who have already had children will ask, "And what about me? Why am I feeling so sick? I'm already an experienced mother. Why can't I get out of bed in the morning without using the bucket; why can't I even brush my teeth without spitting up?" Many men remind their wives that it was exactly the same the first time around, but pregnant women don't like to hear that fact. As is the case so often in life, the positive memories of the first pregnancy have remained in the foreground, and the mother of several children may will have repressed the initial problems. She surely does remember, but that doesn't help her in this situation. In my opinion, this is because she knows, she recognizes, that the new child will be a completely different child, causing her a completely different kind of discomfort. Maybe the pregnant woman is already subconsciously asking herself, "How will I manage with two?" Or she has realized that, while she can raise her children, she can't change their natures. This new being in her belly will be different, but in what way? What qualities will it have? Perhaps the mother would like to maintain the symbiosis – as we refer to the first trimester of pregnancy – as long as possible, but knows it will come to an end, an entirely independent child will develop and she will have to let go of it.

Thus there are perhaps many plausible psychological explanations for the nausea and the new circumstances women find themselves in.

As a midwife, all I can do is offer food for thought and, more than anything else, listen. I'll never be able to answer all the questions that come up, and I don't see that as my job. But an open ear and the confirmation that many women feel the same way in early pregnancy are already a help.

The woman in the early stage of pregnancy is happy to hear that she doesn't have to walk around with a blissful smile on her face like the ladies in the advertisements, if that's not the way she feels. Actually, in the majority of cases, this woman describes her condition as miserable. I try to explain to the young mother that she can communicate her situation to the people around her already at this early phase, and should even stay home from work when it's necessary. If a woman already has a child or children at home, she will need the help of Grandma or her partner in that situation. In the mother's relationship with her older child, it is often now that she really lets go for the first time.

Unfortunately, so many women suffer so greatly from nausea during pregnancy that it takes on the dimension of an illness; sometimes only a stay in hospital brings about an improvement. Often, however, a "change of scenery" is the only therapy, i.e. not medication, but just a change of surroundings is necessary.

Many women complain not only of vomiting and nausea, but also of the accompanying loss of weight. This can usually not be avoided, however, and ceases by the twelfth week of pregnancy at the latest, when, on the contrary, the expectant mother begins to gain weight. Look at the positive side of this weight loss: it is an opportunity to rid the body of harmful substances which would otherwise only burden your child by way of your milk.

Of course it is advisable for the expectant mother to consult with a midwife before an acute state of vomiting – referred to as emesis – sets in. Natural medicines can provide a lot of relief, limiting the degree of nausea and vomiting or, in some cases, eliminating the symptoms entirely. It already helps many women simply to chew on a piece of dry bread or drink a glass of milk in small sips first thing in the morning. Others have found that sucking on a slice of lemon helps.

⑤ Homoeopathic Remedies

From homeopathy we know of a number of remedies which provide tangible relief in cases of morning sickness caused by pregnancy: *Arsenicum album, Cocculus, Ipecacuanha, Magnesium carbonicum, Nux vomica, Phosphorus, Pulsatilla, Sepia, Tabacum.* Precise instructions for the administration of homoeopathic medicines can be found in the section of the appendix on homoeopathy (p. 438) and in my book *The Homoeopathic Home and Travel Medicine Chest*.

I well remember ...

... a friend who rang me up during the seventh week of pregnancy and told me how badly she was suffering from constant nausea. At that point in time she was already in hospital. But after her discharge, the situation at home was just as bad as it had been before. Her vomiting, dizziness, and lack of appetite were back. I listened to her complaints and then asked her about her mother. "Yes, you know, it's difficult with my mother. She's still trying to bring me up. I'm constantly trying to break away from her but somehow I can't manage. Now she keeps telling me that my pregnancy will probably be just like hers. In other words, I'm confronted with her again, which is exactly what I want to avoid. I just want to finally be ME." When I asked her whether she liked to listen to music, she answered, "Yes, usually I do, but now it doesn't help." I advised her to take the homoeopathic remedy Sepia in an LM

potency. For the two days following, she felt worse than ever, but after three days I received the good news: "I've got my appetite back, I can already eat cheese, and I just took a bath. I feel like a totally normal pregnant woman. I do still vomit in the morning, but I can live with that!" In the background I could hear classical music. Her state had improved distinctly.

⊚ Essential Oils

A very pleasant means of treating nausea and vomiting during pregnancy are essential oils. Smelling salts, sniffed at the onset of nausea, are an age-old, time-tested method. Women in early pregnancy like to use: *bergamot, grapefruit, mandarin red, neroli, peppermint* and *lemon*. When using these oils, it is most important to trust your own sense of smell and choose the aroma most agreeable to you. Incidentally, for many women a heightened sense of smell is the first sign of pregnancy. For that reason, I am quite sure that a pregnant woman can find the aroma that will help her best simply by smelling. Many young mothers love lemon oil when they feel nauseated. In a 10% solution with jojoba wax, neroli helps, as does the refreshing and invigorating scent of grapefruit, to keep your stomach from turning around in circles. Bergamot is a good choice for those who are also suffering from sudden changes of mood. I only recommend peppermint, however – a drop rubbed into each temple or in the form of smelling salts –, if the "patient" is suffering from dizziness/weak circulation and is not already taking homoeopathic medication. All of these oils can also be used in the aroma lamp or added to your morning wash. This will be particularly helpful during early pregnancy. The ideal form of use is to concoct your own natural perfume by producing a jojoba solution containing 10% of your favourite oil and applying this blend to your ear lobes or the insides of your wrists. Since many pregnant women work, or are surprised by a wave of nausea while they're out – e.g. shopping for food –, it is advisable to carry the little aroma bottle with you, like …

… Claudia, who was sure she was pregnant again, judging from her morning sickness. She did not want to take any homoeopathic remedies, but wanted to know whether she could use an essential oil, because she was suffering quite considerably from nausea. I asked her what oils she had in the house and then advised her to choose her own smelling salts by taking a sniff at bergamot, lemon and mint. She decided in favour of mint and from that day on she always had it with her, as she told me later on. She used it for several weeks, whenever the need arose, and it helped her cope quite well.

In the past years, the *Original 𝒟® Aroma Blend Andere Umstände/Expectant 𝒟®* has proven very effective. This somewhat unharmonious-smelling essential oil blend containing lime, neroli, rosemary and sandalwood is often just the right thing in this discordant state. It is likewise used in the form of smelling salts, in the aroma lamp or as a perfume, by mixing a drop of it with a drop of jojoba wax. The mixture I call *Hans guck in die Luft/Johnny-Head-in-the-Air 𝒟®*, available as an aroma spray and useful as an aid to schoolchildren when they're doing their homework, also helps pregnant women suffering from dizziness and nausea. The oils it contains – linaloe wood, litsea, mandarin red and lemon balm, have a calming and encouraging effect and help to maintain concentration. The spray is perfect when you're out and about, whether in the car, on the train or at work. For women who have weak circulation to contend with in addition to morning sickness, the aroma blend *Kräuterkorb/Basket of Herbs* $\mathcal{D}^\circ$ has proven extremely helpful, also in the form of an aroma spray. Even before you get out of bed in the morning, you can put this mixture of peppermint, rosemary, sage and myrtle hydrolat to use by spraying your calves with it. The spray is a welcome refreshment on hot summer days as well.

Cravings

In early pregnancy, women with the abovementioned symptoms almost always mention that they have discovered themselves to have very strange cravings. Late in the evening, from one minute to the next, they'll suddenly want to eat pickles, or they'll crave sausage with onions and vinegar for breakfast. Others can't fall asleep without having consumed a box of chocolates or other sweets though they have never done such things before in their life.

I would like to encourage you to give in to these cravings and the signals your body is sending you, at least to start with. Your body knows exactly what to reject and what will do it good. Giving in to it means trusting yourself. It is clear to me that early pregnancy represents an entirely new life situation, particularly when it is your first pregnancy. Until now, everything has been clear and simple. Now somebody is telling you: *"Trust yourself; your body knows what it wants."* This is, to my mind, one of the first and most important ways of preparing for pregnancy and motherhood. You want to have natural childbirth, and when you breastfeed you will have to leave it to your body to produce the right amount of milk at the right point in time; as a mother you will have to recognize whether the child eats enough, sleeps enough, and whether or not it is sick.

Naturally, cravings are not a sign to start eating nothing but chocolate, but perhaps they're there to tell you: "As the mother of this child, you'll have to do lots of things you've rejected until now." Whether through conviction or repulsion, the child will teach the mother to change her diet and her habits. She'll often have had it "up to here" or be "sick" of everything, but she'll also be open to trying everything once.

If the cravings are too abnormal, I have a few words of advice:

If you have a craving for sour things, eat them – sauerkraut or pickles, for example.

If you crave sweet things, eat products with valuable carbohydrates such as grains – don't fill up on processed sugar. Carrots and fennel are also good choices. Chew everything well, until you can actually feel the sweet taste in your mouth.

If you have a strong desire for chocolate, it could be a sign of magnesium deficiency, which can be remedied by taking magnesium tablets, drinking mineral water with magnesium in it, or chewing five skinned almonds several times a day. When buying and preparing green vegetables, be sure they're outdoor-grown, as those are the only kind which really do contain lots of magnesium.

Heightened Sense of Smell

An interesting phenomenon during pregnancy is the heightened olfactory sense. Cigarettes are a particular problem in this context. There are still lots of people – men and women alike – who can't overcome their addition to nicotine despite their knowledge of the consequences. It is a well-known fact that cigarette smoke is detrimental to unborn children even if the mother herself does not smoke but only breathes in the cigarette smoke of others. And lots of women accordingly cannot bear the smell of it; already the smallest waft of cigarette smoke nauseates them. It would seem to me that this is nature's clever way of protecting the unborn baby, and it is to be hoped that it will encourage many an expectant father to kick the habit. I would like to take this opportunity to mention something which has been scientifically proven: infants who have been subjected to cigarette smoke suffer much more frequently from flatulence and respiratory illnesses. In other words, there is absolutely no excuse for smoking. In my opinion, for the defenceless unborn child and throughout childhood, it is nothing short of constant abuse. The carcinogenic effect of nicotine has long been a proven fact, as has its effect on the infant by way of the placenta, and the danger of premature delivery.

Swelling of the Breasts and Soreness of the Nipples

In response to complaints of swollen breasts and sore nipples, I try to explain to women that their breasts are preparing for the task ahead: in a few months, they will be the child's source of nourishment. For many women, this requires a certain amount of rethinking: their breasts are no longer to be thought of as an "attractive appendage" but as a vital organ. To me it appears quite obvious that our bodies call attention to themselves in exactly the places where changes will take place during pregnancy. When I put it this way, many women understand that a prickling in the breasts is not a pathological phenomenon but a wonderful sign of the fact that the breasts are preparing to give milk.

If the symptoms become unpleasant, it helps many women to wear a brassiere temporarily or constantly. By that I don't mean to say, however, that all pregnant women should wear a bra. The natural friction of the nipples against the surface of the clothing is actually one of the best methods of inurement.

In severe cases, a warm lavender breast bath or a warm lavender compress may provide relief. Both methods soothe and relax the irritated nipples. In cases of swelling of the whole breast, I recommend a massage oil made of lavender and neroli in an emulsion of cold-pressed oil basis, or simply the time-tested *Schwangerschaftsstreifenöl/Stretch Mark Oil 𝒟®*, which also contains rose and linaloe wood oil. Many women also like to use orange blossom, rose or lemon balm hydrolat. Be sure to use hydrolats which are free of alcohol, because they will not dry out your skin but, on the contrary, provide moisture.

Lower Back Pains

Pregnant women sometimes complain of strong sacral pains – the sacrum being the triangular bone forming the posterior section of the pelvis. Often these women suffer from retroversion of the uterus, i.e. the uterus is tilted toward the back. In such cases, the growth of the child and the increasing weight of the uterus puts strong pressure on the sacrum. The best remedy here is to sleep in a prone position – with a small cushion under your tummy to take the strain off the spinal discs – and, during the day, to practice the knee-elbow position as often as possible, or do belly dancing. Physical exercises of this kind help the uterus to straighten up and out of the pelvis, and the unpleasant pressure on the sacrum is reduced.

Another cause of sacral pain is the entirely natural, hormonally induced softening of the joint between the ilium and the sacrum.

✆ Essential Oils

Women suffering from sacral pain are advised to massage the painful area with essential oil blends of jasmine, mandarin red, rosemary and juniper with a cold-pressed vegetable oil base, for example *Kreuzbein-Massageöl/Lower Back Massage Oil 𝒟®*. This Original 𝒟® Aroma Blend has been used with great success for many years now, and also helps persons suffering from sciatica. The scent of jasmine supports the female hormonal balance and helps us to cope better with this "cross" that women in particular have to bear. Mandarin red oil is especially suitable for massages performed with the aim of loosening up the muscles. Rosemary oil supports the blood flow and helps bear the pain. Juniper berry, a strong basic woody scent, is always a boon on account of its purifying effect in connection with rheumatic symptoms. *Kreuzbein-Massageöl/Lower Back Massage Oil 𝒟®* can also be used in conjunction with warm compresses. If you would like to read more about these beneficial applications, I recommend my booklet *Aroma Therapy from Pregnancy to Breastfeeding*.

Medication and Dietary Supplements during Early Pregnancy

In principle it is not necessary to take medication, vitamins or other nutritional supplements during the early phase of pregnancy and if you do, it should be by doctor's prescription only. And incidentally, a well-informed pharmacist can provide you with detailed information on the necessity, effects and undesirable side effects of all medications. Do not recklessly take pills, tablets or seemingly "normal" painkillers, because their active agents will take the quickest route to the growing infant. As you surely know, the basic development of both the sensory organs and the central nervous system take place within the first twelve weeks. The careless intake of medication can cause the infant irreversible damage.

The controversial obligatory dispensation of iodine and folic acid is also a subject of discussion among midwives. As mentioned above, these medications should only be taken on a doctor's advice. My concern here is to inform you that, right now, assuming you are reading this in the early stage of pregnancy, the optimal point in time for folic acid supplementation is already long past: the positive influence of this substance on the neural tube ends in the fourth week of the child's development, when the tube closes. It would therefore be more sensible to begin taking folic acid when you decide you would like to become pregnant, particularly if you have been taking the Pill for a long period. You would be doing a good deed if you passed this information on to your friends who want to have children, as there is still too much ignorance among women on this subject. If you're already past the fourth week of pregnancy, don't worry. The rate of deformities caused by folic acid deficiency is in fact infinitesimally small. And anyway, pregnant women shouldn't have to support the pharmaceutical industry. With the right nutrition you can already cover your minimum daily requirement with 200 g of broccoli (containing 200 µg of folic acid) or 50 g of oat flakes (50 µg) plus 10 g of wheat germ (50 µg). And last but not least, even among scientists there are varying opinions as to the length of the period of heightened need and the amount to be taken: the estimations range between 200 and 600 µg per day.

There is likewise quite some disagreement concerning the intake of iodine during pregnancy. The Federal Republic of Germany is classified as an "iodine deficiency area" but these days iodine supplementation is compulsory almost throughout the food chain – from mineral fertilizers for our vegetables and fodder containing iodine additives to iodized mineral water and the products sold by bakers and butchers. The physician and obstetrician Dr. Friedrich Graf even refers in his writings to "forced iodization" which we can no longer escape. Particularly restaurants and fast-food chains "take care of" our health by using iodized salt. It is a known fact that iodine deficiency can lead to disturbances of fetal brain development, but no mention is ever made of the fact that an overdose of iodine can have a toxic effect. Until 1997, the estimated minimum daily requirement was 100 µg; since 2000 it has been 200 µg. Iodine increases the metabolism of energy, and too much of it can lead to hyperthyroidism or to so-called iodism, a state accompanied by irritations of the mucous membranes, allergies, asthma and auto-immune diseases. In view of these circumstances, every pregnant woman should check her diet carefully, perhaps have her iodine status controlled by her general practitioner and then decide for herself. If you are plagued by symptoms such as extreme weight gain, fatigue, listlessness, dryness of the skin and mucous membranes, hair loss, low tonicity and depression, it is essential that you contact your doctor about iodine supplementation. If you take iodide and suffer increasingly from nervousness, insomnia, palpitations, shakiness, diarrhoea which irritates the skin and/or previously unexperienced allergy-like rashes, stop taking iodide immediately, as in the case of Ms. N. …

… already during the antenatal class I noticed that she couldn't calm down during the relaxation exercise. After the session she asked me what she could do to help her get to sleep and whether palpitations and dry skin were really normal during pregnancy. This caught my attention and I asked her into my consultation room. During the consultation I learned that she had been prescribed iodide. When I asked her how long she had had these symptoms, it quickly become clear that there was a connection. Ms. N. subsequently stopped taking the iodide and when I talked to her a few days later she said, "Everything's back to normal now. I'm so happy we were able to figure out the cause!" I called her gynaecologist, and he told me that he was actually an advocate of general iodine prophylaxis in view of the fact that symptoms such as those affecting Ms. N. were extremely rare, but that he would certainly keep a closer watch from now on. He couldn't resist adding, though, that, as a midwife, I was not authorized to make such decisions and I should send such women to him in the future!

To parents interested in a critical look at this subject, I recommend the brochure "Kritik der Arzneiroutine bei Schwangeren und Kindern" by Dr. med. Friedrich Graf.

If you decide in favour of iodine prophylaxis, it is extremely important that it be continued during the breastfeeding period. Incidentally, 70 g of coal fish or 3–5 g of iodized salt contain 150 µg of iodine, the recommended daily dose. Lamb's lettuce, dairy products and algae are also rich in iodine.

Antenatal Care

Midwife and/or Obstetrician?

An increasing number of women would like to have their antenatal care carried out by a midwife. For pregnancies which progress normally, midwives are just as capable of carrying out the care as doctors, and are authorized to do so. If you would like to have an ultrasound, however, you will have to consult an obstretrician or go to a hospital. For this reason, many women decide to alternate between a midwife and a doctor for their antenatal appointments. In my opinion, a cooperative relationship between a midwife and an obstetrician is beneficial to the expectant mother and she should not be required to choose between the two. Naturally, there are women who want to have the antenatal check-ups done exclusively by a midwife. There is no reason not to comply with this wish as long as the pregnancy is a normal one. At the first sign of any irregularity, the midwife will refer the woman to a specialist. What you should know is that midwives offer midwife-oriented antenatal care, while those offered by doctors are medically oriented. Midwives and obstetricians are both trained in obstetrics, but the two professions are entirely different. Nevertheless, they complement one another well and ideally work hand in hand. Midwives place primary emphasis on holistic care and carry out all the examinations required by the health scheme, including the necessary laboratory tests. Recent studies have shown that pregnancies accompanied by midwives progress at a lower risk than those in the control group of patients in the exclusive care of doctors. What is more, an increasing number of doctors are cooperating with midwives. If you hear about a cooperative arrangement between a doctor and a midwife, you as an expectant mother should find out beforehand whether the midwife merely replaces the doctor's receptionist or really is permitted to practice her profession independently. If you are required to consult the midwife *and* the doctor at every appointment, you are not receiving truly midwife-oriented care.

The "Mutterpass" – Maternity Notes

In Germany, every pregnant woman is given a booklet in which the results of the antenatal examinations are recorded – a "Mutterpass."

During the first antenatal appointment, the expectant mother is questioned in detail about previous illnesses and her general medical history. I have noticed that this session is unfortunately often carried out very superficially with regard to the questions and the answers alike. You should take the questions very seriously and also inform your partner about previous illnesses. He should likewise think about illnesses which have recurred in his family. The doctor and midwife are not asking you these questions out of personal interest or curiosity, but in order to provide the best possible care to mother and child, and to recognize – or rule out – risks at an early stage.

The answers to the questions, the results of the blood tests and the ultrasound as well as all other examination results during pregnancy are recorded in the Mutterpass. From now on, you should always carry this booklet with you and bring it to your appointments with your midwife as well. That way, the doctor and the midwife can both inform themselves as to which examination results the other has recorded. If you give birth in a hospital, the obstetric team there can read about how the pregnancy has proceeded. This is usually the only record available to the hospital. All other files and records of the pregnancy remain in the midwife's/doctor's practice. In an increasing number of German cities, a system is offered whereby one and the same midwife (and sometimes the same doctor) accompany the woman during pregnancy and childbirth alike by means of affiliations between the self-employed midwife and the hospital. Usually, however, this is not the case, and when the birthing woman gets to the hospital she is confronted with a midwife and an obstetrician she has never laid eyes on before. Independent birth centres and home births are a different kettle of fish. Here the midwives attach the greatest importance to getting to know the woman as soon as possible and providing the antenatal care in the midwife's practice or the birth centre. If a doctor is to be present at the birth taking place at home or in an independent birthing centre, he or she should also be involved in the antenatal care.

For the purposes of alternating antenatal appointments with a midwife and an obstetrician, as well as for the hospital birth, every woman should see to it that her Mutterpass is filled out completely, and take it with her to all antenatal check-ups. It contains information which can be of decisive importance for the mother and infant during childbirth, especially when there is no time to inform the hospital personnel about the progress of the pregnancy in detail. This is the case, for example, when the birth goes very quickly. In such situations the mother is not in a position to respond to such questions.

The Estimated Due Date (EDD)

The due date requires a bit of explanation. Babies rarely heed the date calculated by the antenatal care providers. Only four children in a hundred are actually born on the due date. This date is calculated on the basis of the first day of the last menstrual period, to which 280 days are added. If you know the date of ovulation, however, or the actual date of conception, you can calculate on that basis, adding 266 days to the date in question.

Example:	last period was on	18 March
	+ 280 days	
	= prospective due date	24 December
or:	last period was on	18 March
	ovulation according to temperature curve	5 April
	= prospective due date	28 December
or:	last period was on	18 March
	conception was presumably on	27 March
	= prospective due date	19 December

(The next possible date of conception is 13 April but the first ultrasound on 25 April clearly indicates the seventh week of pregnancy.)

My intention in showing these examples is to emphasize that it is advantageous to provide precise information during the first antenatal appointment. Don't be tempted to provide false information in order to extend your maternal leave. When the baby shows no signs of being born on that date, it will be a difficult state of affairs to explain to the obstetricians. Moreover, it is always the mother who has to put up with extensive observation from the calculated due date onwards. This date may serve as a basis for deciding whether the birth must be induced or the child can be left to determine its birth date itself.

Pregnancy accordingly lasts forty weeks, ten lunar months or nine calendar months. I advise expectant parents to talk in terms of weeks as well, in order to avoid misunderstandings. Midwives and obstetricians divide pregnancy into three thirds or so-called trimesters:

first third/trimester   –   1st to 12th week of pregnancy
second third/trimester –   13th to 28th week of pregnancy
third third/trimester   –   29th to 40th week of pregnancy

The outline of the first chapter of this book is also based on this system of division.

Antenatal Check-Ups/Signs of Life

During the antenatal appointments – which normally take place every four weeks – the *fetal heart rate* is made audible from about the twelfth week by means of a small, easily manageable ultrasonic device. This is a very special experience for parents, for until now the child was perceivable only to the mother. Fathers are very excited and as happy as little children themselves when they manage to hear "their" baby. Naturally, the heartbeat is visible in the first major ultrasound examination, but our ears are also important sensory organs and should not be underestimated. I never fail to be surprised at the number of expectant parents who have often *seen* their child in the course of the pregnancy, maybe even have photos and video recordings of it, but have never *heard* it.

In the context of listening to the fetal heartbeat, I like to point out to the parents that they also have to prepare their ears for parenthood. Infants can make quite a lot of noise. Already in the first days and weeks after birth, they can put a great strain on their parents' ears. At the same time, the child's first cries are a sign of life. Everyone can see the newborn infant, but that's not enough. Everyone present at the birth also wants to hear the child yell. I am therefore very much of the opinion that we should take advantage of this offer made by modern technology and – in addition to visual images – provide parents the opportunity of hearing their baby as early on as possible.

It will not be long before the mother begins to feel the child move in the womb. This will take place in about the twenty-first week if it is the first child, and as early as the eighteenth week if it is a later child. Initially it will feel like a gentle prickling beneath the abdominal wall, which you can best perceive by laying the palm of your hand flat across the womb. Many women say they originally mistook the movements for gas. Soon it will become clear, however, that what you are feeling is the movement of the child.

If you know the exact date on which that happens, be sure to inform your midwife because even today – in the age of technical prenatal monitoring – this is a good way of checking the prospective due date, without using machines.

For the mother, the child's first movements are a very special experience – comparable in significance to other developmental achievements later on, such as the child's first attempts to walk or its first words. These movements are the first tangible contact or, in other words, the baby's first perceivable communication, which serves to boost the woman's confidence: I am becoming a mother; a whole little human being is growing inside me.

"Antenatal Package Plus"

In the wake of the most recent health reform, a new and very peculiar system has become popular in many doctor's practices: expectant mothers are supposed to decide whether they would like to book an "Antenatal Package Plus with Extras" or whether the range of tests and examinations traditionally comprised by antenatal care will suffice. The "extras" include, for example, additional ultrasounds and a glucose tolerance test to rule out the possibility of gestational diabetes. I will leave it to my readers to judge the extent to which these practices can be described as normal antenatal care or whether advantage is being taken of women's and young parents' fears and uncertainties. One thing is certain: that every examination result which is "positive" (in the medical sense) causes insecurity and anxiety and, often, sleepless nights. Eventually, the doctors will put everything into perspective for you, but that doesn't erase the fears and worries you have undergone during the previous weeks and months of pregnancy. During early pregnancy, for example, doctors all too often make remarks about "placenta previa" – meaning that the position of the placenta is abnormally low – a condition which, at the worst, can lead to placental insufficiency. The position of the placenta, however, will soon change, because it grows upwards along with the musculature of the uterus, at which point it turns out that all of the excitement and worry was for nought! But the fact that, in such a situation, a great strain is put on the emotions of the mother, the child and presumably the father, and nobody is talking about happy anticipation anymore, but about risks and caesareans, is something the health plans offering the above-described special packages don't mention. The emotional state of the unborn child in the womb is still not a subject of interest to science. Doctors prefer to speak of the fetus as opposed to the child.

A similar example is the often unsystematic search for heightened blood sugar levels in the expectant mother: one woman pays for the special service and a lab result is attained, while the other woman, with the "basic" antenatal package – who perhaps really does run the risk of gestational diabetes – apparently has no right to proper care! Here we are well on the road to a two-class society. The fact that gestational diabetes actually is on the rise cannot be denied, but it certainly should not be overly emphasized in the context of a normal pregnancy, for it will only cause unnecessary fear and anxiety.

Here I would like to point out that, in view of the German antenatal care system, even obstetricians are seriously thinking about how much care is really sensible. In comparison to other European countries such as England, for example, the usual range of examinations comprised by antenatal care in Germany must be questioned. The gynaecologist Dr. Bartholomeus Maris has indicated that it should always be possible to weigh medical necessity against individual preference on the part of the expectant mother. In an article appearing in the *Deutsche Hebammen Zeitschrift* (a German midwifery journal) in December 2004, he wrote: "With regard to both the woman and the doctor, the degree of fear and of the need for a personal sense of safety is often a decisive factor and usually leads to control examinations being carried out to an exaggerated extent." Among other things, his article addresses the wisdom of performing ultrasound examinations after the twenty-fourth week of pregnancy, regular vaginal examinations, the search for bacterial vaginosis, the regular monitoring of the fetal heartbeat as well as CTGs. According to English studies, none of these measures is to be regarded as necessary within the context of routine antenatal care. As a matter of fact, the results of such studies frequently contradict the recommendations made in Germany. It is my hope, however, that – as is also expressed by Dr. Maris – well-informed women will be in a position to decide which offers to take advantage of and which to turn down on the basis of the detailed information provided them by their midwife and obstetrician. In the future, then, ideally, everyone involved – the parents, the midwife, the doctor – will decide together how much precaution is sensible. Instead of hiding behind medical guidelines, they need to realize that sometimes "less is more." In the decision "for or against" an examination, it is my special hope that advocates of the unborn child and its emotional well-being will be heard. The still very uncertain physical consequences of all these measures should also be considered. It should never be forgotten that the many controls are not therapy but merely momentary takes, which – when they deviate from the norm or produce uncertain results – have the power of increasing fear and anxiety rather than allaying them.

Naturopathy and Individuality

At this stage I would like to tell you a bit more about the relationships between individuality, natural medicine, childbirth and the midwife's profession. After all, it is an entirely natural as well as an individual course of events to expect and bear a child.

Women have always adopted the wisdom of nature as their own. Naturopathy is nature's system of treating disease. To practice naturopathy means to understand nature's peculiarities – its joyful processes of renewal as well as its disasters. To learn and know about nature's system of healing also means to entrust oneself to the elements of the earth and not be angry or surprised about its cravenness, crudeness or wisdom. For millions of years, the earth has been taking care of itself, changing, adapting. It destroys and creates, now with brutal elemental force, now with angelic patience and at a hardly noticeable rate in the course of the millennia. Nature heals her wounds – which are often inflicted on her by human beings – sometimes overnight, by simply washing them away with rain. Sometimes, for example, a whole winter passes before the pressure of the blanket of snow erases marks left by human beings, perhaps to make room for healing plants. Sometimes nature needs years to turn deep gashes back into fertile soil where tyres and boots have dug their way into sensitive moorland. And sometimes the earth doesn't heal at all, where, for example, water cascades into valleys unchecked by the rocks and forests which have disappeared so that human beings can build themselves a new road. It seems to lie in the nature of man that we force ourselves onto nature, causing many an action to be doomed to failure from the start.

The knowledge of nature's system of healing requires intensive understanding of nature, and we are often confronted with mysteries that only spiritual thought can help us come to terms with. For despite the efforts of scientists, nature remains a closed book and – like the natural event of childbirth – she demands to be viewed once again with reverence and awe. Human beings want to experience natural pregnancy and childbirth, but are frequently not familiar with – nor do they respect – the possibilities and limitations of nature. We midwives accompany the woman in labour, sense her fears, but also recognize the unsuspected strength that lies within her and try to guide her through childbirth with this feeling of basic trust as our predecessors already did many millennia ago.

I am very grateful to naturopathy, particularly homoeopathy, for it describes and teaches holism. Thus I have learned to provide "my" women with individual care, to see everything as it is, to hear what is really worrying them and to accept that other people have other views and opinions – in other words to understand the women in their entirety. Every human being should be treated and cared for in the manner that is good for him or her personally. This desire for individual care is also justified during childbirth, and leads to fulfilment. Since I have learned to think, act and practice my profession in this way I have come to experience a much greater number of happy expectant mothers, women making informed choices about their childbirths, content mothers and families who feel well provided-for and safe.

Home Birth or Independent Birth Centre

I am always glad when an expectant mother who is considering home birth comes to a midwife's practice for a consultation in the first months of pregnancy. That is the best time for the midwife and mother-to-be to talk about whether home birth is a possibility.

Essentially, if you want a doctor to attend an out-of-hospital birth, you have to look for one who is willing to do so. We midwives will be happy to advise you in the process; perhaps we even know if there is a doctor or obstetrician in your area who offers this service, which is time-consuming and complicated from the point of view of health insurance formalities. What is more, like the midwife, the obstetrician should be a person you trust. But since people have different views and different sensibilities, there will never be the midwife and the doctor who can satisfy the expectations of all involved. Especially the expectant mothers themselves quite often believe that it isn't necessary to have a doctor attend the birth. Usually the reason they cite is: "I remember only too well that when I was giving birth to my last child the doctor didn't appear until the very end, and I really only needed the midwife. SHE helped me. And anyway I know that as a midwife you're allowed to accompany the birth alone." Here I must agree; it's true that when the birth progresses normally, even in the hospital, the doctor usually stays in the background. What is more, at most out-of-hospital births – i.e. those which take place at home or in a birth centre – there is no doctor present because, medically speaking, it is not necessary. We midwives are trained and authorized to accompany normal pregnancies and births on our own. Nevertheless, in 1987 our profession was forced to carry out a bitter struggle to maintain the so-called "calling-in obligation." This is a law which rules that a midwife must be "called in" to attend every birth. She, on the other hand, is only required to call in a doctor if there are irregularities in the course of the birth. For many midwives and parents, it is therefore a reassuring feeling to know that there is a doctor who can be reached by phone. Ideally, he or she knows the birthing mother and is happy to attend the birth when such support is necessary. But in many places, doctors are not willing to come to births conducted outside the hospital, either for reasons of health insurance technicalities or due to lack of experience. Many self-employed midwives have begun to request the presence of a second midwife or a midwife-in-training. As a result, two specialists are present at most births. We have made necessity the mother of invention and come to the conclusion that it is better to make decisions on our own than to have obstetricians present who are inexperienced or afraid of out-of-hospital births. For me as a midwife, my confidence in the capability of the birthing woman to give birth is indispensable. But as soon as there is someone in the room who doubts this capability in particular or the success of the birth in general, it can have such a negative effect on the progress that the birthing mother may have to be moved to the hospital midway through the birth.

In view of these circumstances I would like to take this opportunity to express my sincere thanks to my teachers. Many years ago, a doctor and an experienced obstetrician were the ones who encouraged me to embark on home obstetrics. Unfortunately, specialists such as these have become an absolute rarity and we can only hope that soon there will be more doctors with the courage to provide assistance in out-of-hospital obstetrics, although the outrageous cost of liability insurance presently makes this virtually impossible. For me, the success of an out-of-hospital birth depends primarily on the amount of mutual trust that exists between the parents, the midwife and the other trained professionals present. Expectant parents should not derive their sense of security from machines and titles, but from a feeling of basic trust and healthy common sense.

Partnership

For the pregnant woman's partner, the first trimester of pregnancy is undoubtedly a difficult phase. Nothing can be seen, felt, heard of the child, but nevertheless the child is there. Sometimes the woman is no longer herself. She smells things no-one else can smell, she is much more sensitive, she cries and is elated about one and the same thing. Once a man told me: "I have the feeling she's like a little child herself, totally enthusiastic about everything but insulted at the slightest remark." These words speak for themselves. I myself am not in a position to feel what men feel; all I can do is ask them to try to show their partners understanding and remind themselves that it's a very special situation, it will pass, and it's for a good cause. And I also think that men should get together more often and talk about their experiences as expectant fathers.

Antenatal Screening

Antenatal screening is the term used to refer to examinations carried out to detect disorders or abnormalities in the unborn child at an early stage. The possibilities offered by this branch of medicine are certainly alluring, but they should be taken into careful consideration since, on the one hand, the results are relatively uncertain and, on the other hand, many of the examinations can themselves cause miscarriages or premature births. The statistical figures not only vary from country to country but even from hospital to hospital. You read of a 0.5% rate of miscarriages one day, a 20% rate the next. Regardless of how low or high the rate is, ultimately no statistics in the world can help when a healthy child is sacrificed to an erroneous positive result. Conversely, it can also happen that the child is in fact sick but the illness is not detected by the antenatal screening tests. We simply have no control when children develop differently from the way we want them to. The first question to be posed before every screening test must therefore be: would I consider terminating the pregnancy? If not, then you can confidently turn down all tests; they're not a must, even if the doctors would like to have you think so. Remember that despite all of the diagnostic methods available today, you also have the right *not* to know if there is something wrong with your unborn child.

The Bundeszentrale für gesundheitliche Aufklärung (BZgA; German Federal Centre for Health Education) in Cologne offers an instructional and worthwhile brochure on the subject of "Pränataldiagnostik" (antenatal screening), which provides comprehensive, objective information on examination methods, their risks and side effects, and the names of information centres. The brochure is available free of charge and can also be downloaded on the Internet (for address see appendix p. 460)

Ultrasound Scanning

The measurements carried out within the framework of the first ultrasound scan still provide the most reliable basis for calculating the due date when the menstrual cycle is irregular. And for technically oriented people, the pictures of the unborn child are undoubtedly an exciting insight – if an exclusively visual and somewhat alienating one – into emerging life. Many expectant fathers find it helpful to be present at the first ultrasound – but that doesn't mean that an early scan should be arranged just to give the man something to look at, something he, understandably, cannot (and perhaps must not) even comprehend.

I would like to point out that the process of adjusting to the new situation of becoming a mother or father cannot be replaced by any technology. Parents will experience many situations in which they wish they could look inside the child, but what is really going on in there will remain a secret. Later on in parenthood, there is no way of having your child "scanned" in order to understand it better. In other words, I would like to say that the technology isn't there to satisfy our curiosity but to detect abnormalities and clarify the resulting problems.

Moreover, I must call the reader's attention to the fact that, ultimately, it has not yet been determined whether the heating of the amniotic fluid during an ultrasonic scan can cause late sequelae, particularly if the scan is carried out during the early stage of pregnancy – the stage in which the infant's development is still very much in progress. The so-called doppler ultrasound is being carried out with increasing frequency to measure the flow of blood in the placenta, the umbilical cord and the child as a basis for assessing possible risks. What is more, many women are entirely unprepared for a vaginal examination during the first weeks and because of the penis-like shape of the doppler device experience it can be a very unpleasant, even violative, ordeal. The fact that the device is only a few millimetres from the tiny developing infant is also something to consider. This form of examination has become virtually obligatory in the early stage of pregnancy and serves in doctors' practice everywhere as a reliable form of pregnancy test.

Your obstetrician can provide you with information on the necessity of using this method. You should take into consideration that scientists at the Mayo Foundation in Rochester, New York proceed on the assumption that ultrasonic scanning during pregnancy subjects the infant to a noise level of 100 decibels (!). Young parents should also be aware that routine ultrasound scanning has been abolished in several European countries, e.g. Denmark. In Switzerland only one routine scan is carried out in the course of pregnancy, whereas in Germany, antenatal care still calls for three and the "baby watching" craze has even led to monthly control scans. They are carried out despite the fact that an error rate of some 30% to 40% is cited in medical circles for ultrasound results. This means that false conclusions are drawn about the infant's size and about alleged abnormalities, all of which only serves to upset the expectant parents. They tend to react by having further tests carried out, for example amniocenteses, which can lead in turn to a premature termination of pregnancy. In view of these circumstances, it is well worth your while to think carefully about every "routine" measure. Pregnancy is never a routine, and therefore no antenatal screening should be carried out on a routine basis.

On the basis of the ultrasound, conjectural diagnoses are often made, beginning with the words: "As far as we can tell …," for nothing can be said about the child with certainty. On the contrary, the results depend largely upon how much experience the obstetrician/sonographer has in the use of the ultrasound device and whether the latter is state-of-the-art or an older model. In about the twentieth week, for example, ultrasound scans are used to examine brain and heart structures, detect deformations of the feet and check for Down's syndrome – purposes for which ultrasound is simply not 100% reliable. And for you as parents, how will the situation change? This type of examination only makes sense if you intend to take action on the basis of the results. Otherwise, possible "positive" results mean the weeks ahead will be filled with anxiety rather than harmony. It is often not until the child is born that all the worries dissolve because they prove to have been unfounded.

Other Tests

The same applies to the blood test, the triple test generally carried out in the sixteenth week of pregnancy. It is often performed rather *en passant*, in the process of taking a routine blood sample. Many mothers will consent when the doctor's assistant mentions: "We're going to do a test to see whether the baby is healthy." Only very few of them are aware that, on the basis of the lab results – which unfortunately come out false-positive all too often – Down's syndrome is detected, but only in 60 to 79% of all cases. A positive triple-test result leads to further examinations which the parents had never even considered subjecting themselves to. In or around the twentieth week, for example, a chorion biopsy might be carried out (a test otherwise undertaken in the tenth to twelfth week) although the parents had originally decided against it. By this time the mother can already feel the child moving; she is already halfway through pregnancy and is once again faced with the decision as to whether she wants to keep the child or not. An amniocentesis could likewise have been carried out in the fourteenth week, but at that point the parents had perhaps not considered it. Now, however, startled by the "harmless" blood test and its result, they are suddenly faced with the whole range of questions all over again.

Amniocentesis

In the world of medicine, pregnancies in women age thirty-five and older are classified as "high-risk." What the doctors fail to take into consideration here is that most children are born healthy regardless of the mother's age. Increasingly, women come to the midwife's practice with the question: "Should I have an amniocentesis done or not?" The care-providing obstetrician is required to inform women thirty-five and older of the existence of this test and of her right to have it performed on her. Recently there have even been efforts to have the age boundary lowered. It makes me sad that other women ask their pregnant friends the virtually obligatory question: "You've had an amniocentesis, haven't you? You don't want a disabled child, do you?" For me it's as if an engaged couple were asked whether they had already been to see a fortune teller to find out whether their partnership would last. My initial answer is always: "Slow down." Give yourself plenty of time to think about whether you want this analysis, because – depending on the result – it leads necessarily to a decision for or against the child.

With amniocenteses and other methods, modern science attempts to detect certain handicaps in children. In the range of illnesses they test for, Down's syndrome is presumably the most well-known. One percent of all children born to 40-year-old mothers have this disorder (which is also called trisomy 21); in the case of 35-year-old mothers the rate is 0.2%, in the case of 25-year-olds only 0.08% (source: Schindele, Eva: *Gläserne Gebärmutter*. Frankfurt: Fischer 1990).

Many expectant mothers ask me: "Do you know women who have been in the same predicament? Am I really already at the age in which childbearing is a risk?" I then explain to them that other women have different partners, different living conditions and different children in their bellies. It is therefore essential to discuss these questions with one's partner, because the performance of the antenatal screening require the self-responsible decision of the parents. The result of the test can confront expectant parents with the decision as to whether they want a disabled child or not. Both parents will have to live with the consequences of their decision. I work with the parents to try to answer the following questions: can I bear "differentness," can I deal with children and adults who are different from us "normal" folks, would I be able to cope with my own child being different? I remind the parents that an originally healthy child can also become "different" from the neighbour's children during pregnancy, during childbirth, or later as the result of an illness or an accident. These are commonplace occurrences which tend to be forgotten in the context of researchable and controllable pregnancy. This point of view is certainly not an immediate help to many parents faced with such a decision, but it does give them food for thought about the realities of life. After all, a year earlier nobody would have been thinking about these controls; the woman wouldn't have been 35, her pregnancy not classified as "high-risk." It is certainly not my intention to look down on parents who decide in favour of an amniocentesis, because life with a "different" child, a disabled child, is not easy and our society is not always capable of supporting parents in such stressful situations. Both decisions – pro and con – are justified, but nobody can make the decision for the parents. I have also known parents who regard their disabled children as a gift and are appalled when people ask them why they had it, considering it's no longer necessary these days.

Another important consideration is the emotional strain on the woman while she is waiting for the result of the analysis. Most women have already begun to feel the child's movements very distinctly by the time the lab results arrive. A positive outcome generally means that the woman is permitted to have an abortion at this relatively late stage of pregnancy – usually sometime past the twelfth week. Here we cannot help but ask ourselves: why are women over 35 allowed to terminate the pregnancy while younger mothers are deemed capable of bearing the fate of having a disabled child? Who presumes to act here as a judge over life and death?

When parents decide against a disabled child the story isn't always over. On the contrary, after the abortion many women find that the inner conflict has only just begun; they can be burdened by emotional problems for years. For, as mentioned above, the woman must be aware that this child is part and parcel of her biography and she will be reminded of it again and again throughout her life. Whenever she encounters a disabled child, thoughts of her own child will fill her mind. We women are not capable of simply erasing a decision like this from our memories.

The decision which has to be made in such a situation is undoubtedly a very difficult one for a partnership. It is very important to look at the questions from all conceivable angles, calmly, patiently, without time pressure: the examination is quickly performed, but your lives and your relationship will endure for a long time yet. Women often join their partners in making decisions influenced by masculine rationality and forget that their partners can never decide about a woman's feelings. The unborn child at the centre of this decision is in the woman's body; she is pregnant, she feels the change and she will have to undergo the abortion, whether by suction or curettage, performed under temporary anaesthesia, or, in an advanced pregnancy, as foeticide, the killing of the fetus in the womb, which is followed by childbirth in the normal form. The partner should be aware that, if he has pushed·for an abortion, he will be confronted again and again, even many years later, with having influenced the woman. And he will likewise not be able simply to repress his feelings and his memories, because what has happened is irreversible.

As much as I can sympathize with the longing and desire for a healthy child, I find that I must ask myself: can we claim the right to perfect children?

THE SECOND TRIMESTER

The period from the thirteenth to the twenty-eighth week of pregnancy – the second trimester – is one of adaptation, well-being and reorientation. These are the weeks in which the child grows the fastest, since its organs are already fully developed. The uterus has to keep pace in order to provide the active little person inside with plenty of space.

Following the symbiosis of the first three months, reflected by the mother's declaration: "I'm pregnant", the first separation has now taken place, audible in the words: "The child is growing in my womb and already taking up quite a lot of space." The woman perceives very clearly that the child is growing, and now she really is expecting a child.

What is more, the pregnancy can usually no longer be concealed on the outside; the woman's tummy swells unmistakably and her colleagues show more understanding when she doesn't feel well. Apparently it's easier for people to cope with a pregnant woman when the pregnancy becomes visible.

Changes in the Body

As the pregnancy progresses, most women feel the need to adapt their body care habits to the physical changes that are taking place. Many an expectant mother notices that, in addition to the shape of her body, her skin and hair are different. These changes, caused by heightened hormone production, are completely normal. The woman's skin often becomes more strongly pigmented, producing brown spots on her face which have traditionally given rise to all kinds of speculation as to the child's sex. At the centre of her abdomen, a brown line appears, the linea fusca, the central vertical axis of the human body. All skin changes will disappear again a few weeks after childbirth. The hair can change in a variety of ways: from hair loss to abundant growth to change in consistency from straight to wavy. Wait and see what nature has in store for you! I have never witnessed pathological changes in this respect. If you are worried about your loss of hair, homoeopathy will be sure to have an appropriate remedy for you, but it has to be selected individually.

Stretch Marks

In order to avoid stretch marks I recommend beginning with regular massage early on in pregnancy: not only of the abdomen and breasts, but also of the buttocks and thighs, where stretch marks are also common. If you suffer from a congenital weakness of the connective tissue, however, you won't be able to avoid stretch marks altogether. And already existing marks can no longer be conjured away. I can offer you some consolation, however: nearly all stretch marks disappear again in the months following the child's birth, particularly the small, thin ones. The wide "rifts" will get narrower, initially take on a bluish shade and finally, in the course of several months, return to normal skin colour.

✎ Aroma Therapy

To make this preventive treatment as effective as possible, I like to recommend a massage oil blend based on evening primrose, wheat-germ and almond oil and containing lavender, linaloe wood, neroli and rose essential oils. This *Schwangerschaftsstreifenöl/Stretch Mark Oil 𝒟®* is particularly suitable if you have sensitive skin and are plagued by the thought: "I just *know* I'll get stretch marks!" The lavender will give you a sense of calm and clarity: "Everything will be as it should be." The linaloe wood has a relaxing effect, and the neroli oil is a perfect enhancement due to its freshness and power to counter anxiety.

Another blend – *Körperöl entspannend/Body Oil Relaxing 𝒟®* will appeal to women who are not fond of lavender and who are caught up in the stress of everyday life on the job or at home and want to do something for themselves. Here the basis is a mixture of jojoba wax, almond and wheat-germ oil, "flavoured" with chamomile Roman, neroli, rose and cedar wood.

In this connection, I am reminded of the following situation. A pregnant woman came to my midwife's practice "Erdenlicht" in a state of quite some stress, and said:

"… I don't have much time, but I have to ask you a few questions; it's about the skin of my abdomen, it's so taut." In order to shorten her waiting time, I recommended that she take a sniff at some of our oils and try them out if she liked. It was for me an unforgettable experience when she came into the consulting room firmly gripping a bottle of Body Oil Relaxing 𝒟® *and saying: "This is terrific; the smell is so pleasant, I have already applied it to my tummy." When I asked her what she found particularly pleasing, she answered: "My life is so stressful that I really don't have time for 'smearing' products on myself, but I'm going to take this with me, it really appeals to me, I can't stop smelling it. I am absolutely sure that I will take the time and treat myself and my child to a little daily massage session, this oil is just so pleasant." And it was really true: this woman, who usually made a very nervous and irritable impression on me, suddenly seemed much calmer. Of course I had to explain to her that she couldn't just take that bottle with her but would have to purchase one on her own.*

I have been having experiences like this one with essential oils for many years. For me they are proof that even people who are under a lot of stress and strain instinctively choose the right oil. The body can't be fooled! I think it's wonderful that a mere aroma can make a person's mood so positive, without my having to contribute much as a midwife. Providing help with aroma-therapy products gives me so much joy and so many satisfied faces. And I would like all mothers to share in this, because midwives and mothers have a lot in common: always being there for the family, listening when there are problems, providing equilibrium: simply *giving* in every situation.

This is why it is so very important for a pregnant woman to take some time for herself now and then, and care for her own body, because after the child is born everything will revolve around the child. But the mother will have her memories of the wonderful moments and hours of time she had for herself – a gift she owes this very child. And what is more, I am certain that massage helps to establish much closer contact to the baby and develop a more positive attitude towards the physical changes brought about by the pregnancy – the growing belly, the swelling breasts, etc.

Another pleasant body oil that is helpful in cases of dry skin is hazelnut oil with rose and linaloe wood essential oils, available as *Körperöl trockene Haut/Body Oil Dry Skin 𝒟®*. It has a relaxing and calming effect. For women who have already gone through pregnancy and childbirth before, I like to recommend my time-tested *Rosen-Körperöl/Rose Body Oil 𝒟®*. In addition to rose oil it contains rose geranium, which helps to strengthen the connective tissue, and the blend of wild rose oil and jojoba wax not only constitutes a high-quality basis for this product but also aids in preserving the elasticity of the skin.

☯ Fatty Oils

Massage oils are helpful for various reasons. For one thing, the expectant mother receives loving attention. The masseuse treats certain pathways of energy (meridians), and is entirely justified in using her intuition to do so. Energy blocks can be dissolved, and both body and soul benefit from the treatment.

For another thing, the skin is warmed when the oil is rubbed into it, causing the essential oils contained in the blend to penetrate the skin barrier faster and – provably – enter the blood stream within ten minutes. Their beneficial mechanisms are thus quickly available to the body. Depending on the consistency of the basis oil and the intensity of the massage, the essences can make their way through the skin and into the deeper layers of tissue within one to two hours. It is thus very important that not only the essential oil additives but also the basis oil be selected with care.

Only first-cold-pressed fatty oils should be used, preferably from organically grown plants. So-called mineral oils (petroleum extracts) are of inferior quality and should not be employed. They are incapable of passing the skin barrier of the human being, and can therefore not transport essential oil into the body to carry out their healing effects. In fact, mineral oils block the pores of the skin and actually form a barrier. Since we would like to achieve a therapeutic effect in addition to the benefits for the skin, only high-grade fatty vegetable oils are suitable as a basis for a body or massage oil, as is the case with the *Original 𝒟® Aroma Blends*. Only these oils are fully absorbed by the skin, allowing them to make their way into the connective tissue, the lymph channels, the musculature and the blood. They serve as conveyor substances for the essential oils, which are thus introduced into the organ systems. Moreover, the fatty oils can also possess healing qualities themselves; they differ greatly in character and are therefore put to a wide variety of uses.

For more detailed information on fatty oils such as jojoba wax, almond, nut and other oils used in aroma therapy as bases for essential oil blends, see my book *Time-Tested Aroma Blends*.

Antenatal Classes

The majority of pregnant women still seek contact to a midwife in the phase between the eighteenth and the twentieth week of pregnancy. And that is the ideal point in time to register for an antenatal class. You should begin with the class between the twenty-fourth and – at the latest – the twenty-eighth week. These classes, which last from eight to fourteen weeks, are offered to women and couples by midwives and women who have specialized in antenatal care.

As in the case of all other consultations and aids for pregnant women in the Federal Republic of Germany, the class teachers are reimbursed directly by the health insurance company for the cost of the class. In many places, however, the class participants are required to make an additional contribution, since the fees paid by the health plan do not entirely cover the cost of the class. Unfortunately, we midwives often cannot communicate our extensive range of information within the fourteen class sessions and have to offer additional information sessions, independently of the class. The costs of the latter have to be borne by the parents.

In my opinion, the attendance of an antenatal class is particularly important for women expecting their first child. Until now, the woman's life has usually revolved around her job; from now on, though, becoming and being a mother are going to be her profession. During this transition, midwives provide support and, in a certain sense, help. In the old days, within the framework of the extended family, a young mother had often already experienced her sister's or other relative's pregnancy, childbirth and breastfeeding. To meet the demands placed upon us by our profession, we midwives try to compensate for the loss of the extended family and stand by young mothers with our experience and expertise.

But women who are pregnant for the second, third, etc. time are frequent visitors to midwives' practices as well. They are a great enrichment to antenatal classes, because by telling of their experiences they help "first-timers" to overcome their fears. Among other things, they confirm my motto that

First of all, things don't always happen
Second of all, the way parents expect, but
Third of all, sooner or later entirely of their own accord!

They convey to first-time mothers that it's worth the effort to listen carefully, to prepare, and above all, to learn the breathing exercises. Mothers who already have children at home are glad to have this one hour a week in which to devote themselves entirely to the new child. Certain words and thoughts are only truly absorbed the second or third time around. The group session is restful and relaxing, a time and place to think, talk – and perhaps find answers to questions – about previous births, and a very welcome opportunity to make contact with other women. Often the weekly session represents the first experience of what it means to leave the older child at home to be put to bed by its father – in its own way an important preparation for the changes in family habits that will be brought about by the advent of the younger sister or brother.

Preparation for Couples

Many couples want to prepare for the birth of their child together. There are mid-wives who offer classes in which the expectant father participates in every session. If you are interested, you will be sure to find a class like this in the vicinity of your home. A woman can naturally also attend the class with a good woman friend, prefer-ably one who has already given birth. I would like to encourage all expectant parents to talk openly and honestly about the subject of "preparation and childbirth as a cou-ple." As the years go by, I am becoming more and more convinced that many men decide to attend the antenatal class and the birth itself because they feel enormous pressure to do so, rather than being honest with themselves. After all, the most im-portant thing for the expectant mother is to have someone accompanying her who trusts her completely. What is more, she must also come to realize that she must give birth herself, no matter who is ultimately at her side. Like midwives, expectant fa-thers must become aware that the goal of the class is not to train a group of obstetri-cians. The fathers shouldn't have to act as an assistant or see to it that the birth pro-ceeds correctly, and they certainly will not have to take the midwife's place. All they really have to do is just simply be there and experience becoming a father. It is always good to have experienced fathers in the class, who then pass on their experience to other men from a man's point of view. I am always grateful to them for that informa-tion, since, as a woman, I am simply not able to convey a man's emotions.

In all my years of working in antenatal care I have tried out various types of classes and have come to the conclusion that it is best for expectant mothers to attend a class exclusively for women. In these sessions, women gain a much better sense of their own bodies, and we midwives can convey their role as mother to them more con-sciously. For parents who would like to attend a prep class together, our midwife's practice "Erdenlicht" offers expectant fathers the opportunity of attending three in-tensive preparation sessions. This gives the women a chance to practice their exer-cises; the men benefit from only having to plan three evenings. For parents who al-ready have children it's easier to find a babysitter for three evenings than for eight: most couples classes comprise eight to twelve sessions. Sometimes neither variation suits a couple's schedule, but there are a number of midwives who offer weekend "crash courses" – two concentrated days of preparation for childbirth and parent-hood.

It has been our experience that it works better to concern ourselves with the role of the man during the birth in the framework of three long evenings. During a two-hour evening session, we can convey that – in addition to a massaging hand – time, calmness, patience and simply being there will be the most important aids. I devote myself especially to creating an awareness of the fact that already the accompanying person's presence alone is a big help. Most fathers want to learn what they can "do" to help their wives during childbirth. This isn't possible – they can't actually "do" anything at all. They will never be able to take over some part of the job of giving birth. But they have a very important job of their own – to convey to the mother: "You can do it!" In the antenatal classes, we want all parents to realize that the birth of a child is a tremendous physical achievement on the part of the woman, that women are "designed" to give birth, that we must place our confidence in the woman's ability to carry out this achievement. A woman must always try to "ride the storm", to swim on the surface of the waves, as it were, but not fight against them, or she will go under. If the birthing woman is capable of accepting the pain of the contractions and go along with it and does not try to resist that pain and the course of events in general, she will be in a position to achieve and experience the birth. With the use of the correct breathing techniques, she will manage it, especially if she receives support from the people accompanying her. We midwives make it our business to teach these breathing techniques to the expectant parents – "affirmative" breathing, with an emphasis on exhalation. If the woman's partner succeeds in breathing along with her, in conveying to her during the strong contractions that she can say "Yeeeeeeeeeeeeeeeeeeees", that she can let it all out, her voice, her feelings, her child, everything "aaaaaaaaaaaaout", that is the best support a woman can wish for.

Giving positive support is the first and foremost task of any person accompanying a birth.

Midwives and mothers alike rave about the new and effective enhancement of traditional antenatal classes by birth preparation in water. The woman learns to use the buoyancy of her body in the water to attain optimal relaxation, the bath provides excellent support to the metabolism, and pregnancy-related disorders such as the accumulation of fluid in the tissue (oedema) are reduced or never come about to begin with. Moreover, gymnastic exercises in the water help to guard against postural problems and prevent backaches.

The Antenatal Class Curriculum

During the fourteen weekly sessions, we midwives attempt to convey everything we consider important from the point of view of our profession. This includes explaining, discussing, describing and practising the following:
- pregnancy-related ailments in connection with pointers on nutrition and helpful physical exercises
- the contents of the "Mutterpass"

- body perception exercises, posture exercises
- "letting go" and "delivery"
- learning and practising breathing techniques
- breathing exercises for the first (dilation) stage and the birth
- positions for the second (expulsion or pushing) stage
- stages and mechanisms of labour
- childbirth and postnatal period in the hospital
- preparing the breasts for nursing
- information on the first weeks of breastfeeding
- the woman during the postnatal period
- the care of the baby
- the use of natural medicines in pregnancy, childbirth and the postnatal period

Unfortunately, it is impossible to cover all of these topics within the fourteen hours covered by the health fund. For this reason, additional classes on infant care or the use of naturopathic aids are offered to expectant parents. You should attend an infant care class as early as possible – before you start shopping for your baby.

I also urgently recommend that midwives include breastfeeding (also see p. 370) in their antenatal class curriculum – or have the parents read the related chapter in this book.

Natural Pregnancy

In the context of her first contact with a midwife – whether in the framework of a consultation, an antenatal appointment or the first session of an antenatal class – the expectant mother learns that pregnancy is a physiological process, i.e. a natural occurrence. Pregnancy and childbirth are not illnesses, but rather a phase in the life of a woman that is not only wonderful but also leaves an indelible mark. Every pregnancy and every birth is an absolutely unique experience. Being pregnant with this child cannot be compared with a previous or later pregnancy, because that was, or will be, a different child. And a woman will not experience pregnancy in the same way her girlfriend, neighbour or mother did – the women who try to help her with all kinds of good advice: "When I was pregnant the contractions always started much too early and the pills I had to take never helped. So I just asked a midwife; she gave me some herbal remedy. I still have some, you can have it, then you can start taking it right away when your contractions start early. You'll see, it'll be the same with you; after all most women have that problem these days."

Women often tell me about apparently well-meant counsel of this kind. Most of them already know what I then confirm for them: that it is a big mistake to take such advice to heart. Because now you are pregnant with *this* child and have to adjust to the development of *this* pregnancy, which will be entirely different from what other women have experienced. Because they had *different* children! And of course it is also extremely important to be aware that so-called "herbal remedies" are not always completely harmless. On the contrary, their effect – especially during pregnancy – is not to be underrated. Due to the fact that naturopathy takes a holistic approach to healing – i.e. takes the entire human being into account and not only the organ affected by the illness – a natural medication will have the desired effect for a specific woman in a specific situation. Even if a different woman exhibits the same symptoms, that medication may have no effect at all, or, on the other hand, lead to a worsening of her condition. During pregnancy, please therefore always be very careful about well-meaning advice from friends and other people. Always ask your midwife, your attending physician or your pharmacist whether it is really advisable for you to take such "herbal" medication.

I would like my readers to know that the great majority (ninety percent) of all pregnancies and births proceed normally. Thus the expectant mother is not a patient – but a pregnant woman. I would like to point out in this context that many of the ailments that accompany pregnancy are not pathological, but just the child's own special way of calling attention to itself. In an entirely natural way, these ailments help the woman to adapt to her changing situation. An ache in the groin, a pain in the sacrum or the problem of getting to sleep are necessary reminders of the fact that, when this child is born, your everyday life will change. Nature gives us several months to get used to the idea that changes are on the way.

Natural Support

Expectant mothers often ask about natural means of coping with the discomforts brought about by pregnancy.

⑤ Herbal Medicine

Pregnancy does not actually require any measures or medications to support it, but since time immemorial women have always sought to do everything in their power to ensure the child's well-being – an important prerequisite for a birth which is free of all complications. From this point of view, I can understand the requests of present-day women as well. My first recommendation here is a tea blend which has been proving its usefulness for two decades now – *Schwangerschaftstee/Pregnancy Tea*. Among other things it was my good experience with this blend during my own pregnancies that convinced me of its value. It consists of stinging nettle, lady's mantle, raspberry leaves, Saint John's wort, lemon balm leaves, yarrow and horsetail.

Lady's mantle (*Alchemilla vulgaris*) tea is an age-old means of supporting the hormonal balance. The raspberry leaves help pregnant women by loosening the muscles, particularly in the pelvis minor. The entire metabolism receives support, and the intestinal excretory process is also stimulated. Stinging nettle and horsetail stimulate renal excretion. Saint John's wort has a nerve-strengthening effect, and lemon balm a calming one. Stinging nettle leaves improve the absorption of iron in the blood, especially when a few drops of lemon juice are added to the tea. Yarrow supports the co-agulation of the blood – an important consideration during childbirth, in view of the danger of haemorrhaging.

Initially, I myself found it hard to believe that a blend of herbs could be so effective. In the past years, however, an increasing number of women swear by this tea. They confirm to me that digestion problems disappear, retention of fluid in the legs de-creases, the iron content of the blood increases without their having to take an iron supplement. This is particularly good news for women who react to iron supplements with constipation and stomach aches. The expectant mothers who drink this tea re-port that their circulation and their mood are stable. But even if many womens' expe-rience with this tea has been positive, I would like to remind my readers that miracles always take time! What I mean is: if a bodily function gets "off track" or has been ir-regular for years, a spoonful of herbs won't help within a few days. But if this tea blend is taken regularly from the sixteenth to twentieth week of pregnancy onward – three cups a day suffice – then the above-mentioned bodily functions will be posi-tively influenced well before the various threatening problems even have time to de-velop, and the body will maintain its equilibrium during pregnancy. You should try to ensure that the tea is concocted from organically grown herbs so as not to burden the organism unnecessarily with environmental pollutants. I would also like to stress that, contrary to widespread opinion, a daily dosage of approximately 0.5 g of sting-ing nettle by no means has a diuretic effect which could cause damage to the kidneys or even increase the occurrence of oedemas. The often-repeated belief that pregnant women should stay away from stinging nettle tea is based on erroneous information regarding the formation of oedemas due to the phytooestrogens it contains. The phy-tooestrogens in stinging nettle – the beta-sitosterols -, however, are not water-soluble, and what is more, they are not present in the leaves, but only in the root of the plant. The pregnant woman need therefore have no qualms whatsoever about drinking this tea blend during pregnancy, even if she has already suffered – or is presently suffer-ing – from gestosis (a toxemic disorder of pregnancy) – since the abovementioned negative effects cannot possibly occur.

Nutrition and Dietary Supplements

If you have special questions concerning your diet, I would like to recommend that you consult a nutritionist. Otherwise a healthful, balanced, diversified diet provides you with ideal nourishment during pregnancy. To the extent possible, the fresh fruit and vegetables you eat should be certified organically grown. animal proteins, and meat should be enjoyed in moderation, the meat only from sources you know are reputable. Liver should be avoided due to its high vitamin A content. Moreover, you should consume enough dairy products or suitable alternatives to cover your calcium requirement. Two teaspoons of cold-pressed vegetable oil (e.g. olive or sunflower oil) a day supplies you with vitally essential fatty acids. Whole-grain products contain iron, zinc, starch and above all high-quality carbohydrates. The latter are broken down by the system much more slowly than white flour and therefore do not stimulate the pancreas to secrete an excessive amount of insulin. Whole-grain products are therefore also a means of preventing diabetes. By eating muesli consisting of rolled oats, sunflower seeds, flaxseed, nuts and wheat germ along with milk or yoghurt every morning, you already supply yourself with a large proportion of vital nutrients at breakfast time. To guarantee sufficient intake of proteins, I would like to cite another piece of advice which is quite easy to put into practice: eat twice as many potatoes as eggs (on a weekly average) or add a generous dash of whole milk to your scrambled eggs. And if you eat nearly three times as much salad and fresh vegetables as meat, you are on the right road to giving your child everything it needs. And you don't have to have a nutrition chart on your kitchen wall, but can continue to plan your diet by "rule of thumb."

After eating, pregnant women should take a break on the sofa, followed by a short walk. As in every life situation, exercise is one of the most important prerequisites for a healthy metabolism. Pregnant women are also affected by the general increase of diabetes in our society. In addition to reducing refined sugar and flour, regular exercise can contribute greatly to preventing this illness. And don't forget that taking a walk in the fresh air increases the oxygen content of your red blood cells, ensuring that your overall system is well-supplied despite the natural reduction in haemoglobin content during pregnancy.

The guidelines I have mentioned surely form a good basis for a healthy diet during pregnancy, not only for the expectant mother but also for her child and her family. Of course I myself am only too well aware that it is not easy for pregnant working women to cope with having a job, eating right, getting plenty of exercise and relaxation, etc. If you open your eyes and ears, maybe you will find a place nearby where you can get a daily meal of fresh whole foods. My readers are surely aware that canned food, microwave menus and fast food are worthless.

Your healthy body sends you plenty of signals and lets you know what will do it good and what it needs at a given moment. I believe that pregnancy is an ideal time to place more trust in your body again, develop a sense of it and its normal reactions. If you feel thirsty, it means: please supply fluid! If you're out and about, don't wait until you get home, but drink something as soon as possible. When I was training as a midwife in the 1970s, it was said that pregnant women should drink no more than one litre of fluid a day, but this assumption has since been proven wrong in a great number of nutrition studies. Like everyone else, expectant mothers can – and should! – pay attention to, and satisfy, their individual needs. This example is a clear indication that, even if they are based on scientific research, new findings should always be critically questioned, and that it makes more sense to master life with common sense. Women were already getting pregnant thousands of years ago and didn't need scientists to bear healthy children. But in former times, women are sure to have been more accustomed to knowing and understanding the language of their own bodies. It is never too late to learn, however, and to get to know yourself with a baby in your womb is a wonderful point in time to liberate yourself from generalizations and become more self-confident as an individual woman.

When you're eating, don't forget that relaxation and pleasure are the best "side dishes." As soon as you enjoy your meal, perhaps chuckle about a story being told by someone else at the table, endorphins are released in your body. These are by far the best anti-stress hormones and as such a wonderful aid to digestion. Perhaps you remember from childhood how you lost your appetite and every bite of food got stuck in your throat when mum chose dinnertime to talk about the bad marks on your school report. But you surely also remember that magnificent feeling of happiness when there was something sweet and yummy – something there was never enough of – for dessert. Treat yourself to a bit of chocolate or a sweet dessert now and then. These goodies contain the amino acid tryptophan, which provably stimulates the release of serotonin, a neurotransmitter and "feel-good" hormone, and you'll be as happy as a child again. Just another proof of the fact that the way to peoples hearts is through their stomachs (that doesn't apply to men only!) and that happy people are healthy, since serotonin also plays a role in the immune system. What is more, I am very sure that if the mother is happy, so is the baby inside her. That's something we shouldn't forget, no matter how many scientific findings we hear about.

Common Minor Problems

Pressure on the Pelvic Floor

Many women who come to consult me during the second trimester, particularly those pregnant with their second or subsequent child, complain of a feeling of downward pressure on the pelvic floor due to the expansion of the uterus. I try to call their attention to the fact that they should exercise the pelvic floor muscles as often as possible: when carrying out certain daily tasks, they should consistently tighten those muscles. I give them specific pointers on how to exercise. I also advise mothers not to carry their small children anymore at all if possible, or at least to ask them to climb onto a chair before picking them up, thus reducing lifting to a minimum. I also suggest that they tell their children who are still in nappies to climb onto the changing table themselves. These pointers will also be helpful after the delivery and later on. An awareness of the pelvic floor muscles and how to cope with them is important throughout a woman's life.

✆ Homoeopathy

If the discomfort of the downward pressure becomes too great, the homoeopathic remedy *Sepia* is often very helpful. *Aletris* is a sensible alternative in some cases. Many women ask specifically for a homoeopathic medication during the consultation. Finding the right homoeopathic substance is not always an easy task but generally takes considerable time and experience.

✆ Aroma Therapy

Many women take the time and treat themselves to a sitz bath with the *Original 𝒟®* *Aroma Blend Myrte-Rosengeranie-Öl/Myrtle-Rose Geranium Oil 𝒟®* mixed with Dead Sea Salt or use *Körperöl kräftigend/Body Oil Strengthening 𝒟®* as a means of firming up the lower abdomen. As always, it is important to stop carrying out the treatment when the symptoms have disappeared.

What is more, both the baths and the body oil should be discontinued no later than five weeks before the estimated due date. As is the case with all naturopathically oriented measures, I advise women to consult me as to whether they should carry on with the treatment if there are any changes in their condition or if new symptoms appear. It is always encouraging to note the sensitivity with which pregnant women perceive their bodies. In my opinion, the greatest advantage of using natural medicines during pregnancy is the immediacy with which undesired reactions can be recognized.

Ligament Pain

The uterine ligaments have to accommodate the growth of the uterus by stretching and softening, often causing quite some pelvic pain. We can imagine the uterus like an "inflated" captive hot-air balloon anchored in the pelvis with the uterine ligaments. When the child is very active inside this "balloon", the ligaments are jerked and pulled, producing a sensation much like sore muscles. The expectant mother often feels this pain in the lower back or in the groin.

✆ Homoeopathic Remedies

Homoeopathic medications such as *Aletris, Clematis* or *Helonias*, administered in medium potencies, can be very helpful.

✆ Aroma Therapy

Pregnant women often find very pleasant a massage or an oil compress with *Massageöl entspannend/Massage Oil Relaxing 𝒟®* in the area of the groin. This aroma blend contains the essential oils fennel, chamomile, lavender linaloe wood, mandarin and neroli; I also like to call it "uterine ligament oil." Due to its strong oestrogenic effect, fennel oil is a suitable ingredient for this relaxing blend. During pregnancy, the body itself produces considerable amounts of oestrogen, which aids in maintaining the pregnancy.

Varicose Veins

One of the most frequent maladies accompanying pregnancy are painful varicose veins: here it is particularly important to take action right away, because an extremely painful inflammation of the vein can develop quite rapidly.

In order to prevent varicose veins and keep the condition of already existing ones from worsening, the following pointers should be observed:
- integrate *regular leg exercises* into your daily routine in order to support the flow of blood by contracting the muscles. These exercises are taught in antenatal classes.
- *put your feet up* regularly in the course of the day. At night, sleep on a bed which is slightly elevated at the foot end.
- shower your legs with alternating hot and cold water in the morning and, especially in the summertime, administer cold *affusions to the calves* several times a day. When applying cold water, it is always important to adjust the temperature so that the water feels cool – the actual temperature can vary greatly from person to person. The jet of cold water should furthermore always be administered in an upward direction.
- Make sure your *diet* includes plenty of fibre and reduce animal protein; in general, take measures to ensure good digestion and regular bowel movements. One way of achieving this is with the regular consumption of cold-pressed vegetable oils such as olive oil. The high content of unsaturated fats in these oils have a strengthening effect on the immune system, aid digestion and prevent the calcification of the vascular walls. As in so many contexts, coping with varicose veins is also a question of nutrition. Even if I am otherwise of the opinion that healthy pregnant women don't have to watch their weight, this advice has to be modified with regard to varicose veins. Every superfluous pound puts a burden on the legs and, with them, the varicose veins.
- In addition to all of these applications, well-fitting elastic stockings are always an important means of taking pressure off the veins. If you go to a pharmacy or specialized shop, make sure you are fitted for the stockings in the early part of the day. Even better, have the salesperson explain how to carry out the measurements and do it yourself before you get out of bed in the morning. This will guarantee that the stockings really fit properly. The stockings should always be donned in the morning after putting your feet up for ten minutes. Otherwise the pain will worsen because the blood has already pooled in the veins.

Vulva varicose veins, i.e. varicose veins in the vaginal region, are particularly unpleasant. Many women don't like to talk about this condition, because it pertains to the intimate zone. The pain is further aggravated by the worry – or even fear – that these veins will cause problems during the birth. There are lots of rumours about these varicose veins bursting. I have never seen this happen, and even if it did, the doctors know how to put everything back in order – so there's no cause for panic. In contrast to the abovementioned pointers on coping with varicose veins in the legs, here you should see to it that you never wear *restrictive stockings, knickers or trousers!* Loose, so-called harem pants are suddenly pure pleasure to wear. *Exercise the pelvic floor muscles regularly*, avoid sitting for long periods if possible or use a "knee" or "kneeling" chair so that the veins in the pelvic girdle are not blocked. Most women with varicose veins prefer to sit on a fitness ball, which ensures constant movement. With regard to *diet*, the same pointers apply as for varicose veins in the legs.

Herbal Medicine

When the symptoms are acute, the application of *Ringelblumensalbe/Calendula Ointment* or a gel containing *horse chestnut extract* can be very helpful. In general, *Schwangerschaftstee/Pregnancy Tea* has a supportive effect on the veins. *Venentee/Vein Tea*, a blend of buckwheat herb, butcher's broom, horse chestnut leaves, sweet clover and lemon zest, can't make the symptoms disappear entirely, but has long proven its value in the therapy of veins. It supports the metabolism and has an anti-inflammatory effect. I recommend drinking a cup of *Schwangerschaftstee/Pregnancy Tea* in the morning and in the evening, and enjoying *Venentee/Vein Tea* in between times.

Homoeopathic Remedies

There are a number of very helpful homoeopathic medicines: *Arnica, Hamamelis, Pulsatilla, Lachesis, Lycopodium, Sepia* and *Zincum*. As always, a midwife or doctor possessing experience with homoeopathy should be consulted. In the case of constitutional remedies, it is particularly important not to administer too low a potency.

Aroma Therapy

Aroma therapy provides an extremely effective means of treating varicose veins, as I know from a great deal of experience. For this purpose I use a calendula-almond-oil base containing the essential oils lavender, lemongrass, myrtle, yarrow, juniper berry and cypress: available as one of my *Original D®* Aroma Blends, I like to refer to this *Lavendel-Zypressen-Öl/Lavender Cypress Oil D®* as "Varicose Veins Oil." For best results, massage it onto the legs every morning from the bottom up. Ideally the skin should be dampened with water first in order to support its natural moisture level. Or you can use the *Lavendel-Zypressen-Öl/Lavender Cypress Oil D®* emulsion, to which myrtle hydrolat has been added. In cases of low blood pressure it is advisable to add a drop of essential *Rosmarinöl/Rosemary Oil*.

When the pain caused by varicose veins is acute, it has proven extremely helpful to make a compress with a teaspoon or tablespoon (depending on the size of the affected area) of refrigerated milk curds ("quark") mixed with a bit of *Lavendel-Zypres-*

sen-Öl/Lavender Cypress Oil $\mathcal{D}^\circledast$ and apply it to the painful zone. The same effect can be achieved with Retterspitz External, a German-made product. This remedy causes many women irritations to the skin, however. Alternatively, put a leaf of white cabbage on the painful area after applying the oil, and leave it there until it wilts. This is likewise a method of preventing inflammation. *Hamamelis-Myrte-Balsam/Witch-Hazel-Myrtle Balsam* $\mathcal{D}^\circledast$ can also be applied pure or in a blend with quark.

At this point I could fill reams with stories about varicose veins, always ending with the sentence: "I never would have thought natural medicine could provide any relief; I tried so many different things!"

I remember one woman, a hair stylist …

… who already suffered from pain in her legs simply on account of her profession, and now, during pregnancy, had developed burst capillaries beneath the surface of the skin. They aren't painful, but they're a bother because they're somewhat unsightly. A few weeks after the application of the Varicose Vein Oil, she reported to me: "Just imagine, even the burst capillaries are disappearing." It seemed rather incredible, but I saw it with my own eyes: the reduction was clearly perceivable.

Or …

… Ursula, with big fat varicose veins on one leg, which caused her quite some pain every evening. She told me: "You won't believe this, but already after the second evening my leg hardly hurt anymore. Now I never forget to use the oil, because if I do, I have to pay for it that very night." After a week there was another new development: "Since I started using the oil every morning, I have the feeling my circulation has become much more stable. Otherwise I often had days where I felt tired and drained. My doctor told me at the time that this was related to my low blood pressure. But now that's gone too. Can this all have to do with the oil?" I was able to confirm to Ursula that her problem had indeed been one of circulatory instability. Whether or not the improvement had been brought about by the oil, I was not able to say at the time. Today, however, with the knowledge I have gained in the meantime about the way essential oils work, I would say yes, it was the effect of the Varicose Vein Oil.

Or …

… Christine, a colleague of mine, said: "Inge, every midwife who works in the hospital should have Varicose Vein Oil. Since I've been using it, I no longer have pains in my legs. The birthing women and my fellow midwives also benefit if I am capable of standing at the birthing bed for hours without a problem.

The stories go on and on. It always makes me happy to learn about such success – it gives me a boost and encourages me to pass my knowledge on to others, and to find even more ways of helping people with essential oils and aroma blends. With regard to relieving discomfort and creating a sense of well-being, the potentials and limitations of aroma therapy have yet to be thoroughly explored.

Haemorrhoids

I can report on similar successes in the treatment of haemorrhoids. Many women suffer from this malady during pregnancy and come to me for advice and help. I also recommend that these women exercise the muscles of the pelvic floor regularly in order to stimulate the circulation in that region. As for diet, the same pointers apply as for varicose veins.

Herbal Medicine

In cases of haemorrhoids I once again call attention to *Schwangerschaftstee/Pregnancy Tea* and the regular consumption of organic *fatty vegetable oils*; here again, the treatment is the same as for varicose veins, because both problems – haemorrhoids and varicose veins – are caused by vein blockage. This tea blend supports the organism's overall metabolism as well as its natural detoxification processes.

Hametum®-Salbe – an ointment containing Hamamelis virginiana – or cool sitz baths with *oak bark* are likewise helpful.

Aroma Therapy

I have found essential oils to be even more effective than herbal medicines for treating haemorrhoids. In the *Original $\mathcal{D}$® Aroma Blend Hamamelis-Myrte-Balsam/Witch-Hazel-Myrtle Balsam $\mathcal{D}$®*, the essential oils lavender, myrtle and cypress are combined with a high-quality preservative-free ointment basis. If you have even just one of these oils on hand, you can mix one or two drops of it with salt and take a cool sitz bath. In cases of acute pain, relief is provided by an ice cube with a pinch of salt and a drop of the essential oil on it, wrapped in a gauze pad and placed on the haemorrhoid. Alternatively, you can spread the ice cube with a thin layer of the balsam. A more pleasant treatment is a teaspoon of quark mixed with approx. 0.5 cm of *Hamamelis-Myrte-Balsam/Witch-Hazel-Myrtle Balsam $\mathcal{D}$®*, likewise wrapped in a gauze pad and placed on the painful haemorrhoid/s.

Homoeopathic Remedies

Naturally, there are also helpful homoeopathic remedies such as *Acidum muriaticum, Arnica, Collinsonia, Hamamelis, Lycopodium* or *Nux vomica*. Because the symptoms are usually of a purely physical nature, I recommend the lower potencies. As a first-aid measure, any pregnant woman can begin by taking *Hamamelis*. As always, if this does not bring about any relief, a specialist in homoeopathic medicine should be consulted.

Urinary Tract Infections or Cystitis

Not infrequently, I am asked to provide help and advice for infections of the urinary tract. The cause of the discomfort should always be determined by a doctor. Often women don't even have any physical symptoms yet, but come to me or ring up about the doctor's diagnosis: bacteria in the urine. They want to know: "Do I really have to take the antibiotic I've been prescribed? How else can I cope with the problem?"

If it is not an acute or chronic infection which is at the root of the problem, but a pregnancy-related excretion of bacteria by way of the urine, I can provide a number of pointers and pieces of advice upon request.

I must begin by explaining that, along with the rest of the body, the bladder and kidney system is affected by the pregnancy. Changes in the hormonal balance not only bring about vasodilation (widening of the blood vessels) in the form of varicose veins and haemorrhoids, but also a widening of the ureter or urinary duct. Germs and bacteria can therefore make their way into the bladder much more easily, and consequently it is important to observe certain rules of bodily hygiene, particularly in connection with urine tests.

The regular prenatal examinations always include a urine test. It is very important that the urine sample tested is from the middle of the urine stream. In other words, first release a small amount of urine into the toilet, then put the container in the urine stream and collect one to two ounces; the bladder can then be emptied into the toilet. This way, every woman can exercise her pelvic floor muscles and has an excuse to drink lots of fluid, at least on the day of the appointment. By observing these measures, many a "positive" urine test result is negated. The reason is that the bacteria are usually located near the opening of the urethra and are washed into the toilet before you collect urine in the container.

As far as bodily hygiene is concerned, it is advisable to wear cotton panties and change them frequently. In cases of constantly recurring cystitis, it also helps to wear panties made of pure silk, since silk is an animal protein fibre and therefore has an anti-bacterial effect. It is likewise important to avoid perfumed soaps and so-called feminine hygiene products, since they contain preservatives and disinfectants which can disturb the healthy balance of the vaginal ecosystem. Bacteria can grow more easily as a result, a problem also brought about by shaving the pubic hair. Panty liners are also inadvisable since they impede the flow of air and, what is more, they're often scented.

The regular passing of water helps to avoid disorders of the bladder. You should not wait until the bladder is full and the urge to pass water is too great. In this context we can once again witness how the body protects itself during pregnancy, because women always say they have never had to go to the bathroom as often as they do during pregnancy. Another worthwhile bit of information is that passing water after having sexual intercourse is a good way of reducing or preventing bladder problems, because it washes off any germs that may have found their way into the urethra from the rectum, the adjacent tissue or your partner.

Here again, the food factor should by no means be ignored. A diet rich in sugar creates a "sweet" environment in which the bacteria thrive. Eating acidy foods or taking Vitamin C, on the other hand, increases the acidity of the urine's pH balance and the germs lose their "breeding ground".

Remember that, as already emphasized above, it is absolutely essential to drink plenty of fluids during pregnancy. A bladder which is constantly rinsed out will be much less susceptible to infection, and a healthy bladder moreover prevents infections that might affect the kidneys. Many kidney problems begin during pregnancy, and should be avoided if at all possible.

(◎) Herbal Medicine

A good remedy for bladder disorders is *Kamille-Hauhechel-Tee/Chamomile-Restharrow Tea*, containing bearberry leaves, birch leaves, golden rod, restharrow, chamomile flowers and dandelion root (only half parts of chamomile, dandelion and golden rod). Drink three cups of this tea a day in sips, in addition to at least two litres of water. Bearberry leaf tea only helps, though, when the urine is alkaline. In this case you should therefore avoid acids such as those in red teas and fruit juices. You can determine the pH level of your urine yourself with a test strip from the chemist's. By the way, a pinch of baking soda (sodium bicarbonate) in your tea aids the transition from acidy to alkaline.

(◎) Homoeopathic Remedies

Homoeopathy treats these problems with: *Apis, Berberis, Cantharis, Equisetum, Pulsatilla, Sepia* and *Solidago*. To tide you over until your next appointment with your midwife, you can take *Berberis* in a low potency.

(◎) Aroma Therapy

In the past years, I have found the *Original 𝒟® Aroma Blend Sandelholz-Sitzbad/Sandalwood Sitz Bath 𝒟®* extremely helpful. Like all of my aroma bath additives, it is produced on a basis of Dead Sea Salt in order to obtain a stronger disinfectant and healing effect. It also contains the essential oils of bergamot, lavender, rose and yarrow. Prepare a warm sitz bath with this blend. If you happen to have sandalwood oil on hand, you can also prepare a sitz bath with three drops of the oil, mixed with two tablespoons of salt. Relief can also be obtained by soaking a handkerchief with two drops of sandalwood and one drop of Roman chamomile mixed with a teaspoon of St.-John's-wort oil and using it as a compress.

Many women have followed these pointers and words of advice and were soon relieved of their discomfort. I do not know the extent to which they were able to avoid taking the antibiotic which had been prescribed them, but that is not my concern here.

I remember one woman only too well …

… who called me up in tears on a Saturday morning. She complained of acute pain in the area of the kidneys and a strong burning sensation when urinating. She couldn't reach her doctor. She did not want to follow my initial advice that she ring up a hospital or an emergency doctor. She asked if I knew of any alternative. In my concern, I listed several possible means of finding relief: she should lie down

with a hot-water bottle on the painful area, but on the side that didn't hurt. She should drink the abovementioned tea blend in addition to large amounts of other fluids, and take the homoeopathic medicines Berberis and Cantharis in constant hourly alternation. As soon as her husband had come home from the pharmacy with the salt/essential oil blend she should immediately take a warm sitz bath. I also urgently advised her to see a doctor if the symptoms had not substantially improved within half a day. That evening she rang me up and, to everyone's delight, told me that the burning sensation when passing water was almost gone, the kidney pains had become quite bearable within two hours of the warm bath and the use of the hot-water bottle, and had disappeared entirely in the course of the day. I was relieved and very grateful that nature provides us with such wonderful remedies.

Gaining Weight

In order to help expectant parents understand why women gain so much weight, I would like to list the kilos needed just for the child and the growing uterus: by the end of pregnancy the child will weigh between 3,000 and 3,500 g, and will be swimming in about 1,000 g of amniotic fluid. The unborn baby receives its nourishment from the placenta, which then weighs about 700 g. The child, amniotic fluid and placenta are swathed in a uterus whose muscles develop from 70 g to 1,500 g. After its birth, the child must be fed by the mother's breasts, which also gain in size and weight – as much as 500 g – in the course of the pregnancy. A weight gain of approximately 6,000 g is accounted for by physiological accumulations of fluid in the tissue and the blood.

It is therefore entirely normal to gain between twelve and fourteen kilograms during pregnancy. During the first two trimesters, a weekly gain of 300 g is normal; in the third your weight will increase by about 500 g per week.

A balanced, varied diet (as described on Page 47) certainly provides the best basis. I would like to propose that a healthy pregnant woman has no weight problems. Naturally, I am aware that there are women who gain much more weight. When I ask women if their weight varies in the course of their menstrual cycle, I am often told that they often weigh up to an additional kilo before their period. What this means is that women with a tendency towards hormone-related weight vacillations will also gain more during pregnancy.

As I have often witnessed, many expectant mothers suffer terribly when they are constantly "picked on" about their weight. They have to come to terms with getting fatter themselves and can hardly bear being regarded so critically by others. They have no understanding for people who already start reminding them early in pregnancy how difficult it is to lose weight again after childbirth. Sadly enough, they often have to listen to these words of wisdom from men. Not infrequently, it makes them extremely unhappy. Everything just gets worse and more hopeless, and they start "swallowing" their discouragement and frustration about gaining weight all the more. When a mother complains that her doctor will surely scold her again for gaining weight at her next antenatal check-up, I try to cheer her up by telling her that she's not pregnant for the doctor but for herself and her partner and the child, and that she should take care of her own health and that of her child. A few kilograms more may serve as a good reserve during the breastfeeding period – a phase in which she should by no means lose weight. Rapid loss of weight during the lactation period would promote the excretion of toxic substances such as heavy metals, pesticides and dioxins, representing further contamination of the milk. I often have the feeling our bodies are preparing for the time that is to come and want to help us themselves. The most important thing in any case is not to make a big deal out of weight gain. Eat a balanced diet and trust your body and your child – both of them know what you need and will send you plenty of signals. Learn to listen to your body and react accordingly.

Naturally, this doesn't mean you should start eating for two! There are situations in pregnancy in which excessive weight gain can also lead to illness. One such illness is high blood pressure; another, as described above, varicose veins.

The opposite condition – *too little increase of weight* – can also be a problem. Women with this condition naturally suffer as well. They live in constant uncertainty as to whether it will harm their child and are afraid it might be undernourished or born underweight. I can allay their fears immediately, however. The child takes all it needs from the mother, and might come out just a bit less chunky than other newborns. I can well remember a woman who had only gained four kilos, and had a child who weighed four kilos at birth! Other women who have gained twenty-five kilos give birth to children that weigh "only" 2,500 g. Although they seem paradoxical, phenomena such as these are nothing out of the ordinary.

Homoeopathic Remedies

If you are worried about gaining too little weight, it may be possible to find an appropriate homoeopathic remedy within the framework of individual consultation.

Aroma Therapy

It has helped many women to rub *rosemary hydrolat* into their skin in the morning or to sprinkle a drop of *Rosmarinöl/Rosemary Oil* onto a damp washcloth and wipe their body with it. Rosemary stimulates the appetite as well as the circulation if the problems are caused by low blood pressure. Persons with high blood pressure should by no means use rosemary oil. In this case, an alternative is to take a frequent sniff of your favourite aroma, for example *grapefruit*, to stimulate your appetite.

I have seldom been confronted with questions about insufficient weight gain and therefore have little advice to pass on. I am convinced, however, that a solution can be found within the framework of consultation with a midwife. In any case, all pregnant women – no matter what their problem – should always seek contact and have the opportunity to relate their concerns to at least one health professional. It sometimes happens to me that a woman will leave the consultation room without a suggestion for treatment or a remedy, but says: "Just talking about the problem did me so much good, I feel much better already." It doesn't always have to be a certain tea, a certain oil, a certain remedy – often just attention helps.

Sciatica

The second trimester is unfortunately also often accompanied by severe sciatic pain. Due to the growth or position of the child and with it the increasing weight of the uterus, strong pressure is exerted on the sacroiliac joint. Of course it is no longer possible to sleep face-down, but, as in the first trimester, it helps to assume the knee-elbow position as often as possible, or to do belly dancing. Physical exercises of this kind take the pressure off the muscles, the child may change its position and the unpleasant pressure in the sacral area decreases. Another cause of this pain is the entirely natural, hormone-related softening of the sacroiliac joint. When unctions and homoeopathic remedies fail to bring relief, I advise pregnant women merely to find a good reflex-zone or craniosacral therapist. Many midwives nowadays know how to carry out these treatments or are versed in belly dancing. I am constantly amazed by how quickly women feel better after such treatment. I always advise my fellow midwives to collaborate with good physical therapists – after all, we usually have our hands full just with the tasks of midwifery. I would like to encourage all mothers suffering from these problems not to shy away from the costs of these manual therapies, because they really spare you a lot of pain. Often enough, the pain is not merely caused by a harmless irritation of the sciatic nerve, but by a seriously herniated disc. This was the case with Ms. B. …

… one Saturday morning I got a call from Ms. B. She sounded quite desperate and asked me if there was anything I could do about her indescribable back pains in the twenty-eighth week of pregnancy. She told me that she had been riding her horse since the beginning of pregnancy. When dismounting, she felt a sharp pain in her back. She had to drive her daughter to a friend's house, and when she got there she could hardly get out of the car. She managed to get home, and her concerned husband took her to the hospital. When she arrived there, she was suffering from severe pain. The ultrasound, CTG and results of the vaginal examination were all normal and gave no cause for concern. Ms. B. was admitted to the hospital, and the pain diminished somewhat through the pain relievers and the rest she got there. On the morning of her call, she had been discharged with the diagnosis "sciatica". By the time she got home, the immobility and pain were as bad as ever. In total desperation, she rang me up to ask if there were any globuli she could take; the doctors were at their wits' ends. I urgently advised her to do everything she possibly could – even though it was Saturday – to find a physical therapist who treated pregnant women and would be willing to take a look at her back and correct the spine. For me, the tele-diagnosis was clear: a slipped vertebra! Five hours later I got a second call from Ms. B. with a cheerful voice, free of pain: "Thank you so much for your advice; I can walk, sit and run again without any discomfort! Why didn't the doctors think of this super simple treatment?!" It probably hadn't really been all that simple, but it had been extremely effective. I am repeatedly amazed – and grateful – that there are human beings with such healing hands. Again and again, it is glaringly obvious that the most important thing is to perceive the person in his or her entirety – on all levels. It's really a shame, though, that doctors and healers know so little about one another, and cooperate so little. This woman ultimately didn't care whether the health plan would cover the costs or not. The days she had spent in the hospital were certainly more expensive and all for nought. But now she was free of

pain, free of anxiety, and full of good hope once again, and on a Saturday! Nevertheless, I advised Ms. B. to take Rhus toxicodendron.

◎ Aroma Therapy

See "The First Three Months", p. 24f.

◎ Homoeopathic Remedies

Homoeopathy can frequently be applied effectively in cases of sciatica during pregnancy. Possible remedies are medium potencies of *Arnica, Bryonia, Pulsatilla, Sepia, Kalium carbonicum* and *Rhus toxicodendron*. As always, good familiarity with the remedy's characteristics is necessary, or a reportorization must be conducted, leading to a simile.

Partnership and Sexuality during Pregnancy

During my consultations, the subject of sexuality during pregnancy occasionally comes up. During the second three months of pregnancy, many women find sex quite pleasant. Due to the dilation of the blood vessels, the circulation in the pelvis is good and the woman greatly enjoys physical love. The bond with her partner is reinforced; a need for sensual affection and attention develops. But parents are often worried that "it" is in some way detrimental to their child. I can only allay their concerns: if the father and mother are happy, so is the child. The baby is lying in the soft uterus, well protected by the amniotic fluid. If you like pleasure and lovemaking, it will not harm your unborn child. Otherwise nature would certainly have "put a kibosh" on sexual intercourse during pregnancy. Here again, I have confidence in the female body. It is entirely possible that a lack of desire for sex is a natural protective mechanism. Unexpressed problems in the relationship might also be the cause, however, in which case it is advisable to talk to your partner about it or seek the help of an experienced therapist or counsellor. In conversation it is often possible to identify the fears, worries or false expectations that lie at the root of the lack of sexual desire. In general, every couple can rest assured that there is no reason to abstain as long as the pregnancy proceeds normally and nothing to the contrary is mentioned during the antenatal check-ups. It is also quite worthwhile to use massage to find new means of showing affection and tenderness. For men and women alike, pregnancy can represent a wonderful opportunity to rediscover one's body and experience its reactions. Intimacy is part of life, and also has its rightful role in the context of giving birth.

If problems or questions come up with regard to sexuality or partnership, I would like to encourage you to confide in your doctor or midwife.

The Home Birth

Parents who have decided in favour of a home birth should contact a midwife in the twenty-sixth to twenty-eighth week of pregnancy at the latest. I have often experienced parents who say they had been planning to have a home birth since the very beginning of the pregnancy. But they only remember to look for a midwife during the final weeks, and she must then disappoint them because she is already booked up during the period in question. Midwives cannot take on an unlimited number of home births, because the latter require an intensive form of accompaniment. What that means for the midwife is: to get to know the expectant mother as well as gain a sense of her partner, or even the whole family, in order to be able to judge whether they are aware of the responsibility they are assuming for the unborn child. Then she accompanies the parents through the pregnancy, is on call and provides help for several weeks before the due date, attends to the mother during the postnatal period and is once again available and present. Only several weeks after the delivery, when life with the newborn child has found a certain routine, is the midwife's job over. For all of these reasons, a home birth midwife can only care for a limited number of women at a time. I would like to recommend that all expectant parents set out in search of a midwife early on in the pregnancy, because midwives don't sit at home and wait. And, finally, midwives want to be able to plan a holiday with their own families now and then, just like everyone else. More and more midwives have joined to form teams to ensure that you will be cared for even if "your" midwife is on holiday or attending further training.

Prerequisites

Naturally, a home birth can only be jointly embarked upon if certain conditions are optimally fulfilled, and if it has been determined in the course of intensive preliminary talks that the pregnancy is free of risk and progressing entirely normally. Nevertheless, possible complications must be discussed, since parents must be aware that the trip to the hospital can suddenly become unavoidable at any moment throughout labour. They have to prepare for a hospital birth as well as the home birth they have decided to undertake. Both parents must be aware of their need for safety in connection with the birth; they must decide whether they feel up to the responsibility. The decision in favour of a home birth is and must be a very personal one, which no-one can make for them. They have to think about how they will come to terms with suffering and disability or birth defects. All expectant parents must go through a process of realizing that a child can be born with an illness or disability, or stillborn. Nowadays, these tragedies are accepted by society if they occur in the hospital despite the employment of all medical and technical aids. But if the child is born ill, disabled or dead at home, this event is not accepted by society, which accuses the parents of failure to carry out possible remedial measures.

All of these subjects must be discussed with the parents. Certainly the reader will now understand that, in addition to the other necessary and usual examinations and provisions, preparations for a home birth are very time-consuming.

The desire to give birth in the safety of one's personal surroundings is justified in our present-day, supposedly so easy-to-plan world. When all of the aspects of the home birth have been carefully considered and the necessary preparations have been made, this form of midwifery will certainly once again find its place in our society. Just like any others, parents who want their child born at home have a right to understanding and care. Midwives who agree to accompany home births are naturally well trained and aware of the responsibility they bear. To the same degree as our colleagues in the hospital, we home-birth midwives are invested in keeping the risk accompanying childbirth as low as possible, and to take the wishes of the parents and the needs of the expected children into account to the greatest possible extent.

Independent Birth Centres

In many cities in Germany, midwives have joined to establish independent birth centres, a type of institution geared to meet the widely varying interests of the parents and the midwives. Accompanied by self-employed midwives, family-oriented natural childbirth is carried out in a home-birth-like atmosphere. The midwives are spared the strenuous and time-consuming drives from one woman to another – a factor of particular relevance in today's large cities –, and can plan their on-duty time better. The parents are presented with the opportunity of a self-determined delivery outside their homes, where they might be worried about disturbing their neighbours. They can acquaint themselves with the midwives who will be on duty in the month their child is due. It is generally necessary, of course, to register at an independent birth centre well in advance, since the midwives can only take on a limited number of births. As in home-birth obstetrics, making the acquaintance of the midwife at an early point in time can help to prevent risks. When a risk situation occurs unexpectedly during pregnancy or childbirth, the midwives will have you admitted to a hospital of your choice or in the immediate vicinity. In many places, independent birth centres collaborate with doctors, and many such centres offer the assistance of a second midwife on a regular basis. Unfortunately, the cooperation with doctors is complicated for legal reasons having to do with liability. In many independent birth centres, for example at "Erdenlicht", the midwives have accordingly decided to offer care conducted exclusively by members of their own profession. As parents, you can by all means place your confidence in these experienced midwives in the certainty that we know exactly when it is necessary to call a doctor or have the birthing woman transferred to the hospital. In the past, the doctor has often merely confirmed our assessment of the situation, and valuable time has been lost. Transferring the birth to the hospital as early as possible helps to reduce the likelihood of complications in the further course of labour – as opposed to relying on possibly less-than-competent medical help at the birth centre. In Germany, it is simply a reality that well-versed obstetricians practice their professions in hospitals. The rural family doctor and obstetrician with the vast range of experience has become a rarity. As expectant parents, you must be aware that the independent birth centre offers you no more "safety" than having a home birth. The midwives are equipped with oxygen, a suction device and emergency medications but will nevertheless take you to the nearest hospital if complications arise. Independent birth centres are not intended as competition to hospitals or home-birth midwives, but as a place where natural, self-determined childbirth can be carried out in a familiar environment with as little use of medical or technical aids as possible. After delivery, the young family leaves the birth centre and experiences the postnatal period at home, where they have the further regular assistance of a midwife.

It remains to be hoped that political steps towards supporting such projects will continue to be taken, since in the past plans to open independent birth centres have often failed for lack of financial resources. In order to ensure the subsistence of birth-centre midwives, parents are presently compelled to finance the birth of their child on their own, as – due to the lack of a legal basis – most health insurance schemes do not consider themselves in a position to bear the attendant costs. In many places, though, the health insurance companies cooperate and take over a proportion of the operating expenses.

Incidentally, the annual quality reports of the "Gesellschaft für Qualität in der außerklinischen Geburtshilfe e.V.", which can be downloaded on the Internet under www.quag.de, testify to the high standards of obstetrics outside the hospital. Their statistics show that childbirth is possible with a very low rate of episiotomies, an extremely low proportion of caesarean sections (under 5%) and a nearly 100% rate of spontaneous delivery. I therefore advise expectant parents to inquire about the respective statistics in the hospital of their choice, in the independent birth centre, or with the self-employed midwife – the comparison is worth your while.

Twin and Multiple Pregnancies

When reading this book, the parents expecting twins or multiples will probably think: this is typical; she only talks about one child, but we're having two/three, etc. I will therefore now discuss several special situations in some detail.

Not infrequently, parents of twins report that their friends and acquaintances have trouble coming to terms with the news that they are expecting more than one child. The tidings of the pregnancy initially reap an enthusiastic response, but as soon as they mention twins, the excitement turns into dismay and alarm. Even for you, the thought of having two children at once might have taken some getting used to. You'll vacillate now and then between courage and confidence on the one hand, doubt and fear of what the future will bring on the other. Your friends will feel the same, with the difference that they will express those feelings more openly, whereas you, as parents, will try to come to terms with the reality from the beginning and emphasize the positive aspects. So brace yourselves for comments like: "Oh, God! Two at once! I'd be at my wit's end!" As the mother or father of these children, however, you will certainly have the strength to do justice to your twins. You will go through emotional and physical lows, just like parents of singles. Please remember that, already now, in the uterus, the children are experiencing that they are not alone. The two of them have already become accustomed to sharing space, nutrition and attention. But think of them as individual personalities nevertheless and don't be surprised if the two children don't call attention to themselves in exactly the same way. Try to discern which child is doing what at a certain moment; see whether you can learn to distinguish between their positions and their behavioural patterns. This may help you to adapt to having two distinct little persons to take care of after the birth. Particularly in the case of fraternal twins, you will notice very quickly that they do not resemble one another more than other brothers and sisters. And the latter can differ enormously in their development and their behaviour. Many people even claim that siblings like to contrast with one another. Wait and see how your twins will behave; maybe they'll be different from the others after all.

The twin or multiple pregnancy will resemble the single one in many respects, but the discomfort and pain may have different emphases. You will become rounder, more corpulent and more in need of help. In many cases, multiple pregnancies are associated with greater risks. Your gynaecologist is likely to want to conduct the antenatal check-ups more frequently, in order to determine anomalies early on. But make sure that your pregnancy is not labelled "high-risk" merely because you are expecting twins. If nature allows a woman to conceive twins, then nature will also make it possible to carry and give birth to them. Naturally, you should avoid unnecessary strain from the very beginning and rest as often as possible so that your body has the strength to provide for the children sufficiently. As soon as your job becomes too strenuous, talk to your doctor about it and ask him to issue a notification of illness for your employer. Rest and the ability to distribute your work over the course of the day are good prerequisites for a complication-free pregnancy.

One of the most common discomforts of early pregnancy are certainly lower back pains (see p. 23 f.). This is hardly surprising, since the uterus, larger than usual from the beginning, often puts a strain on the sacrum. Things will improve as the uterus and your abdomen continue to grow. Until that time, you can take the load off the sacrum by sleeping in the face-down position. As the pregnancy progresses, it will be advisable to assume the knee-elbow position regularly. In general, I would advise all women undergoing multiple pregnancies to get themselves a special cushion for pregnant women which can also be used later for breastfeeding. Your midwife will surely be able to give you more detailed information.

Even if you have most of your antenatal check-ups carried out by your doctor, you don't have to go without consultations with a midwife. By the way, it is advisable to make contact with a midwife as early as possible so that you will have someone to turn to in unforeseen situations. You should register for an antenatal class which you can attend from the twentieth week on since twins are often born before term.

Mothers expecting twins often complain of bladder and kidney problems (see p. 54 f.), because the children take up so much space. Again, it is important to pay attention to your posture and sleeping position and avoid lying on your back to the extent possible.

Premature contractions occur frequently. You should try not to react with extreme anxiety, however, because actually it's no wonder that it takes the uterus some time to adjust to the children's growth and stimulates the circulation by means of increased contractions. (Also read the section on "Assessing Contractions", p. 92 f.) In my opinion, expectant mothers of twins and multiples should have *Toko-Öl/Toko Oil D®* on hand and gently massage their abdomens with it at the first sign of heightened contractions. It is also advisable to drink the "midwives' tea" Valerian in cases of premature contractions. Keep some in the house. If you don't end up using it, it's better to have bought it for nothing than to have your first premature contractions on a weekend when the pharmacy is closed. A warm bath in the evening with 500 – 1,000 g of Dead Sea Salt in the bathwater is also quite pleasant. Towards the end of pregnancy, the night-time is as burdensome as going for a walk, a circumstance easily explained by the weight and size of your womb. Many pregnant women suffer from shortness of breath, insomnia and strong downward pressure. For these discomforts there is unfortunately only one thing I can say to console you: this pregnancy, too, will one day be over.

Fathers-to-be of multiples will surely have to comfort their wives now and then, help them with the housework, even get them to go for a little walk on occasion, although walking becomes quite cumbersome and strenuous towards the end of pregnancy. But remember that your wife will have to accomplish labour and childbirth – and is capable of doing so. I am quite convinced that nature only assigns the task of a multiple pregnancy to women who are capable of carrying it out.

Particularly mothers of multiples must be prepared for a stay in the hospital since serious premature contractions have to be treated medically. Premature contractions certainly don't always mean premature birth, however. I know of several mothers of twins who carried their children to term and experienced normal spontaneous childbirth, the only difference being that two children were born instead of one. But regardless of whether premature or punctual, the beginning of childbirth, the task of coming to terms with the contractions, the delivery and breastfeeding will all be topics of relevance for you. Among twin and multiple pregnancies, the proportion of caesareans is understandably higher, but the operation certainly isn't always necessary. My older colleagues can still remember so many good and spontaneous deliveries and shake their heads about the fact that so many caesareans are carried out nowadays.

There should be no doubt that twins can be breastfed just as single infants can, even if it takes some time to find a routine. In any case, even in the case of twins, breastfeeding is much simpler and more practical than bottle-feeding. In your preparations and thoughts, you should take into account that the children often have to stay in the hospital longer since they are frequently born earlier and more lightweight. (You should therefore by all means pay particular attention to the section on "Premature Childbirth" on p. 98 f.) Like mothers of singles, you will continue to receive the help of your midwife until you are able to cope with breastfeeding on your own. Even if your children have to stay in the hospital the first few weeks, you should call a postnatal midwife soon so that she can provide you with help and advice on using a breast pump. And when the children come home, she will give you the benefit of her experience and soon you will figure out the most efficient and practical way of breastfeeding two children. The midwife will also help you bathe your children the first few times, or maybe she'll know of a midwife-in-training who would be happy to come by and assist you from time to time. If necessary, the midwife will also see to it that the health insurance company finances family assistance.

No matter how excited you are about the birth, as parents of multiples you should not forget to organize the subsequent period beforehand, since the first few weeks following childbirth are much more suspenseful and out-of-the-ordinary than the birth itself. You as the father should see to it that your wife has plenty of help – not only during pregnancy but for many weeks after the birth, your help, that of a relative or paid help. Actually, I have come to the conclusion that nobody organizes and plans as well as parents of multiples. But they do have to acquire that ability.

I neither wish to play down nor to exaggerate what it means to become parents of twins or multiples; it is surely both – double the joy and double the burden.

Self-help groups for parents of twins and multiples are surely the best source of insights into the processes of pregnancy, childbirth and the postnatal period. These groups have been welcome in our midwives' practice from the beginning and are very popular among the pregnant women and their partners.

THE LAST THREE MONTHS

Development/Sensory Organs

The last twelve weeks serve the child as a period of preparation for life outside the womb. The child's *development* has been concluded. It will soon be viable; it is now putting on a protective layer of fat and its *sensory organs* are developing into a perfect system. The baby participates actively in the mother's life. With its behaviour, it often communicates to her that it is feeling good or that something is bothering it; often it may be telling her with its powerful kicks: what I'm *hearing* out there is a bit too loud! By being still, it can perhaps signal to the mother – who might be experiencing something exciting – "I won't get involved; that has nothing to do with me!" The child can now perceive sound very clearly; it hears everything, it lives with its mother and her surroundings. It can enjoy music but also be frightened by loud noises. Scientists have proven many times over that, after birth, children recognize music which has been played to them regularly during pregnancy. If the baby has just been sleeping and there are suddenly loud, piercing noises to be heard in the mother's surroundings, it will wake up and announce its aural perception with strong movements. I cite these examples as a way of showing that the mother-child union has become very intense. The child's *sense of smell* is also completely developed and is waiting for its first encounter with air in order to begin using the sensory cells which have already been in place since the seventh week of life; from the moment of its birth it will begin to store all olfactory impressions in its memory. It has likewise been proven that the *sense of sight* already functions in the uterus and the child reacts to light and dark. It is not pitch black in the child's surroundings but slightly crimson in the sunlight – to the extent that the mother can enjoy the sun – since light penetrates our muscles. When the sky is overcast, the light is dim or the mother is indoors, the shade the child perceives is more of a bluish red. Under the blanket it's dark, in the uterus as well. No agreement has yet been reached on the extent to which the central nervous system is capable of processing the sensory stimuli – i.e. the degree to which pain can be perceived. For Frédérick Leboyer and Michel Odent as well as other scientists, however, there is no doubt that pain is perceived, for the necessary brain cells, the neurons, already develop in the fourth week. It is well known that babies can sense displeasure or snuggle cosily in their parents' arms after delivery. What greater proof do we need that the conduction system functions perfectly?

The expectant mother now shares her everyday life with her child in every respect; she talks to it and reacts to its needs. Remarks such as: "Let's rest for a while; I think you need to calm down!" are nothing unusual. On the other hand, the mother often misjudges the boundaries of her new body form. She bumps things with her tummy and spills things on her blouse during meals. It becomes increasingly clear to her that she has a big belly, but that her belly belongs entirely to her child. Women often tell me: "The child has taken over possession of my middle. It's beginning to get uncomfortable." What they mean is: not their circumference, but the child is beginning to cause them discomfort. With its movements it exerts an influence on the mother – she'll sit down, for example, without actually wanting to. For the child's sake she will take up a sleeping position she is totally unaccustomed to. With its signals, its vigorous movements, kicks in the area of the stomach or the kidneys, the child is capable of letting the mother know that her present pose isn't good for it, that the circulation in the placenta is insufficient, or simply that, if she turns over on her other side, it will have more space in her womb.

The unborn child can no longer move like a fish in water; that phase is over. It is continually growing in size and weight. At the beginning of the eighth month (of ten lunar months) it weighs about 1,400 g/3 lbs., by the beginning of the ninth this number has already increased to 2,100 g/4 lbs. 10 oz. and by the beginning of the tenth to 3,000 g/6 lbs. 10 oz. Due to the cramped quarters and its increasing weight and size, the child has greater difficulty turning somersaults. From about the thirty-fourth week of pregnancy on, this type of movement becomes very strenuous for the child and it therefore prefers to content itself with merely turning from one side to the other. At this point in time, nearly (!) all children assume the position which is favourable for childbirth, namely with the head down. The medical term for this is cephalic presentation.

In the final weeks of pregnancy the child is already capable of sucking its thumb inside the womb. It is highly probable that children don't learn this habit but are born with it. It also learns to drink before birth, making sucking movements with its lips very similar to the breathing movements of a fish. The amniotic fluid it swallows often goes down the wrong pipe and the mother feels the child's hiccoughs as a rhythmic knocking against her abdominal wall. With these sucking and drinking movements, the child is preparing to suckle at its mother's breast.

In these months the mother becomes very tangibly conscious of the fact that a little person is growing there with all its individual characteristics and habits, and already strongly influences its surroundings. The baby is already part of family life; it hears its brothers and sisters talking, singing and shouting. Even the dog's bark is a familiar sound.

Working Women/Maternity Rights and Benefits

For working women, the reactions of others to her pregnancy play an ever greater role. Colleagues – men and women alike – who have never even given her a nod before now, stop, pat her tummy and greet the child with a cheerful "Good morning! Already up?" Many pregnant women are shocked; others are pleased about this solicitousness. In antenatal classes I point out that perhaps there is still something of a herd instinct, or a protective instinct, in our society.

Unborn children, newborns and toddlers can put the biggest sourpusses into a good mood. Such people open up to the unborn baby with friendliness and love in the knowledge that children can be the most wonderful reason for living and should grow up in a friendly and peaceful environment.

I hope that every pregnant woman is treated with understanding and consideration at her place of work. Any expectant mother who is treated otherwise should inform herself about the laws in effect in her country for the protection of women in her condition. These laws stipulate certain rights, for example concerning breaks for rest. They were enacted in order to provide expectant mothers with social protection. Your health insurance scheme will be able to provide you with the most up-to-date information.

At the beginning of pregnancy, many women think they can work as long as they feel like it, even all the way up until childbirth. They believe: "Pregnancy is not an illness." That is true, of course, but from about the thirty-second week of pregnancy onward, most pregnant women find themselves longing to go on pregnancy leave.

Every woman has a right to pregnancy leave, which – in Germany – begins six weeks before the estimated due date. At work it becomes more and more difficult for the expectant mother to meet the professional demands placed on her, what with the baby in her womb, her increasing weight and her shortage of breath – an entirely normal "symptom" of late pregnancy. This condition is caused by the fact that the uterus grows all the way up to the costal arch of the ribcage and the maternal lungs have less and less room to breathe. The child fills every centimetre of space it can conquer. And accordingly, it participates everywhere, influencing and restricting its mother in all kinds of situations. The baby plays ping-pong with her bladder, as a consequence of which she is constantly running to the bathroom, interrupting her work to do so, which is bothersome. Due to the fact that the constantly growing child leaves less and less space for her stomach, the mother has to eat smaller and smaller portions all the more frequently, a circumstance not always looked upon kindly by the people she works with. The child inside her succeeds in having the mother distracted by every pram being pushed along by a proud mother outside her office window. A pregnant woman pauses to listen when she hears a small child crying and thinks about how it will be when her own child throws such a temper tantrum in a department store someday. In her thoughts, she sees herself reacting much more sensibly than the mother who was just in her department as a customer and immediately gave in to her child's whims. (In two years, when she's the mother of a hard-headed toddler, she may see things quite differently!)

Preparation for Childbirth

The expectant mothers who have registered for an antenatal class now find their own situation reflected in the group. They learn that other working pregnant women have the same experiences at their jobs. The women encourage one another to talk to their employers and tell them that certain aspects of their everyday work have become too strenuous. Or they gather the courage to call in sick for a week if the strain becomes too great. In many professions, particularly nursing, pregnant women are simply no longer able to keep up with the physical strains and demands. It is also always nice to see how the atmosphere in the antenatal classes changes from rather reserved at the beginning to cheerful and happy-to-see-one-another-again within a few weeks. Lasting friendships often develop out of these classes. Many toddler groups and mother groups began in our courses and still exist to the very present.

Changes in the Woman's Body

Fetal Movements

For many expectant parents, the changes in the woman's body are associated with a sense of apprehension: in some very noticeable ways, her body has become a stranger. In the final twelve weeks of pregnancy, her belly becomes round as a globe and grows upward all the way to the ribcage.

The child braces itself against the mother's ribs with such vigour that she says: "I'll bet my ribs are covered with bruises, they're so sore!" All pregnant women now perceive the fetal movements very clearly. The movements are even plainly visible to others. Sometimes the child's need for activity is no longer experienced as something purely playful, since now the movements can literally be painful.

In my consultations I often encounter women who complain about painful fetal movements. Particularly very slender and petite women often suffer from the stretching of the abdominal wall and the forceful movements.

Like Mrs. S. …

… somewhat shyly, and with tears in her eyes, she told me: "I hardly dare say this, but my child is hurting me so much! I have the feeling my entire insides are bruised and crushed. I can tell you that, can't I? You know, at home, nobody understands me. Everyone says I shouldn't think such a thing, a child can't hurt its mother with its movements, I'm just imagining it. But believe me, it's really bad, I can hardly stand it any longer!" I gave Mrs. S. Arnica pills. Several days later, she told me her condition had only improved briefly. But now everything had gotten much worse, since now she had so much pain in the area of the navel that she really couldn't stand it anymore – but she figured there was nothing that could bring her relief after all. By this point she made a very impatient, almost hysterical impression on me. I thought she might lose her composure any minute, and I gave her Cimicifuga. The

very next day, Mrs. S called me, and with great relief in her voice, reported to me that the pain was gone and she felt better than she had felt for a long time. Two weeks later she received another dose of the medication and was free of her severe navel pains for the remainder of the pregnancy.

When I find the right remedy, I'm very happy about the success of the homoeopathic treatment. But it's really not always easy to find the right medication on the first try.

Umbilical Sensitivity

Many a woman worries when her navel protrudes outwards. Sometimes it looks quite amusing when it shows through her clothing like a little head. But often the navel hurts. In any case, it is very sensitive, since for years it has been retracted, and thus protected, and now it is exposed to the constant rubbing of the clothing. I can console all pregnant women who have such a bothersome protruding navel by telling them that it will return to its normal position again after childbirth.

In some cases, however, an umbilical hernia can occur. Usually this condition requires no special treatment, to say nothing of surgery. In these cases, your doctor will surely be able to advise you.

⑤ Aroma Therapy

Lavender is very good at providing relief in cases of umbilical pain. Apply either the essential oil *lavender extra*, ideally diluted *10% in jojoba wax* (1 part oil to 9 parts wax), or *Massageöl entspannend/Massage Oil Relaxing 𝔇®* to the navel. You can also apply a damp lavender compress at body temperature to the painful spot. Relief is also brought about by massaging the navel several times a day with a drop of *chamomile Roman 10% in jojoba wax*, or applying this blend with a compress. *Dammmassageöl/ Perineum Massage Oil 𝔇®* and *Entspannungsbad/Relaxation Bath 𝔇®* are likewise very helpful.

Abdominal Girth

The growth of the child in the twenty-eighth to thirty-fourth week of pregnancy is tremendous, and you can almost watch your abdominal girth increasing. It often measures as much as 100 cm/39" and more by the end of pregnancy. Try measuring your circumference shortly before the birth. Later on it will be fun for the mother and child alike to reconstruct the size of your belly during pregnancy by holding a measuring tape around your waist. Unfortunately, this measurement is no longer routinely taken at the prenatal appointment. It's also well worth the effort to take pictures. For the parents it is quite impressive to re-experience and remember the pregnancy with the aid of the photos, later, when the big belly has disappeared. In the antenatal classes it's always interesting to see the expectant mothers comparing their bellies. And parents always enjoy it greatly when a midwife uses a doll to demonstrate how the child has to roll itself up in the mother's tummy, and how they sometimes do stretching exercises or try to straighten out in the uterus. These exercises are visible on the surface of the mother's belly as shapeless bulges.

Linea Nigra

The so-called *linea nigra* – which literally means "dark line" – is one of the more remarkable visible changes the body undergoes during pregnancy. By the third trimester, the woman's vertical middle axis is very strongly pigmented and takes on a dark shade of brown. As the uterus grows, this line extends all the way up to the bottom of the ribcage. For many women, however, it only becomes clearly visible after childbirth. Due to the enormous stretching of the abdominal wall, the intensive pigmentation only shows clearly when that wall slackens again. The line will fade again in the course of several months following childbirth. The epidermal pigmentation can neither be avoided nor influenced, neither during pregnancy nor during the postnatal period. Neither oils nor or massages can prevent this entirely natural process; it is simply part and parcel of pregnancy.

Preparing the Breasts for Breastfeeding

The *breasts* of a pregnant woman undergo major changes. The sensitivity of the nipples accompanying early pregnancy has perhaps decreased somewhat, but the pigmentation of the areola – the ring of colour around the nipple – has increased. The areolae have become darker and larger. The size and weight of the breasts themselves have likewise changed. In most cases the breasts become substantially heavier. This is the reason many women believe they should wear a brassiere – a measure which, however, is not always absolutely necessary. In my opinion, a pregnant woman should decide for herself what she needs and what she finds helpful. Naturally, her maternity bra should be elastic, fit well, and made of a breathable fabric such as cotton or silk.

I have already mentioned the importance of massage for the body in the section on stretch marks. And massage is all the more important for the expectant mother's growing breasts. I recommend that you simply use whatever oil you have chosen for your belly. Massage your breasts vigorously, applying uniform pressure, from the outside towards the nipples, with astral and circular movements. This is the foremost manner of preparing your breasts for nursing your child. In the framework of this regular massage, every woman has the opportunity to get to know her breasts and become conscious of the fact that they are a very important organ, and not merely a symbol of sexuality.

Further Means of Preparing the Breasts

- Wash regularly with cold water and a coarse washcloth.
- Dry yourself with a coarse towel.
- In the process, rub your nipples with the flat palm of your hand.
- Use a soft brush to brush the skin in astral and circular movements from the outer edges of the breasts to the nipples, gently brushing the nipples as well.
- Take hold of the erect nipple with your thumb and index finger and roll it vigorously between your fingers.
- Placing your fingers on the outer edge of the areola, pinch your nipples together repeatedly in imitation of the pressure exerted by the baby's jawbone.
- Then massage your breasts with good-quality massage oil (e.g. *Schwangerschaftsstreifenöl/Stretch Mark Oil D*®, containing the essential oils of lavender, linaloe wood, neroli and rose on an almond, evening primrose, sunflower and wheat germ oil basis).
- Try to express a drop of the colostrum or foremilk by clasping the breast with your hand and stroking it in a forward direction, applying slight pressure and pressing it together vigorously when you get to the outer edges of the areolae. This will serve to unblock and activate the milk ducts and help to prevent breast congestion in the early breastfeeding period.
- Finally, you can apply a slice of lemon to each nipple to make the skin tough and resistant.
- If possible, enjoy a sunbath with bare breasts and try going without a brassiere for a few hours a day – the normal rubbing of the clothing is the simplest means of acclimatizing your breasts.

Please begin slowly and cautiously with the toughening-up process. Add one more of the measures mentioned above to your programme every several days and only do as much as your skin will tolerate well. In my experience there have been women who subjected themselves to a week of the "harum-scarum" method and then come and told me their breasts were bleeding. Needless to say, that is precisely how *not* to prepare your breasts for breastfeeding. Treat this sensitive skin with caution and sensitivity. And remember, even if you are pregnant for the second or third time, your nipples require preparation every time – a change of hormones has taken place, making your nipples sensitive all over again.

I am aware that many women, including health-care professionals, consider this type of toughening unnecessary, even brutal. As a midwife, however, I am confronted almost daily with breastfeeding problems, and most of the women affected tell me they did not prepare their breasts for nursing. So my advice to every pregnant woman is: don't start too early, but do prepare your breasts for breastfeeding! Your child won't take into account whether you have acclimatized them or not. And there is nothing more unpleasant than embarking on the breastfeeding period with sensitive, sore breasts. Take this important organ seriously. Literally take your body, with all its changes, into your own hands, and prepare it for what is to come.

If the preparation procedure is painful despite all your caution, apply a drop of *lavender extra 10% in jojoba wax* to your nipples several times daily, or moisten them with *orange blossom* or *rose hydrolat*, two substances with soothing and healing properties. *Rosenbalsam/Rose Balm 𝒟*® is also very helpful.

Flat and Inverted Nipples

With this "toughening-up" method, even so-called flat nipples will begin to become erect. Be convinced, already during pregnancy, that your child will know how to cope with your nipples. After all, it's your child! But you can work on preparing your nipples – don't just placidly rely on the possible problems solving themselves of their own accord before you begin breastfeeding. And please don't think what many women unfortunately think: "The midwife or the nurse will help me out when the time comes." Hospital professionals can't work wonders overnight. In order to achieve an ideal nipple form for breastfeeding with flat nipples, it is necessary to carry out preparatory measures for several weeks. Maybe your partner would even enjoy helping you; as the father he is sure to be interested in his child's obtaining the best nourishment possible. And that is breast milk, which is not only cheaper and more practical than bottle feeding, but the only nourishment really suitable for a human baby. Think about the fact that animals aren't raised on human milk or the milk of any other species besides their own. No rabbit can be fed with a mare's milk, but human infants are fed with cow milk, which Mother Nature actually intended for calves.

I am certain that flat nipples can be changed with the above-described treatments. But if not even the slightest change is discernible within a few weeks, or if you actually have true *inverted nipples*, i.e. nipples which sink down into the breast tissue, it is essential that you begin wearing *breast shells* several weeks before childbirth, or begin using a Niplette. Both can be obtained from your local pharmacy. But first ask your midwife which of the two methods she recommends. In the first few days to weeks of breastfeeding, the mother should wear the shells or Niplettes for a few minutes before nursing, and only remove them in the instant the child is searching for the nipple and attempting to latch on.

If the above-described treatment of the nipples is successful, they are sure to be extremely sensitive, and daily application of *Rosen- und Melissenbalsam/Rose and Lemon Balm 𝒟*® is extremely soothing. Another helpful and usually sufficient method of making the sensitive skin of the formerly flat or inverted nipples resistant is to apply sage tea, which has a slightly astringent effect. In the course of your daily body care, dab your nipples with this tea regularly. Naturally, it should always be freshly brewed. Sage tincture is often recommended, but I would advise you against using it. It is very strong and can even cause uterine contractions.

Sometimes women tell me that, after they have carried out their nipple preparation exercises, they notice a slightly increased tendency of the uterus to tense up. If this is the case, stop your treatment session, especially if the contractions are rhythmical or painful. A brief tensing up of the uterine muscles is nothing to worry about if it decreases through the application of abdominal breathing exercises, supported by lying down and relaxing. If you react with premature contractions, on the other hand, you must discontinue the nipple treatment for good.

Colostrum during Pregnancy

Incidentally, during pregnancy your mammary glands may frequently secrete a few drops of colostrum. Individual drops, or even large yellow spots, can show up on your clothing. Some women therefore have to start wearing breast pads during pregnancy, while others wait in vain for a drop of foremilk.

The secretion of colostrum is experienced differently by every woman and in every pregnancy. The amount of fluid that "leaks out" is completely unrelated to the quantity of breast milk you will produce later on.

Apropos "too much colostrum", I recall the following incident …

… Angelika was pregnant with her second child and greeted me one day with a smile. She had a tiny jar with her and asked me if she could demonstrate her new stretch mark lotion, with which she had been treating the skin of her belly for several days, to excellent effect. At first I couldn't understand why she kept grinning. She insisted that I try a bit on my hand. I was amazed by the cream's golden colour and smoothness. My reaction was: "It's very pleasant, but you won't get very far with this amount." But my curiosity had been aroused and I wanted to know how she had concocted this ointment. With amused pride, she told me that, for quite some time now, she had had plenty of foremilk. It was simply too precious just to let it soak into her clothing. She used the milk collection shells she had saved from when she breastfed her first child, collected the colostrum and mixed it with wheat germ oil. The result of this blend was the ointment she had shown me. Now it was my turn to laugh, and both of us were pleased as punch about her inventiveness and her unique and precious stretch mark cream.

Common Minor Problems

Iron Deficiency

During the consultation session, many pregnant women ask for advice on how to cope with iron deficiency. The women are worried and uncertain, because the haemoglobin (Hb) level is often marked in red in their medical records. The simplest means of determining iron deficiency anaemia is with a blood test. At the antenatal appointments, a drop of blood is taken from the tip of the middle or ring finger. The haemoglobin, of which iron is the chief component, is then measured.

The expectant mothers have usually already been taking iron pills for quite a while, prescribed to them by their obstetricians. When this therapy does not bring about the desired results, or when the side effects such as constipation, stomach-aches and nausea get too unpleasant, the women come to see a midwife and ask her for advice.

The first thing you should know is that a decrease in the Hb level is normal around the twenty-fourth to twenty-eighth week of pregnancy, because this is the phase in which the child has its biggest growing spurt. The mother can usually confirm that this is the case, because her abdominal girth is likewise increasing constantly. The growing child gets every bit of nourishment it can from the mother. This means that the maternal cardiovascular system – including the formation of blood cells – must be mobilized to the utmost.

Surprisingly, however, the Hct (haematocrit) level remains relatively constant. The Hct level indicates the percentage of red cells in the blood. Red blood cells are re-sponsible for transporting oxygen, while iron content enables the blood to absorb oxygen from the air we inhale. It is also normal for the Hct level to decrease during this stage of pregnancy. As long as these values do not go under 10.5 g/dl and 32%, it can safely be assumed that neither the mother nor the child will suffer from a defi-ciency.

Nevertheless, in order to avoid anaemia (iron deficiency), the levels must be checked regularly. Every textbook on obstetrics says that treatment should be under-taken when the Hb level is below 11.2 g/dL (assuming a normal level of approxi-mately 14 g/dL). Here it is important to take the individual into consideration, since every person has his or her own normal levels. As a rule, it can be assumed that iron substitution (iron intake) must begin when both values fall, or when the related phys-ical symptoms are discernible.

But I would also like to point out that mistakes can be made during the taking of a blood sample and in the lab. It is important to make sure the woman's fingers are warm and well supplied with blood before the sample is taken. If the level deter-mined is conspicuously low, you should request that the test be repeated a few days later – especially when you haven't noticed any of the symptoms that might point to a deficiency, such as fatigue, listlessness, concentration difficulties and general weak-ness.

If treatment is necessary, it is possible to carry it out by natural means.

⑤ Herbal Medicine and Nutrition

As a preventive measure against iron deficiency anaemia, I can warmly recommend *Schwangerschaftstee/Pregnancy Tea*. As mentioned above, this tea blend suffices in many cases to raise the Hb level. It can be further enhanced by mixing in *sorrel* and *parsley root*. These two roots, as well as *stinging nettle leaf*, which is contained in the blend, are known for their extremely high iron content.

In this context it is very important to mention that the tea should be drunk with a few drops of lemon juice. Our bodies require vitamin C (ascorbic acid) in order to make better use of the iron introduced in herbal form. You must not forget that the body of a woman requires 33% more vitamin C than usual during pregnancy.

Among other things, this vitamin is responsible for stimulating the bone marrow function, and red blood cells are formed in the bone marrow. It is also a known fact that vitamin C deficiency can lead to bleeding. If you suffer abnormally from bleeding of the gums during pregnancy, you should check your vitamin C intake. At the same time, I would like to warn you not to go overboard: taking too much vitamin C can lead to diarrhoea, which in turn can trigger premature contractions. The intestines are directly adjacent to the wall of the uterus and any intestinal hyperactivity could suddenly turn into labour pains. As in the case of other substances, it is also true of vitamins that they are helpful if taken in moderation, and damaging if taken in excess. This is actually a rule of thumb for nearly all naturopathically oriented aids.

As far as *nutrition* goes, you should see to it that your diet includes foods that grow and thrive in the earth's crust, because that is where iron is to be found, and only there can it be absorbed. Beets and carrots have the highest iron content. The intake of these two vegetables, either raw, gently cooked or as vegetable juice, will surely lead to verifiable success before long. And again, don't forget the vitamin C which is necessary for the absorption of the iron.

All dark-coloured berries, particularly elderberries, but also raspberries and black currants, have a high iron content and are very popular in the form of juice.

Many women have told me that they took *Floradix* (a juice made of herbs containing iron), which they purchased at the organic food store or pharmacy, and that their iron levels went up rapidly as a result.

Nuts likewise exhibit a high iron content. Pistachios, for example, contain 7.3 mg per 100 g of fresh nuts, followed by almonds with 4.1 mg and Brazil nuts with 3.4 mg. They are also very valuable on account of their high proportion of unsaturated fatty acids as well as their high vitamin E content. Nuts are outstanding suppliers of energy and should by all means have their place in your diet during pregnancy. But remember: nuts should always be eaten consciously as a foodstuff and not just as a snack, since 50 g of Brazil nuts (well chewed) along with one to two apples, for example, can substitute an entire midday meal! Here as well, make sure you purchase organic-quality products, since otherwise you will be exposed to many heavy metals and other environmental toxins.

Pumpkin seeds (12.5 mg) and sesame (10 mg) contain even more iron than nuts. Other good sources of iron are all rolled grains (grain flakes), wheat germ, soy flour and cocoa. Of all the various types of grain, millet (sorghum) has the highest content: 9 mg per 100g of dry goods. As is widely known, a portion of meat is always a good supplier of iron. Particularly blood sausage (also called black pudding) – a food which has largely gone out of fashion – should not be underestimated in view of its 16.8 mg iron content. The only product with more iron is brewer's yeast, with 17.5 mg.

One of the most important things to consider in this context, however, is that, as an expectant mother, you should avoid black tea. Like all foods containing phosphates, including alginates, which are used as additives in processed foods, this beverage virtually destroys the effects of all your efforts to raise your haemoglobin level.

⊙ Homoeopathic Remedies

Naturally, there are also homoeopathic remedies which can be prescribed, such as: *Ferrum metallicum, Ferrum phosphoricum, Phosphorus* and *Pulsatilla*. As always, please ask a midwife or doctor with training in homoeopathy which of these substances would be best for you.

Heartburn

A rather minor problem which often occurs during the final trimester of pregnancy is heartburn – it is not harmful, but it can be quite disagreeable. Often heartburn prevents women from being able to take an afternoon nap and fall asleep at night; sometimes it causes discomfort with every downward movement of the body. Gastric acid gets into the oesophagus and causes that bothersome burning feeling, which is extremely unpleasant. This condition is caused by the hormonal situation of the pregnant woman as well as the increasing pressure exerted by the growing uterus. The stomach is literally "forced into a corner." It is therefore better to eat several smaller meals than a single big one at lunchtime.

⊙ Herbal Medicine and Nutrition

Heartburn can also be caused by sweet dishes or *irritants* such as coffee or black tea. If this is the case, these foods and beverages can simply be avoided.

In cases of heartburn, it has proved very helpful to take a sufficient amount of *magnesium* or chew shelled almonds.

The discomfort can also be avoided or alleviated by drinking *fennel tea* in small sips after meals.

If the heartburn occurs first thing in the morning, it is often helpful to drink a bit of milk or chew dry bread. You should be aware, however, that milk can also cause heartburn. If you are not able to solve the problem with these suggestions, you might try out the time-tested naturopathic principle of giving the symptoms "some of their own medicine". In other words, in cases of excessive gastric acid production, eat acidy foods – e.g. oranges, pineapple, tomatoes, etc. – or drink the juice of those foods.

Conversely, in many cases fruit juice and fruit can also cause heartburn if too much is consumed. Let me remind you here of the important rule: a little can help to heal, a lot can throw even a healthy state off balance. The habit of drinking one or more litres of fruit juice a day can lead not only to over-acidity but also to itchiness of the skin and haemorrhoids.

Gisela told me an interesting story about a cousin of hers who suffered from heartburn. The cousin's doctor recommended that she take a teaspoon of mustard after every meal. With this treatment, the problem was entirely overcome!

Probably the most effective method of treating heartburn is to drink potato juice. Unfortunately, this advice usually meets with the most rejection. Many women cannot imagine that the juice of raw potatoes is even edible (or, in this case, drinkable). Of course it is rather time-consuming to make the juice. Fresh, unpeeled potatoes – red if possible – are grated and the pulp is then squeezed out in a clean towel. If taken two or three times a day, this small amount of rather unpleasant-tasting juice is guaranteed to help bind the excess gastric acid. If you want to save yourself the effort of pressing the juice yourself, you can ask for bottled potato juice at your health food shop.

Doctors often prescribe acid-binding substances, but these medications also bind iron, magnesium, minerals and other medications, preventing their absorption by the body. Please be aware of these reciprocal effects and, if you are unsure, ask for information at your pharmacy or doctor's office.

I can also recommend cornsilk tea, which has relieved many women of the discomfort of heartburn. It is most effective if drunk in the morning on an empty stomach and before meals.

🌀 Homoeopathic Remedies

Naturally, homoeopathy also has various helpful remedies at its disposal: *Magnesium phosphoricum, Sodium phosphoricum,* possibly *Mercurius solubilis.* Taken in a low potency, *Magnesium phosphoricum* is nearly always a successful treatment.

The subject of heartburn reminds me of an experience I had in the early years of my career …

… when expectant mothers complain of heartburn, they are often comforted by their women friends or mothers telling them that they will certainly have a girl with thick black hair. In the vernacular, it is thus the child's gender and appearance which causes heartburn.

Many years ago, a mother was radiantly happy about her pretty little girl, who had very long black hair. Amazed and somewhat incredulous, soon after the birth she asked me: "You know, I already knew it would be a girl with lots of hair, because I always had such terrible heartburn, but now I want to ask you, as a professional midwife: tell me, how can that long hair have tickled my stomach, way up here, from way down there (she pointed at her pubic bone, since her child had lain in the uterus with its head pointing downward, like almost all babies)?" We were both highly amused and delighted about the fairy tale of the black-haired girl.

Itchiness of the Skin

A form of pregnancy discomfort which is unfortunately becoming more and more of a problem is itchiness of the skin, which can be – but is not necessarily – accompanied by a rash. Many women experience itchiness on the entire surface of their skin, others only in the area of the abdomen, usually with a worsening of the symptom towards evening and at night. Often it suffices to take a cold shower and use sheets made of a fabric with cooling qualities. Many expectant mothers, however, develop not only slight itchiness, but a truly problematic and unpleasant irritation of the skin, accompanied by a rash in the form of little red spots or even "weeping" patches. The condition can be so severe that the woman can hardly sleep and her nights are agony.

As always, I endeavour to view this topic from the holistic perspective. Thus the question must be asked: "What is irritating you to such an extent that you'd like to jump out of your own skin?" Very often, the woman will actually burst out with a spontaneous: "It's no wonder! At work and at home, for as long as I've been pregnant, I'm supposed to be the wonderful, loving woman who is blissfully awaiting her child and as soon as I get the slightest bit upset, I'm told it's not good for my child!" In such cases I encourage the woman to speak her mind and not repress her feelings of displeasure or resentment, because sooner or later, it will start to itch. Such consultations can help a women learn not to blow up to such an extent as to intimidate the child in her womb, but to make the people around her understand that even a pregnant woman doesn't have to say amen to everything. Moreover she can learn that, as a mother, it is important not to lose her temper in such situations, but to express her opinion with composure and self-confidence. This is particularly important in connection with a first child, and at the same time a wonderful preparatory exercise in becoming confident and sure of oneself in one's new role as a mother. Try to encounter others with respect, because that treatment will bounce right back at you like an echo. Stick to your own intuitions and opinions, and form your own views on pregnancy-related subjects. As a mother, you'll have to do this sooner or later anyway, and it won't help to explode.

Of course it is very important to begin by making sure that there are no substances to which the woman is reacting because they don't agree with her. Check whether the skin problem is related, for example, to a new skin cream, a new type of tea or increased consumption of fruit. As described on page 164, the skin could be reacting to raspberry leaf. Or the woman could be allergic to the wheat germ oil which she has been applying to the skin of her abdomen in order to supply it with plenty of vitamin E so that it will cope with the stretching it is being subjected to. Another cause can be the use of a skin product containing paraffin followed by a plant oil with essential oils in it, e.g. *Schwangerschaftsstreifenöl/Stretch Mark Oil* $\mathcal{D}^*$. If this is the case, the essential fatty acids and essential oils cannot make their way down to the deeper layers of the skin, since paraffin oil reduces cutaneous respiration, and the natural substances become overactive in the outer layers. Clothing made of non-breathable fabric can likewise prevent the evaporation of the essential oils, causing increased blood flow in the skin and leading, in turn, to itchiness. Nevertheless, these questions as to the possible causes are often responded to with "no" in every case. As described in the section on "Nutrition and Dietary Supplements" (see p. 47 f.), the woman may be getting too much iodine. This possibility should certainly be checked.

Here it is very important to point out that the consumption of fruit and fruit juice should be reduced to a normal level, red teas should be avoided, and more bread and carbohydrates in the form of pasta consumed in order to increase the body's alkaline reserves. As I have experienced again and again, paying attention to the acid-base balance appears to be the right approach for relieving itchiness of the skin. During pregnancy, many women start eating a lot of fruit and taking vitamin supplements as well. Two thirds of the women who consult me confirm that they do so only because they consider it sensible, but not because they have a craving for fruit. Coffee consumption should also be watched, since the coffee bean can also contribute to over-acidity, another possible cause of itchiness. And we must not forget that, to a certain extent, itchiness of the skin is entirely normal during pregnancy due to the high proportion of female hormones. There are women who suffer from this problem during their premenstrual phase, but then for only half a day at the most. During pregnancy, the liver has to work hard to break down the hormones which are produced in abundance every day, and is pushed to its very limits. For this reason, it makes sense to reduce other substances which put a strain on the liver – for example medications, preservatives, alcohol, animal fat and protein – as well as to take any measures necessary to ensure regular bowel movements, and to eat plenty of fibres so that the intestines excrete well and are thus capable of supporting the function of the liver. It is furthermore important to eat your main meal in the middle of the day and not, as is unfortunately quite customary, in the evening. Eating a lot towards night-time is another factor which puts a strain on the liver. Incidentally, it is interesting to note that women like to eat pretzels during this phase of pregnancy. Pretzels, which are dipped in lye before baking, are alkaline. Remember: it is important to take the body's cravings seriously.

Naturopathy also provides remedies for itchiness of the skin:

Homoeopathic Remedies

The important major miasmatic remedies of homoeopathy such as *Syphilinum*, *Medorrhinum* and *Psorinum*, as well as *Sulfur*, *Graphites* and *Mercurius* should be prescribed only by medical professionals possessing experience with homoeopathy, since it is absolutely necessary to conduct a complete anamnesis before recommending them. But I have often achieved terrific success with *Lycopodium*, *Calcium carbonicum*, *Staphisagria* and *Rhus toxicodendron*. The time-tested remedies *Acidum sulfuricum*, *Caladium*, *Cantharis* and *Urtica urens* should not be overlooked in this context, where they have likewise often proved helpful.

Even if I share the opinion of the classical homoeopaths who are against complex remedies, I would like to mention one which can really make a difference in especially acute cases, at least until the anamnesis has been carried out: *Sulfur compositum*®, which is manufactured by Heel. Taken between meals and allowed to dissolve slowly in the mouth, one to two tablets a day provide substantial relief.

But when the real simile has been chosen, things can progress as in the case of Ms. M., ...

... a blonde woman with a cheerful temperament was waiting to see me. In the consultation room, the mood changed rapidly. I saw her badly scratched wrists and as she told me about the ordeal she was going through she undressed to show me her abdomen. The condition of her skin there was just as bad as that on her arms. The detailed recording of her medical history confirmed my initial impression that a major homoeopathic remedy was called for: Ms. M. received Syphilinum in a high potency. We arranged that she would ring me in a few days and also heed the abovementioned measures in the meantime. Already on the phone, she was able to report that her skin was much better and she had been able to get some rest at night. To my own great surprise, Ms. M. was completely free of symptoms three weeks later, and her skin had completely healed when I saw her in my practice. Recently – many years after the above-described episode – she reported to me that an herbalist had prescribed the same remedy to her again, in an even higher potency, and that she had never had any problems with her skin since.

If homoeopathy was always that successful, more health professionals would surely work with it. Unfortunately, there are stories of a much different tenor, as in the case of Ms. S. ...

... a woman who made a very nervous impression asked to speak to me at the pharmacy. She told me about her rash and I was alarmed at the sight of her abdomen: her entire belly was covered with small, red, weeping pustules. Her dermatologist and gynaecologist had recommended cortisone creams to her, but she didn't want to take them. Here as well, I carried out an anamnesis and then tried to find the right remedy for her. Unfortunately, she had no reaction whatsoever, neither to the first substance nor to the second one we tried. She didn't want to go and see an experienced homoeopathic doctor, because she had already consulted one to no avail. Then she followed my advice and bought silk underwear as well as raw silk fabric to cover herself with in bed. After bathing her severely irritated skin with hibiscus tea every evening, at least she was able to get to sleep again at night.

⟨ ⟩ Aroma Therapy

Fortunately, itchiness of the skin can be alleviated with the help of aroma therapy. Even I am still amazed when women tell me that their skin has improved substantially by these means, and that the problems have decreased. The *Original D® Cistrosen-Mischungen mit Immortelle/Labdanum Blends with Immortelle* on an evening primrose oil basis are particularly suitable for the care of itchy skin. I originally developed these blends for children with neurodermatitic skin, but in more recent years many of my colleagues have also successfully recommended its use during pregnancy. Both the body oil and the bath salts have a relaxing, clarifying, soothing effect. I advise women who are suffering from itchiness of the skin to begin with a *Cistrosenbad/ Labdanum Bath D®* every evening or, in severe cases, in the morning and at night as well, and to enhance the blend with an additional 500 to 1,000 g of Dead Sea Salt. Naturally, after the bath it is important to shower thoroughly so that no salt crystals remain on the skin. After bathing, but also independently of the baths and ideally a few times a day, *Rose* or *Lemon Balm Hydrolat* is a wonderful means of soothing and moistening the skin. Moreover, *Melissenbalsam/Lemon Balm $\mathcal{D}^*$* and *Rosenbalsam/Rose Balm $\mathcal{D}^*$* have proven their value outstandingly in cases of severely itchy skin as well as patches which have been further irritated by scratching …

… and in this context, I can recount an almost unbelievable story about Ms. B. from Cologne. She was in the hospital in the thirty-second week of pregnancy and over night she broke out in an inexplicable rash. Completely at a loss about what to do, she called me on the phone. I was rather at a loss myself in view of the distance and advised her at least to try spraying Rose Hydrolat $\mathcal{D}^*$ on her skin repeatedly. Several days later she received the Rose Hydrolat $\mathcal{D}^*$ by mail and three days after that she gave me another call: within twenty-four hours her condition had improved and remained stable. In a letter I received from Ms. B. at a later date, I learned that she had had no further problems with her skin for the duration of the pregnancy.

Cramps in the Calves

Cramps in the calves are another bothersome, usually harmless problem that can rob expectant mothers of their sleep. When these cramps occur at all, it is usually at night. And they can be so unpleasant that the pregnant woman has to get up and walk around. There is many a father who can tell you a tale about cramps in the calves during pregnancy, because they are often woken and asked to administer a calf massage. Naturally, a massage is very helpful. And it gives the man the feeling of being involved in the pregnancy. But if the woman's partner is not available, she can also try using the foot of the bed or the wall: brace your leg against either with the entire sole of your foot, keeping your leg absolutely straight. If you can manage it despite your big tummy, it also helps to grab hold of your toes and pull them upward. These stretching exercises will be sure to loosen the cramp.

Nutrition

Here again you can help yourself with dietary means, since the problem is caused by a magnesium deficiency. As you know from the preceding chapters, the best way of obtaining magnesium is by drinking mineral water containing that element or chewing shelled almonds. And don't forget to include plenty of fresh green field-grown vegetables in your diet.

Homoeopathic Remedies

The homoeopathic remedies which are most likely to help are *Magnesium phosphoricum*, *Cuprum aceticum*, and perhaps *Sepia* and *Viburnum opulus* as well. Here again, *Magnesium phosphoricum* is a kind of homoeopathic "first aid" which often suffices.

◎ Aroma Therapy

A very suitable aroma-therapy product for this condition is *Massageöl beruhigend/Massage Oil Calming* 𝔇* which contains chamomile Roman, lavender, linaloe wood and marjoram. You can use this essential oil blend in the evening, either to rub it into your calf muscles or to take a warm footbath, in which case you would mix in honey or (dairy) cream. Many women report that *Lavendel-Zypressen-Öl/Lavender Cypress Oil* 𝔇* (see p. 47) has also led to a substantial reduction of cramps in the calves. *Massageöl entspannend/Massage Oil Relaxing* 𝔇* and *Allgaeuer Öl/Oil of Allgaeu* 𝔇* have also been found to be very helpful.

Insomnia

In connection with the various discomforts of pregnancy discussed above, I have repeatedly mentioned that they are accompanied by insomnia. Pregnant women are full of stories about how often and how long they were up and about the house the last few nights. Often they start working or rearranging their furniture at night. When they talk about their sleepless nights at the antenatal classes, I can't help smiling. Naturally, the women ask me what's so funny. I respond by trying to explain to them that they should think about what their child is trying to tell them.

I believe that the unborn children are preparing their mothers for the restless nights to come. It's very considerate of them to let us know that there may not be any more sleeping through the night for the next few years. It seems fairly obvious to me that it is not the mother's organism that has problems sleeping at night, but that the child keeps on "misbehaving" until the mother shifts her position, or maybe even gets up. This behaviour brings mother and child closer; they protect one another mutually. The mother avoids the development of cramps in the calves or bladder problems by getting up. The child is provided for better by the placenta, since the blood flow in the placenta increases when the mother moves around.

In the postnatal period, many women report on how their children actually do keep waking up at the "usual time" every night and want to be nursed. I advise expectant mothers to wake their husbands now and then in these cases, and tell him that their child is awake and that in a few weeks it might be his turn to get up and change the nappies. This is a good way of preparing the father for the coming postnatal phase and his role as a father. And apropos of insomnia, sometimes the fathers are the ones who complain about not being able to sleep because their wives have developed a whole new quirk: they snore. The pregnant women are very embarrassed about this, but I can console them quickly by telling them that this supposed bad habit is caused by pregnancy and very widespread. It is a completely natural reaction, because the child is taking up so much space that the volume of the lungs is restricted. Pregnancy hormones are a further cause, since they cause the expectant mother to begin breathing through her mouth. Among other things, I consider this development to be clearly linked to the natural process of "opening up". The connection between the mouth and the pelvis as well as the interaction of both with the opening of the birth canal are topics the woman therefore learns quite a lot about in the antenatal class.

Of course I also advise the women to do everything in their power to get back to sleep, regardless of why they woke or were awakened. After all, later on the child will be getting her up whenever it wants to and as often as it wants to. These natural disturbances don't have to be rehearsed in detail during pregnancy.

Breathing and relaxation exercises are very helpful for getting to sleep, and are likewise practiced in the antenatal class. But even simple yawning exercises often bring about the desired effect. If the woman nevertheless has great difficulty falling asleep again, a warm footbath or a hot cup of herb tea – ideally the tea discussed below – often helps.

Herbal Medicine

If the insomnia is caused by cramps in the calves, *Hebammentee Baldrian/Midwives' Tea Valerian*, consisting of valerian, hops, St.-John's wort, marjoram, lemon balm and thyme, is a suitable remedy. If the problem of being awake at night recurs regularly, it is advisable to drink a hot cup of this tea in the evening before going to bed in conjunction with taking the magnesium supplement or the homoeopathic remedy.

Aroma Therapy

Another very helpful relaxation aid in the evening is to take an *Entspannungsbad/Relaxation Bath $\mathcal{D}^{\circledR}$*, containing the essential oils chamomile Roman, lavender, mandarin, rose geranium, sandalwood and cedar. Depending on your preferences, you can add a couple of spoonfuls of honey or cream to the Dead-Sea-Salt-based blend. Another time-tested product is the blend *Luftikus $\mathcal{D}^{\circledR}$* (found in the $\mathcal{D}^{\circledR}$ *Aroma Blend* catalogue under *Kinderdüfte/Aromas for Children*), which is likewise mixed with honey or cream for a full bath. When your "thinking machine" tends to switch itself on at night, it helps to make a moist warm neck compress with one or two drops of the blend mixed with a fatty plant oil. An equally helpful aroma blend is *Geborgenheit/Safe Harbour $\mathcal{D}^{\circledR}$*, which is made of benzoin Siam, iris, jasmine, lemongrass, lemon balm, orange and vanilla extract, which I developed especially for such situations. It has a rather intense and flowery scent and is suitable for the evening bedroom aroma lamp, or – even more so – for an evening aroma bath.

Dreams and Anxiety

Frequently, however, sleep disorders do not have organic causes, but are related to the emotions. Restless nights certainly often come about on account of unpleasant dreams. Particularly in the final ten weeks of pregnancy, expectant mothers dream about the birth and are ridden with anxiety in the wee hours of the night. There is anxiety about the child, anxiety about the birth, fear of having a disabled or in some way abnormal child, even fear of encountering death – or simply anxiety about motherhood, about not being able to meet the challenge, etc., etc. The women – and surely the expectant fathers as well – frequently have to "process" all of these often unspoken anxieties and fears at night. But even during the day, these worries can be a burden on a woman or expectant couple. Interestingly enough, the women who have already had children before are usually the only ones who speak openly and honestly about their anxiety. Perhaps they have learned to talk about these things in the course of their previous experiences with childbirth. But these mothers very often confirm that they truly were not troubled with these worries during previous pregnancies. Now, however, after having given birth to two or three children, the fear of having a disabled child becomes much stronger. These women intensely dislike being told: "You surely don't have any questions, you know the ropes, you already have children." For them it is as if no-one wants to hear about their fears and problems. I can well remember this situation during my own third pregnancy, further aggravated in my case by the fact that, as a midwife, I was extremely well informed about everything that could happen. But pregnant women want to be taken seriously during every pregnancy. In our society, many people prefer not to think about subjects such as fear, death, disablement, abnormality, etc., but during pregnancy they can no longer be repressed. Often it is difficult to talk about them, especially for men, who for centuries have been brought up to ignore fears – or interpret them as signs of weakness. In the antenatal classes, a discussion about anxiety and what causes it is often a touchy situation, which many women – and midwives – would like to avoid. In my opinion, however, it is very important to talk about this topic, even at the risk of stirring up long repressed memories. For during childbirth, unprocessed fear can become an obstacle to labour or even lead to a standstill.

I would like to encourage all expectant mothers and fathers to make a point of talking to the midwife, the attending physician or a psychotherapist if these unprocessed fears become a problem, for instance in the form of nightmares. The first time a couple consulted me on this subject, it was a sign of the trust they placed in me as a midwife. Naturally, I first had to learn to cope with this aspect of pregnancy, but I realized that I am often the only person who has access to the parents. I would like to encourage all of my fellow midwives to give parents the feeling that we are prepared to lend them a willing ear for their worries and fears. At the same time, every midwife should be aware of her own limits and let the expectant mothers/parents know if the talk exceeds her psychological competence. What I would like to communicate to expectant mothers and fathers is that the midwife may not be in a position to conduct a psychotherapeutic session but they should nevertheless tell her about the problems, particularly if she will be attending the birth. Openness and trust are the most important prerequisites for the birth-giving process. In any case, the midwife will discuss various possible ways of coping with your anxiety, particular if the experiences that lie at the root of these worries and unresolved problems date back to a much earlier time. Maybe the midwife can recommend a counselling service or a therapist. If the fears are directly related to the coming birth or uncertainty with regard to coping with the child, the midwife herself is in any case the best person to talk to. For it has always been the midwives who are at the woman's side as she goes through the pains of childbirth, and who are therefore very familiar with the fears of a woman in labour.

Homoeopathic Remedies

In the case of fear and anxiety, it is often very helpful to consult a midwife with experience in classical homoeopathy who tries to find the true "simile", i.e. the ideal remedy, chosen especially for you as an individual. Some possibilities are: *Arsenicum album, Calcium carbonicum, Coffea, Ignatia* and *Kalium carbonicum*.

Aroma Therapy

Agitation, anxiety, insomnia and unpleasant dreams can also be resolved well with essential oils, however, since aromas are known to have a direct effect on the subconscious, and thus on the part of the brain which is responsible for our emotions. The simplest oil has proven again and again to be *lavender* with its clarifying effect. It is important, however, to use lavender extra – Lavandula officinalis var. vera – since the substances contained in other types of lavender are unsuitable for pregnant women.

But the lovely rose, the precious iris or the relaxing sandalwood are also helpful. I like to recommend the *Original ℌ® Aroma Blend Sprachlos/Speechless ℌ®* to women who have been confronted with death and have not been able to process the experience. These oils have proven extremely valuable aids when diluted 10% in jojoba wax and used in the form of a perfume.

Remember, though, that a talk with a psychotherapist can also be a great help.

Bach Flowers

Bach Flowers are another very useful naturopathic method which I particularly like to recommend in cases of sleep problems and anxiety. Good possibilities are: *Aspen, Mimulus, Rock Rose, Red Chestnut* and *Cherry Plum*, or simply the well-known *Rescue Remedy* or "first aid" drops – which, incidentally, should not be missing from any family medicine chest. Many midwives are knowledgeable about Bach Flower therapy. Otherwise you can ask at your pharmacy for advice.

Digestion

A positive – and indeed absolutely necessary – by-product of the abovementioned means of preventing anaemia is the healthy functioning of the intestines. Nearly all women report that after they begin drinking *Schwangerschaftstee/Pregnancy Tea* and eating red beetroots, they have absolutely normal and regular bowel movements. All the herbs and other foodstuffs stimulate the mucous membranes of the intestines, a healthy intestinal flora is restored, and the bothersome topic of constipation is a thing of the past. I have already discussed the importance of this for the function of the uterus on page 77 in connection with nutrition and vitamin C. There is a disorder known as pregnancy constipation caused by sluggishness of the bowels. But in most cases the problems merely come about because the intestinal contents are restricted in volume due to a lack of space or the child's position. The bowels react by increased peristalsis (movement) as a means of upholding their function. In the process, however, the uterine muscles are also stimulated and react with increased contractions (muscle cramps). Initially mere "false contractions", in some cases they can turn into true premature labour pains.

Once again, I am reminded of something that happened years ago …

… Mrs. Ü. was sent to hospital by her doctor for tocolysis (a labour-inhibiting infusion), having developed severe pains in the thirty-second week of pregnancy. I was still working as a midwife in a hospital and was on duty. I didn't succeed in ruling out regular, effective contractions. But because the pain seemed unbearable, I hit upon the idea of asking her about her peristaltic motion (bowel movement). She was visibly relieved when I took this aspect seriously – she had already been constipated for several days. After a successful enema and a tocography (recording of the uterine contractions) of several hours, she was permitted to leave the hospital again that evening. The pain was gone, the uterus had calmed down, and the anxiety about having a premature birth had disappeared.

Haemorrhoids

I have already discussed the topic of haemorrhoids in the section on "The Second Trimester" (p. 53 f.). Here I would merely like to point out how important it is to keep an eye on all your bodily functions. Constipation, for example, can often lead to haemorrhoids. Never forget that a healthful diet will help you to avoid all such problems.

Antenatal Care

From the twenty-eighth week of pregnancy on, the antenatal check-ups usually take place at intervals of two to three weeks. Women quickly become accustomed to the routine: urine test, blood pressure measurement, a stab in the finger with a sharp instrument to provide blood for the Hb (iron level) test, climbing onto the scales to be weighed, being hooked up to the CTG machine (which measures the fetal heartbeat and uterine contractions), being called into the doctor's room for a talk, a vaginal examination and an ultrasound check, and finally: "everything is fine, see you again in three weeks or fourteen days?" On the whole, the examinations carried out by the midwife usually take about half an hour, since the initial getting-acquainted talks have now developed into a relationship of trust and many questions can be answered in the antenatal class. In each case, it is decided whether the woman is to come every three, four or even two weeks – or it is left open. Every pregnant woman can come for a check-up spontaneously, whenever she considers it necessary. There are no set rules that have to be followed, only the guidelines established by doctors and health insurance plans. Although the situation is different in many of our neighbouring countries, in Germany there is no limit to the number of antenatal check-ups covered by the public health insurance schemes.

Vaginal Examinations

I am often asked by pregnant women why it is necessary to have a routine vaginal examination within the framework of the antenatal appointments carried out regularly by the doctor. The woman will say that her girlfriend who goes to a midwife for the prenatal now and then doesn't have to go through this ordeal. Or her neighbour, who goes to a different gynaecologist, likewise rarely has a vaginal examination.

In these cases I try to explain that there are differing views as to the necessity of these examinations in obstetrics. Many midwives and obstetricians or doctors consider them indispensable as a means of determining whether the cervix has changed. Others are of the opinion that they help the woman become accustomed to vaginal examinations, which must be carried out frequently during childbirth. Due to lack of routine, many women are supposedly very tense and experience a great amount of pain during the procedure. As an expectant mother, you are once again called upon to voice your opinion and think about what you need for your own peace of mind.

Self-Examinations

For very many women, the examination of the cervix through the vagina is an extremely unpleasant experience which they will never become accustomed to and therefore don't need or want to "practice" for the birth. Actually, the fact that some attending obstetricians and doctors conduct this examination regularly, and others only when necessary, does give pause for thought. In my opinion, every woman has the right of codetermination, and she should exercise it. I always try to explain to expectant mothers that they have to speak up, since the doctor can't be expected to tell by the expression on their face how they want the antenatal examinations carried out. Naturally, a woman who has been accustomed to doing so in the past can continue to examine her cervix manually by herself. Many women have always done this, but don't tell the attending physician out of a sense of shyness or because they are ashamed. Women who have had an intrauterine coil as a form of contraception are often familiar with this type of self-examination – having had to check regularly whether the coil is in place. For these women, the cervix is nothing strange or unusual. But the majority of women have never tried to touch their cervix. I would like to encourage them to get to know their bodies. I can't see any reason at all why a woman shouldn't be able to assess her own body, her own condition. Any woman who is familiar with the so-called NFP (natural family planning) method developed by Rötzer is an expert on her own cervix. What is important here is to inform your midwife or doctor immediately if there is a change or if you have any questions, so that a professional examination can be carried out and a conclusion drawn. Systematic self-observation will give you an increased sense of responsibility for yourself, and the doctor will not be the only one making the decisions. The antenatal examinations can then take on a cooperative quality. But it can also happen that an abnormality is noticed during the manual examination by the obstetrician, not having been discovered by the woman herself. The attending health care professional will take into consideration how the pregnant woman feels and what she says about her growing girth. By manually examining the uterus (in order to determine whether its size corresponds to what is normal for the respective week of pregnancy) and ascertaining the "fetal lie" – the baby's position –, the midwife or doctor will easily be able to recognize a hypersensitivity of the muscles, which could conceivably be a sign of premature contractions. In this case, every expectant mother is sure to agree to a vaginal examination and will be relieved afterward if the cervix is found to be normal.

Effacement of the Cervix

In our midwives' practice we hear far too many worried accounts of diagnostic findings related to the cervix. Almost every day, concerned women come to the antenatal classes and expect answers to questions such as: "Is it really true that I can't take part in the gymnastics anymore? I'm supposed to rest a lot now, since my cervix has shortened. Is it true that the baby will be born prematurely if I'm not careful?" or: "Apparently I have 'shortening of the cervix'; what should I do, how serious is this condition?" Truly, we midwives could fill entire reams with questions like these – with stories of women who don't know how they should react, who sit in front of us, filled with tension and anxiety, or break out in a crying fit on the phone, or those who are so upset and afraid that they don't know if they're coming or going, and are sad because they supposedly can't come to the class anymore. I begin by trying to console the woman and telling her that many expectant mothers go through exactly the same thing during pregnancy. I explain that the doctor surely didn't mean it as drastically as all that, but simply as a way of impressing upon her that she should take it a bit easier in general. Women in the third trimester should consider carefully whether they really still have to keep all of their professional and private appointments and dates. Maybe they can stay home from one social obligation or another. Maybe the children's room doesn't have to be renovated right now after all. This diagnosis can also be intended as a reminder that the pregnant woman should simply be easier on herself and really take a break on the sofa every afternoon. And finally, I tell them about other women who were in precisely the same situation ten weeks ago and are now longingly awaiting their baby, which is already five days past the due date. With the help of drawings and our knitted model of the uterus (!), I explain how the cervix can and must change in the course of pregnancy in order to prepare for childbirth.

These explanations usually help to calm the expectant mother down, and she often asks again whether she can perhaps attend the antenatal class after all. If the woman has not yet begun a course, I describe what she will learn in our midwives' practice "Erdenlicht": she'll sit there and concentrate on her child, breathe, relax, find relief for her aching back, sciatica or shortness of breath with a few simple exercises. Mothers who have already been to a few sessions should decide for themselves whether they want to continue coming or not. They almost always say: "Well, I'm going to have to give birth to my child, and I'm certainly not going to learn the breathing techniques at home on the sofa. And anyway, if I have to go all the way to the doctor's practice for the antenatal check-up, the hour with you won't hurt me. On the contrary, I'd miss coming to the class." Naturally, I couldn't agree more with this logic. The advice of doctors to the effect that the woman should no longer participate is really old hat, rooted in a day and age when pregnant women were told to do rigorous physical exercises and jog around a gym. For years, we midwives have been trying to inform people that our courses are not damaging in any way, and surely do not comprise any contraction- or labour-inducing exercises.

CTG: Cardiotocography

From the twenty-eighth or thirtieth week of pregnancy on, many doctors carry out a CTG (cardiotocogram) regularly at every antenatal check-up. The recorder, or cardiotocograph, helps to assess premature contractions and the pattern of the child's heart rate. It is an absolutely pain-free method of examination for mother and child alike; the heartbeat and possible contractions are recorded by means of ultrasound. Many pregnant women do report, however, that the unborn child reacts to the sound and becomes extremely active. We will presumably never know what this procedure truly means for the child. For the doctor, it is a good means of checking the uterine contractions and the baby's heartbeat without personnel expenditures; what is more, the results are recorded on paper, which serves as proof that the procedure was carried out. The midwife, for her part, sits down with the expectant mother and lays her hand on the mother's abdomen to see whether changes in the form and hardness of the uterus are detectable. The amount of time required for this method is the same as that for a CTG. Unfortunately, many examinations these days have to be documented on paper in order to satisfy legal requirements if the occasion should arise. The midwife's method does not comprise an automatic recording. Please take these considerations into account if you are of the opinion that such technical and/or mechanical aids are unnecessary. Talk to your doctor about it if you decide to take responsibility yourself and are aware of the fact that the CTG is nothing more than a fifteen-minute check-up, the necessity of which still has not been proven beyond the shadow of a doubt. Remember, the CTG is not a form of treatment, but merely a "snapshot".

It is important to me to convey to my readers that you will be alone with your child twenty-four hours a day for the three weeks until the next antenatal check-up. I can well understand the desire for examination and confirmation. Women would like to be reassured: "Your baby is fine and healthy." But there is absolutely no means of constantly monitoring the child in the uterus or after its birth. I regard it my obligation to point out to a mother that – with regard to her child – at some point every woman has to rely on herself, her feelings, her instinct and her common sense. She should place her confidence in her child and trust that she will be able to sense whether the child is alright. Sooner or later she will realize that she could always be worried about her child, whether it is still unborn inside her, a newborn in its cradle, a crawler heading for the stairs, a toddler in the sandbox, a kindergarten kid and, later, a school kid setting out for school by itself every morning. There is no machine that protects and oversees our children. All that helps is faith, trust and positive thinking. Without that attitude, motherhood would be much too strenuous and virtually impossible if all we thought about were the possible dangers lurking behind every corner and waiting to jump out at us and our children. If a mother thinks positively, then she will be able to enjoy even the smallest occurrence with her child, whether it is still in her womb or has already been born. The child senses directly whether the mother is confident or fearful. With regard to the feelings surrounding it, its powers of perception are much more finely tuned than our own. It is in the first years of life that the human being's intuition is the strongest, and the most vitally important. In other words, the baby perceives intuitively whether it can feel safe and good or whether it is in danger. It takes years for a child to learn to recognize danger – presented by a person or situation – on the conscious level.

Assessing Contractions

Preterm Labour/Tightenings during Pregnancy

Every method of monitoring has its disadvantages: it doesn't always come up with positive results, but can also draw our attention to problems. For example, it can happen that preterm labour is diagnosed as the result of a CTG. Time and time again, women come to my practice, distraught and worried, and tell me: "Just imagine, I'm already having contractions and I don't even notice them myself. What if I don't notice the labour pains either?! Will I just wake up one morning with a baby between my legs, not knowing how it got there?" At this point I have to explain to the woman that the contractions which occur during pregnancy and true labour pains are as different as night and day. Contractions during pregnancy often go entirely unnoticed. Many women say they merely feel their tummy tightening or slight pangs in the groin. Many mistake them for the fetal movements. And as a matter of fact, it can happen that the uterus cramps up in reaction to vigorous movements on the part of the child as a way of telling it to calm down.

Labour Pains

Labour pains, for their part, are clearly recognizable. They recur in a steady rhythm – the abdomen gets hard and tight for at least forty seconds, initially in conjunction with menstrual-type pain. As soon as the contractions become effective, i.e. possess the power of opening the cervix, the woman will remember what it means to "breathe" a contraction with a long, affirmative yeeeeeeeeeeeeeeeeeeeeeeeeees! It is completely impossible to sleep through the birth of a child. And what is more, the female body sends out plenty of other signals which make it clear to the mother: "These aren't pregnancy contractions anymore; these are labour pains." I will go into this topic in more detail in the section on "The Signs of Labour" (see p. 204 f.).

Contractions

The word "contraction" comes from the Latin *"contrahere"*, meaning "to draw together". Midwives explain to the expectant mother that the uterus "practices" contracting throughout pregnancy, all the way up until childbirth. By drawing together and hardening its muscles, it is virtually telling the child: "This is how it will be when you get too big for me and have to make your way to the outside world". I remind the mothers to do their breathing exercises. These contractions support the circulation of blood in the uterus, an important prerequisite for supplying the placenta well so that the child will grow. Now and then, of course, there are uteruses which "overdo it" and practice too much.

Ten contractions a day are normal. But if a woman is having as many as twenty or more such contractions a day, she should tell her doctor. The latter will examine the woman to see whether the contractions have brought about changes in the cervix and whether there is any danger of premature labour. Often that is not the case. It is relatively easy to tell whether the contractions you are having are premature labour pains, because in the latter case the abdomen feels very hard and spherical. This feeling goes on for about forty seconds; then it softens again.

Unfortunately, the cervix does not always bear up well under the strain of these "exercises" and gradually begins to open. Often the findings say: "cervix partially effaced". Or even: "soft and slightly dilated". Then, of course, it is important to be extremely careful, because according to the medical textbooks this is not supposed to happen until the thirty-sixth week of pregnancy. Many uteruses ignore the rules, however, and urge the child out too early. Then there really is a danger of preterm birth.

Preterm Labour/Tocolytics

True premature labour can only be stopped by means of intravenous therapy with medications designed to inhibit contractions, so-called tocolytics, frequently Fenoterol, a muscle relaxant. Studies published in the summer of 1992 show, however, that it is usually not possible to delay labour for more than forty-eight hours.

The effect or success of oral anti-contraction medication in the form of pills is very controversial due to the fact that they have substantial side effects on the mother. A study entitled "Bryophyllum in der Behandlung der vorzeitigen Wehentätigkeit" (Bryophyllum in the Treatment of Preterm Labour), carried out at the anthroposophically oriented Herdecke Community Hospital in 1985 and published in December 2002 in the *Weleda Hebammenforum*, proved, however, that the administration of the Weleda product "Bryophyllum 50%" is an outstanding method of treating preterm labour pains without side effects.

Naturopathic Methods of Treating Tightening

Many expectant mothers are very concerned about the frequent uterus "exercises"; in some cases they are actually suffering from these pregnancy contractions. Unfortunately, the latter are all too frequently mistaken for "preterm contractions" and treated with a Fenoterol. As described above, this step should only be taken in the case of *genuine* premature labour. Fortunately, there are naturopathic means of coping with this situation, used successfully now for at least two decades and increasingly recommended by doctors. It is interesting to note that, despite the increase in antenatal check-ups, the premature birth rate has not decreased. It is understandable that parents, midwives and doctors are all keen on recognizing the danger of premature labour in plenty of time and preventing it from happening, but it is simply not up to us to decide what child is to be born when. No matter how difficult it is to accept the fact, the life of a child cannot be planned.

Herbal Medicine

When "false" contractions – also called Braxton Hicks contractions – occur, the first thing a pregnant woman might try is drinking *Hebammentee Baldrian/Midwives' Tea Valerian*, containing valerian, hops, St.-John's wort, marjoram, lemon balm and thyme. You should drink two or, at most, three cups of this blend in the course of the day and supplement it in the evening with magnesium. Incidentally, herbal teas are always more effective when drunk warm.

Homoeopathic Remedies

Homoeopathy makes frequent use of *Caulophyllum, Kalium carbonicum, Pulsatilla, Sepia, Viburnum opulus.* I would like to point out once again that, in such situations, you should be sure to consult a midwife or doctor trained in homoeopathy. In this field, comprehensive knowledge is absolutely essential for treating the patient successfully with the most appropriate remedy! And the success of homoeopathy, when it is attained, is always quite amazing.

⑥ Aroma Therapy

The essential oils with a tocolytic (contraction-inhibiting) effect are: *lavender, linaloe wood* and *marjoram*. One of the *Original D®* Aroma products which has become widely known and is even used in hospitals is the "midwives' alternative oil" *Toko-Öl/Toko Oil D®*, containing precisely these essential oils. It can contribute decisively to relaxation in cases of hyperactive uterine muscles. In view of its effectiveness, you should really only use this oil on the advice of your midwife. Ideally you massage your abdomen with it with upward, stroking motions and as you do so, explain to your child that it really would be better if it stayed inside you for quite a while yet. Don't underestimate the effect of such "dialogs", because, as you know, the child is capable of hearing and feeling inside the womb. Just as couples in love have a non-verbal connection to one another, the connection between the mother and her unborn child is likewise intensive and close – even if you, as an expectant mother, are not always aware of the fact. After all, for you the child is still a tiny unknown creature. But for the child, you are a big, well-known person, the only one the child knows. It hears and understands you perhaps more than you'd sometimes like.

Toko-Öl/Toko Oil D® owes its effectiveness not only to the calming lavender extra and the strongly relaxing linaloe wood with its high ester content, but also to the marjoram, which has a very pleasant antispasmodic effect on the uterine muscles. On the emotional level, marjoram has the reputation of helping regain stability once the balance has been lost, and of being extremely effective in cases of emotional emergency. In my opinion, this quality is the very reason marjoram counteracts increased contractions or beginning labour pains so well, because a pregnant woman burdened by fears of preterm contractions is surely in just such a state of emergency. This condition is often worsened by the CTG and such careless statements as "Oh, you're having contractions." Or: "Your cervix is partially effaced; you'd better see to it that your child isn't born prematurely." Fear and worry can lead to tension which, in turn, have the power to bring about true labour pains sooner or later.

I well remember Stefanie:

… she came to consult with me in the thirty-second week of pregnancy, and asked me: "What do think of this: the CTG shows that I'm having regular contractions and they want me to take a tocolytic. But I remember from my first pregnancy how shaky these pills make me feel. On the one hand I don't want to take them; on the other hand I don't want to risk having a premature birth. Surely you can give me some advice." When I asked her whether she could feel these contractions, she said, "Yes, of course, my abdomen often gets hard and now and then I feel a pang in the area of the sacrum." The first thing I did was to look at the findings of her last antenatal examination, to see whether the cervix had been conspicuous in any way, but it was normal. I then advised her to massage her tummy gently with Toko-Öl/ Toko Oil D® regularly every morning and evening and perhaps even take a lukewarm bath with this oil as a supplement, and to drink Hebammentee Baldrian/Midwives' Tea Valerian during the day. I made her promise to lie down as often as possible and let her daughter go for a walk with Grandma alone sometimes. I was insistent in my effort to make clear to Stefanie that the moment she detected

that these pregnancy contractions were getting painful and rhythmic, she should take the pills immediately. A week later, Stefanie came to the antenatal class, radiant and cheerful again: "There's no other way to describe it – that oil works wonders! It is so pleasant, I care for my tummy so affectionately, which I never felt the need to do before, and my uterus is as soft as a jelly bear. The moment I do too much or haven't used the oil anymore, the tightening returns. The CTG they carried out today detected only one single contraction. But I didn't tell my doctor that I wasn't taking the pills." I was very happy for Stefanie, but I told her she should by all means come clean with her doctor, otherwise naturopathy would never be acknowledged and taken seriously. And anyway, honesty is always the best policy.

Many doctors and hospital midwives have experienced – and will confirm – the amazing effectiveness of *Toko-Öl/Toko Oil D®*. Fenoterol infusions can often be reduced or never required to begin with.

Herbs, Spices and Essential Oils to be Avoided

I gained even greater insight into the effectiveness of herbs – and respect for their healing powers – when Sabina told me: …

… "I have no idea what's wrong with my uterus; it keeps getting hard. Thank goodness at my last antenatal check-up it was determined that the cervix has not been affected by any contraction activity. I was very worried that these were genuine premature labour pains." A short time later, when we were talking about various herbal applications in the antenatal class, Sabina asked, "A neighbour recommended drinking verbena tea regularly during pregnancy; then labour wouldn't last so long. What's your opinion on that?" Something went "click" in my head and I asked her, "Have you been drinking that tea for a long time?" "Sure, this time I'm doing everything I can to keep it from being such a mammoth birth", Sabina answered. I responded by advising her to stop drinking the tea immediately because I assumed there was a connection between it and the constant hardening of her abdomen. From my experience in the area of aroma therapy, I knew that verbena should not be used during pregnancy because the oil has a contraction-inducing effect. The following week, Sabina was all smiles again: "My hard tummy is gone! It was already better two days after I stopped drinking the tea. I'm gradually beginning to think I should learn more about the effects of herbs."

To provide a bit of background, I should mention that Sabina is a nurse by profession and had always been sceptical about the effect of herbs and homoeopathic remedies. What is more, in this case she had fallen prey to the frequent confusion between verbena and lemon verbena. Her neighbour had presumably recommended lemon verbena, known in France as verveine. An exquisite lemony oil is extracted from lemon verbena by distilling the leaves of the Lippia citriodora (also known as Aloysia tripylla) from France and the kindred species Aloisia herrerae from Peru. But these verbena types are not to be confused with the little plant whose Latin name is Verbena officinalis, "genuine verbena". Both plants belong to the verbenaceae genus, which is why they are often mistaken for one another. And as we saw above, these mistakes truly can have consequences, since Verbena officinalis has been scientifically proven to contain verbenalin, which has a labour-inducing effect.

For me, such experiences always serve as proof that naturopathy is not to be underestimated. In the course of the years I have become entirely certain that pregnant women and small children in particular react very sensitively to herbs and essences.

As I result, I have become more and more careful, often look things up in old books on herbs as well as in scientifically acknowledged literature, and often have to voice clear warnings in conjunction with the use of certain herbs or essential oils – particularly when the pregnant woman has been treated naturopathically for several years and reacts sensitively as a result.

In order to *avoid* "false" labour contractions, also known as Braxton Hicks contractions, I recommend that, until the thirty-sixth week of pregnancy, expectant mothers *not* use the following herbs and spices, in any form – neither as essential oils in the aroma lamp nor as massage oils: *basil, ginger, cloves, verbena (Verbena officinalis), cinnamon, camphor, Japanese mint* and *thuja. German mint* can be tried out cautiously.

Pregnant women should be especially careful with *ginger, cardamom, cloves, oregano* and *cinnamon*, since these have a strong warming effect and contain camphor, among other things, giving them a contraction-inducing effect. In the Christmas season, they abound in tea blends and cookies of various kinds. Every year in the weeks before Christmas, my theory is massively confirmed with statements from pregnant women such as: "Yes, you're right, my tummy is often hard these days." Or they say: "Maybe that's why I don't really have a taste for mulled wine, punch and gingerbread this year, because I have to be careful about premature contractions." Remember that the popular Yogi® teas usually consist of these spices.

I have become convinced that cravings or distastes for certain foods during pregnancy – and presumably throughout life – are the best signals our body gives us. What is more, on the basis of many years of observation and experience, I would like to postulate that many early and premature contractions are brought about by spices and herbs or are a sign of an infection in the gastrointestinal tract. I can only recommend to all expectant mothers: "Don't take anything without consulting an herbal medicine specialist first." Unfortunately, according to one widespread opinion, "If it's herbal, it's harmless!" This opinion appears to me to be irresponsible and superficial. Belladonna is also a plant, but we all learn in school how poisonous it is.

We certainly won't be able to trigger a miscarriage within a few days by using certain spices and herbs. But like pieces of a puzzle, ignorance and doing the wrong things can become elements of a complex process. And moreover, the unborn child and the mother should be spared even the slightest pregnancy contractions. In this way, good circulation of the uterus is ensured and fear and worry can be avoided. These two components form the foundation of a healthy pregnancy and the child's healthy growth in the womb.

If your child should be born prematurely despite all naturopathic or medical treatment, contact a midwife near you. She will understand the circumstances and attend to you accordingly, and perhaps she knows how you can get in touch with a group of parents who have gone through the same thing. There you will likewise find help and understanding for your situation.

High-Risk Pregnancy/Hospitalization/ Preterm Childbirth

The antenatal check-up routine, however, can suddenly change when unusual findings are made. A normal pregnancy can turn into a high-risk one from one day to the next. In these cases, the midwife will send the woman to her general practitioner or the obstetrician will have her come in more regularly; in some cases the pregnant woman will be hospitalized.

As one of her health-caretakers during pregnancy, I as the midwife have the task of providing the pregnant woman with information and consolation. In almost all cases, the "risk" turns out to be nothing serious. It is even rumoured that many pregnancies are classified as "high-risk" for reasons having more to do with health-system accounting procedures than anything else.

Hospitalization

Of course, there really are situations during pregnancy in which hospitalization cannot be avoided. When there is a danger of a true preterm birth, the only means of delaying it for as long as possible is with an anti-contraction infusion. In spite of all the technology and medical possibilities we have at our disposal, we will not always succeed in outsmarting nature. The preterm birth rate has not decreased, and will presumably never go down to zero. Many children take the risk of a situation between life and death and surely hope fervently that they have better chances of surviving outside the womb. Despite all the efforts made on the outside to inhibit labour, they will simply be born too early. But perhaps there is also many a child who decides against life by these means and hopes that its incapacity for life will be accepted. (On this subject, please also read the section on "Stillbirth", p. 253f.)

There is certainly plenty more to be said on the subjects of high risk, the threat of preterm birth, illnesses of the mother and child, etc. but to discuss them would go beyond the scope of this book. My intention here, rather, is to describe the normal course of pregnancy, childbirth and the postnatal period, taking naturopathic aspects into account in the process. In the case of premature childbirth or abnormal pregnancies, we turn to modern medicine and all of its helpful knowledge and capabilities. In this situation, scientific medicine offers us the only chance of preserving the lives of both the mother and the child. By saying this, I would also like to communicate that I am not in favour of naturopathy at any price, but advocate a healthy combination of the two approaches. Naturally oriented methods should be used as long as possible, and medically/technically oriented help should be undertaken at the right point in time.

If you as an expectant mother are hospitalized for several weeks during pregnancy, it does not mean you have to go without the assistance of a midwife. Ask to speak to a midwife in the hospital or contact an independent midwife by phone to find out whether she would be willing to provide her services both in the hospital and later at home.

Midwives can accompany and enhance the medical measures by offering the woman "moral support" as well as various naturopathically oriented aids.

Preterm Childbirth

I would therefore like to limit myself here to a few brief remarks on the progress of scientific medicine and medical technology: it can happen that children are born between the twenty-fourth and twenty-seventh week of pregnancy – i.e. at a point in time at which technology represents the little human being's only chance of survival and the parents are faced with an "all-or-nothing" decision: either the most intensive possible therapy with the highest degree of medical-technical effort – or death. Naturally parents in this situation want to decide in favour of life, but it is life with a lot of question marks attached, as well as unforeseeable consequences, and nobody can give the parents a prognosis on their child's long-term development. And not all premature infants have the will to enter into a life-and-death struggle. Sometimes a child chooses to leave this world again, and it lets the parents and doctors know it. The parents can best endure the death of their infant if they take leave of it holding it in their arms and allow it to die in dignity. Unfortunately, many parents who go through this experience are unaware that, even in such an extreme situation, they can contact a midwife, who will then surely be able to offer them encouragement and support. Midwives are trained to deal with *all* obstetrical situations and can generally be reached twenty-four hours a day. But an ethicist, pastor or psychologist from the hospital will likewise be prepared to help the parents and doctor team when they are faced with such difficult decisions between life and allowing the child to die. Since it is impossible to ask the child what it wants, it is important to try to put oneself in the child's position. And our respect for the dignity of the child which has been born much too early demands that we take not only the present moment into consideration but also its future well-being, and protect it from overtreatment and exploitation by outside interests. And that we accept the fact that it was born much too soon and thus, in its own way, decided against life. In the case of a decision in favour of every possible technical measure, the parents must think about the support and accompaniment the child can expect from them and the society.

In addition, it would be a good thing if men and women talked more about the topic of having children in general, and thought about the possibility of these sudden emergencies accompanied by difficult and far-reaching decisions – rather than waiting until the emergency is upon them. And it would be extremely helpful if parents who have experienced such situations were more vocal publicly to make society more aware of the difficult topic of intensive care of premature infants. In my opinion, there is a great deal of cynicism in the fact that prenatal diagnostics works to "weed out" disabled children while premature infant medicine undertakes vast efforts to keep those infants alive – even with the severest disabilities.

Severe Problems during Pregnancy

Many pregnant women are faced with the fact that a pregnancy can be burdened by minor discomforts or problems. Even if there is no need for hospitalization, minor problems or beginning ailments should certainly be taken seriously. Naturopathy usually offers a good means of helping. In order to support our bodies' self-help mechanisms, it is always important to react at the first signs of a problem.

Urine Test Results

If abnormalitiesare detected within the framework of the urine test taken during the antenatal check-up, you shouldn't wait until your next appointment but try to figure out right away what is causing the problem, think about and possibly change your habits. Read the section on "Urinary Tract Infections/Cystitis" (p. ■f.) and begin by checking to make sure you drink enough fluids. If glucose is found in your urine sample, you should immediately omit every type of sugar and sweets from your diet and drink lots of water. As mentioned above, regular exercise is one of the best means of preventing diabetes during pregnancy. Moreover, it is important to know whether there are any incidents of so-called Type 1 or Type 2 (adult-onset) diabetes in your family. If so, you should tell your midwife or obstetrician. If your urine still contains glucose when next tested – despite limitation of sugar intake – the midwife or gynae-cologist will send you to your general practitioner for a blood test in order to check your blood sugar level. Your gynaecologist will then discuss the further procedures with you.

A seriously high blood sugar level during pregnancy requires good, regular medical supervision, which will probably be carried out by an internist.

Oedema (Water Retention)

If you should notice excessive accumulations of fluid, so-called oedemas, anywhere in your body before or around the thirtieth week of pregnancy, it is absolutely essential that you think about the following: what is your daily stress level like; do you have to work hard at your job, are you under stress from other sources? Countless consultations have shown me again and again that oedemas are the kidneys' way of reacting to stress at work or in daily life. When women are hospitalized with severe accumulations of fluid, above all the following is observed: rest already suffices to reduce the swelling and ensure increased elimination of fluid. In other words, a process of normalization begins as soon as the woman is taken out of the environment that is causing the stress. But hospitalization can be avoided if the pregnant woman recognizes on her own that it's time to take a break and reduces her work load to a minimum. The working woman then has to take leave of her professional everyday life; the mother and housewife should ask her husband, mother/mother-in-law or a friend for help, or simply do less ironing, cleaning, baking and cooking. If there is a pregnant mother in the family, there's no reason the family members shouldn't notice that things are going to change on account of the new baby.

Oedema can easily be recognized in the swelling of the feet and calves: your shoes don't fit you anymore, the elasticized upper edges of your socks leave marks on your skin, the skin on your legs, perhaps on your abdomen, feels tight or sometimes even itches. Often a woman's legs will hurt in the evening, since the swelling is usually more massive in the evening than in the morning hours. The skin on her hands also tautens and tingles, and another sign of oedema on the hands is when her rings no longer fit her. Accumulations of fluid can also become apparent in the face. Other people will say: "You've really put on some weight; you look round and chubby from head to toe."

EPH Gestosis or Pre-Eclampsia

In any case, oedemas demand to be taken seriously and properly treated, since they often mark the onset of a pregnancy disorder: so-called EPH gestosis, a pregnancy-specific ailment which calls attention to itself by way of oedemas (E = edema = American English for oedema) and/or the presence of excessive amounts of protein in the urine (P = proteinuria) and/or increased blood pressure (H = hypertonia). Now it is essential to prevent this condition – which represents a danger for the mother and child alike – with all the means at our disposal. Pre-eclampsia is the most common cause of premature birth, although the exact process is yet not completely understood. If the levels are excessively high, the pregnancy must be terminated immediately by means of a caesarean section: the child's well-being is endangered by insufficient circulation, and the mother's by the risk of pregnancy eclampsia (coma and convulsions).

For this reason it is important that you react to oedema in the initial stages and effectively support the kidneys' elimination mechanism as well as the overall metabolism with naturopathically oriented methods.

Naturally, rest and total reduction of stress are the most important measures to be taken in this situation. Give the sofa priority over your workplace, perhaps go and visit your parents or find some way of avoiding that nasty neighbour or those strenuous parents-in-law for a while. Spoil yourself – and let yourself be spoiled by others – like a princess!

⟨⟩ Herbal Medicine

I recommend the following: when you make your *Schwangerschaftstee/Pregnancy Tea* – which you have hopefully been drinking regularly for some time – double the amount of *nettle leaf* and *horsetail* and supplement the blend with *birch leaves*. Drink three cups a day. The tea can be further enhanced with lemon juice or lightly sweetened with honey. Incidentally, I would like to emphasize here once again (as I already did on p. 45 f.) that, according to the present state of scientific research, the nettle leaf contained in *Schwangerschaftstee/Pregnancy Tea* is by no means capable of bringing about oedema, as is often erroneously claimed.

⟨⟩ Homoeopathic Remedies

Homoeoopathic remedies are very helpful in this situation; as always, it takes a bit more time and experience to find the right substance for the individual woman: *Apis, Chelidonium, Lycopodium, Natrium Muriaticum, Pulsatilla, Sepia, Solidago* and *Taraxcacum* are all possibilities.

⟨⟩ Aroma Therapy

In this context as well, I have had very successful experience with aroma therapy. The *Original D® Aroma Blends Hallo-Wach-Bad/Hello-Wake-Up Bath D®* and *Hallo-Wach-Öl/ Hello-Wake-Up Oil D®* have a purifying effect and are soothing for swollen feet. These aroma blends contain the following essential oils: Angelica root, carrot seed, lime, litsea, rosemary and juniper berry. You can either take a foot bath with this essential oil blend as an additive, or use the ready-made bath salts. Unfortunately, people – including health care professionals – who don't know a lot about aroma therapy might tell you "But pregnant women shouldn't use juniper berry!" My answer to this is that a clear distinction must be made as to whether the woman simply takes juniper berry internally because she feels like it or uses it in a foot bath, and whether she is in her first weeks or already in the thirty-second week of pregnancy. Naturally, aside from these distinctions, it is also a question of the amount. In the early stage of pregnancy juniper berry tea should be avoided entirely, as should the use of any bath additive or massage oil containing the essential oil of this plant, since it can have an abortive effect. In the late stage of the pregnancy of a healthy woman without the slightest tendency to develop oedema, a wrongly measured dose of juniper berry oil can lead to a massive irritation of the kidneys. In the case of varicose veins, however, a massage oil containing juniper berry oil can support the liver function so positively that no serious oedema can ensue. The liver is superordinate to the kidneys and plays an absolutely fundamental role in the excretion process. In cases of oedema – which are often caused by liver problems – a juniper berry foot bath accompanied by the intake of plenty of fluid will bring about an improvement quite soon, and promote the excretion process. On the emotional level, juniper berry oil is said to help one let go of things or feelings on which one is dependent. In conjunction with juniper berries, I once read the motto "arouses your energy". This could also refer to getting your metabolism going again and boosting the excretion process. If you are aware of having problems with your liver or have informed a naturopathically oriented professional of the same, it is advisable to make yourself a compress for the upper abdomen using *Karotten-Limetten-Öl/Carrot-Lime Oil 10% in jojoba wax* 𝒟® twice a day for about a week. This blend contains the same essential oils as *Hallo-Wach-Bad/Hello-Wake-Up Bath* 𝒟® and *Öl/Oil* 𝒟®. Rub the oil into the liver region, apply a moist, warm compress to it and take a rest on the sofa.

HELLP Syndrome

This pregnancy-specific illness is a severe form of EPH gestosis, usually occurs unexpectedly and is accompanied by a coagulation disorder.

You should have yourself examined immediately if you have pain on the right side of your upper abdomen, since the HELLP syndrome causes pain in precisely this region, in addition to nausea, vomiting and headache followed by a sudden increase in blood pressure and, in some cases, oedema. You should not attempt to diagnose this condition on your own but consult with a doctor or have yourself admitted to hospital immediately. In such cases, a caesarean section – i.e. the termination of the pregnancy – is almost always the best and most effective measure.

⟨⑨⟩ Nutrition

Another good means of flushing out superfluous accumulations of serous fluid in tissue spaces is *diet:* following the consumption of a large portion of cucumbers, you will experience the diuretic effect – you'll find yourself constantly running to the bathroom to pass water. Cooked potatoes are equally effective. But make sure you buy organic quality, scrub the potatoes carefully and eat your fill of them, with the skins, morning, noon and night. If you're pregnant during the asparagus season, you can enjoy this wonderfully diuretic vegetable every day. Have a meal of potatoes and asparagus with plenty of fresh parsley and chives sprinkled over the top. Other herbs also refine the flavour; try mixing them into a bit of horseradish sauce – which stimulates the function of the liver as well as the immune system.

Another thing not to forget is lovage, an aromatic herb with an intense taste which supports the excretion process and is helpful above all on account of a liver-stimulating effect which is not to be underestimated.

Many women react with increased discharge of urine when they eat fresh pineapple. Be aware, however, that too much of this fruit can cause heartburn (see p. 77 f.).

In the 1970s and '80s, rice diets were very popular. In the course of an entire day, as much boiled brown rice as possible is to be eaten – at least 250 to 300 g. If the cure is carried out for several days, it brings about a major loss of potassium, which must be compensated by eating fresh or dried apricots. This potassium loss is not entirely harmless and leads to severe weakness. It is not known what effect this condition has on the production of amniotic fluid, but it is presumed that an uncontrolled and excessive rice diet going on for several days can lead to the spontanous rupture of the membranes, more commonly known as the breaking of the waters. It is for this reason that I prefer to recommend potatoes, which don't throw the body off balance and which regulate its fluid balance more effectively. Nevertheless, I don't want to advise you against such methods as the rice diet once and for all merely because this method used to be practiced excessively without compensating for the loss of potassium. If you practice this cure with caution, eat apricots, drink lots (!) of water and get enough rest, you will notice that the accumulations of fluid decrease and you feel well. Back in the days of the rice diet's popularity, people also believed in eating very little salt or none at all – a practice since proven harmful – and were unaware of the importance of fluid intake. What is more, rice diets were carried out with white rice instead of brown, as is now recommended.

The topic of oedema reminds me of another story …

… Mrs. G. was pregnant with her third child and her due date was just a few days away. She called me late one morning in a state of hysteria: "I just got back from the doctor's practice. My legs are so full of water that he says it's dangerous for my baby. And to make matters worse, my blood pressure was too high. He said that if the baby isn't born in the next few days, he refuses to take responsibility. What in the world should I do, have you got any advice for me? I refuse to take the medication the doctor wanted to prescribe. He threatened that he would have to induce labour tomorrow if the situation hadn't changed by then. And I was so happy that finally I would have a baby that could come when it was good and ready." (Mrs. G. had had her first two children in the era when programmed labour was common. Now she wanted, finally, to have a child without induced labour, experience everything normally this one last time, as she put it.) The first thing I did was to ask her about the amount of fluid she was in the habit of drinking every day and how often she passed water. She then explained to me that she was very thirsty, but that she followed her doctor's advice and didn't drink more than one litre of fluid a day. "And I run to the bathroom just for a couple of drops; after all, where should it come from when I don't drink anything and sweat a lot at night to top it off", was her reply. I confirmed her doctor's concern but suggested she try out a couple of "alternative methods" just very briefly. I advised her to drink as much of the abovementioned tea as possible, immediately, eat a lot of potatoes with skins and fresh herbs and quark. I told her not to work, but simply to lie on the sofa. She had to promise to get her husband or Grandma to take over on the kids and the housework. She could only achieve something with rest, fluid and potatoes. In addition, she should take Pulsatilla, which she just happened to have in the house, because this was exactly the remedy for her emotional state. And finally, I requested that she call me immediately as soon as she had the slightest physical discomfort or couldn't pass enough water. Since I was aware of the danger of gestosis – which ultimately can develop very quickly into what is almost a life-and-death situation for the child and the mother alike – I decided to go and see Mrs. G. that afternoon. Her husband greeted me at the door and told me that he had just applied for holiday from work. Mrs. G. was lying on the sofa with a pot of tea on the table and a plate of potatoes. She was radiant with joy and immediately told me about her frequent, successful visits to the bathroom. "I haven't 'wee-weed' this much for weeks; it's so satisfying!" I had immediately noticed her

conspicuously bloated face and swollen legs. But I was already somewhat relieved when she told me of her success. Her blood pressure was just under the maximum of what was allowed. I rang up her doctor, who was very glad to hear about my house call. He agreed that, if Mrs. G.'s blood pressure was taken very frequently and she continued to pass water well, the induction of labour could be postponed. He knew Mrs. G. very well and showed understanding for her request. He was rather condescending about my potato diet, but he said: "If that's what you midwives have to do, then go ahead and do it." The next morning, a radiant Mrs. G. awaited me – her face back to its normal appearance, free of oedema – with the words: "You won't believe this, but I'm three kilos lighter. That was certainly a night to remember; I spent most of it on the loo Tell, me does the increased discharge I'm experiencing also come from the fluid and the potatoes?" Of course I could only share her joy about this success; her blood pressure had also gone down a bit. As for the vaginal discharge, I was able to give her wonderful news and tell her that apparently the child was announcing itself. I said, "All that splashing last night was probably too loud for the baby and it has decided to start opening up the birth passage – that is what the discharge means." An examination confirmed my speculation: the cervix had effaced entirely and begun to open. Great joy prevailed in the house of the G. family. The second examination that day only gave cause for more cheer: Mrs. G.'s blood pressure was now absolutely normal; she was still eating potatoes and drinking tea by the litre. But there were no discernible contractions yet. The next morning, however, the happy father gave me a call; I didn't have to come and take blood pressure but could I please come by and attend to the navel wound? The previous night, Mrs. G. had given birth to a healthy daughter; everything had gone very quickly and the parents were just about to leave the hospital. They had decided weeks before to have a birth with an early discharge, i.e. spend the early postnatal period at home.

Naturally, experiences like this are very positive, and women who are accustomed to supporting their bodies with naturopathic means have even better prospects of success. A person who has been living with painkillers and other strong medications for years will not have such experiences. In the area of obstetrics, it is all the more enjoyable to work with natural methods and means, because many of the women who want to have children are young and healthy and usually aware that a lot of medicines are harmful. My fellow midwives claim that, here in Allgaeu, people still have some common sense, and that anyway, the only women who consult me are those who have a healthy attitude. I find it important to point this out to those midwives who haven't had the opportunity to gather such positive experience.

I would also like to call attention to the advice provided by the "Arbeitsgemeinschaft Gestose-Frauen e.V.", an association of women concerned with gestosis. This group recommends not only the intake of plenty of fluid but above all a sufficient amount of salt. They collect and publish studies and investigations, particularly from the U.S., which provide proof that the reduction of salt – still believed in many places to be necessary and desirable – actually triggers a mechanism in the body which increases accumulations of fluid in the tissue. In acute situations, they recommend dissolving 1 to 1 ½ teaspoons of salt in a litre of water. This solution is then to be consumed in the course of the day. I advise enhancing this treatment with a saltwater foot bath, or, even better, a full bath with 1 – 3 kg of salt. This method will bring about an increased discharge of urine within a very short time. I can confidently confirm the correctness of these pointers on the basis of my own experience. I have known women who had already gone through premature delivery by way of caesarean section on account of gestosis. Naturally, they were very careful during their subsequent pregnancy and had obtained information on possible therapies even before getting pregnant. I confirmed to them that salt intake was certainly a good means of preventing gestosis if accompanied by sufficient intake of protein and a satiating diet. The above-named association explicitly emphasizes that meticulous care must be taken to consume satiating foods including a sufficient amount of animal protein. Interested women are advised to contact this association (for address, see appendix, p. 460 f.).

Blood Pressure

Here I would like to go into the topic of blood pressure during pregnancy in somewhat more detail: as already mentioned, there is a close connection between blood pressure and oedema, gestosis and the HELLP syndrome (see p. 100f.).

To begin with, it is always important to be familiar with the levels that are normal for you. It would be very helpful if all women had their blood pressure taken now and then, even when they aren't pregnant. Many women worry about levels which are supposedly too high or too low – without realizing that their blood pressure may always have been that high or low and they felt well and healthy with it. What I mean is that, here as well, individual levels must be taken into consideration. If the individual blood pressure level rises or falls, treatment must be undertaken.

High Blood Pressure (Hypertension)

One blood pressure irregularity is inborn hypertension, i.e. high blood pressure. Your doctor will know the extent to which this condition should be treated, and what medication to use, and will advise you accordingly.

Often, however, there are other causes for the development of high blood pressure in pregnant women, and in these cases reference is readily made to stress-related hypertension.

When women ask my advice on this subject, the first question that comes up is: "What or who is putting you under so much pressure?" The answer is often a long tale of woe. The expectant mother finally has an opportunity to talk about problems in everyday life, at work, in her relationship to her partner, etc. I have the feeling that I'm not just a midwife, but often a midwife, family counsellor and psychotherapist all in one. After a talk of this kind, the pregnant woman usually feels much calmer, sees her problem from a different perspective and finds a way or means of taking the pressure off herself. This is just one more example of a case in which it is not necessary to reach for medication immediately, but where a good talk and the right mental attitude can play a decisive role.

⊚ Herbal Medicine and Nutrition

As you surely know, it is essential that you avoid caffeinated beverages such as coffee, Coke and black and green tea. A diet with a low animal protein content and lots of vegetables and whole grain foods is also very beneficial.

For dyed-in-the-wool tea drinkers, I also have a nice recipe, which I call *Lemon Balm Midwives' Tea, consisting of*: lemon balm, mistletoe and hawthorn. These are time-tested herbs which can be used during pregnancy without any adverse effects. Here again: the most effective way of using this tea is to drink three cups in the course of the day at a lukewarm temperature.

⊚ Homoeopathic Remedies

Many mothers specifically ask what type of homoeopathic remedy might help her. Homoeopathy has various remedies against high blood pressure. As always, the holistic aspect must be taken into account, and a thorough anamnesis with reportorization is indispensable. *Aurum, Apis, Belladonna, Plumbum* and *Pulsatilla* are substances which might come into play here. But please never experiment on your own with them: these are major homoeopathic remedies which, in the case of problems like high blood pressure, must be indicated and administered with the greatest possible degree of precision, and the reactions then carefully observed. For information on the various potentiations of homoeopathic medicines, please refer to the "Basic Principles of Homoeopathy" in the appendix (S. 460 f.).

⊚ Aroma Therapy

In the area of aroma therapy I have had very good experience with *ylang-ylang*. I always associate this oil with a certain attitude I once found phrased as follows in a description in a book: "Let yourself go and enjoy." This is surely the best therapy for high blood pressure: leave everyday stress behind and learn to enjoy life in a state of relaxation. The ylang-ylang extract can be very helpful in that endeavour. By the way, this plant grows in the Philippines. The essence can be used alone or in combination with lavender and pure (100%) lemon balm in the aroma lamp, in a massage oil or a shower gel. The aroma lamp is really only suitable for rooms in which the expectant mother spends time alone. Other persons may not want to have themselves treated with ylang-ylang. There is even a danger that colleagues, for example, who suffer from low blood pressure will suffer from exposure to ylang-ylang, won't be capable of working or will even feel faint. So please take your surroundings into consideration. Since this oil alone has a very strong and distinctive scent, I created a blend which has meanwhile become extremely popular: containing litsea, clary sage, vetiver and lemon in addition to ylang-ylang it is called *Gelassenheit/Serenity ꝺ*° and can be employed as a body oil or aroma perfume. In the former case, it should be administered in the morning by gently massaging it into the skin in a consistently downward (!) direction. Naturally, women with varicose veins should rub it into the legs in an upward direction, the downward direction being reserved for the upper body. In the form of aroma perfume, this blend can be used several times a day, as often as you need it.

I have been able to help other, non-pregnant people treat their high blood pressure with this blend as well: for in the course of conversation, it is not at all unusual for a pregnant woman to ask me if I know of something that might help Grandma…

Low Blood Pressure (Hypotension)

On the other hand, there are many pregnant women who suffer from abnormally low blood pressure. They complain of always feeling tired, getting dizzy when they have to stand for a long time and having to sit down quickly to prevent themselves from fainting.

My first piece of advice is to *exercise* regularly and *go swimming* often. And here again, I repeat my pointer that these women should drink more fluids. For years, I have been telling them not to limit their consumption of salt but keep it at its normal level. Sometimes it already helps to change to a different brand of mineral water with a higher salt content. One or two cups of green tea in the morning will also help you get your circulation going. I frequently recommend ending the morning shower with a *stream of cool water*, to be administered to the body from bottom to top. This treatment is an excellent means of supporting the cardiovascular system, and stimulates the flow of blood beneath the surface of the skin, makes you resistant to illness and activates the body's defence mechanisms. I know it costs a good deal of courage at first, but it has a very noticeable positive effect on your entire condition. In many respects we lead lives of luxury, and it is very important to subject our bodies to fluctuations in temperature. Back in the days when there were no central heating systems or pre-heated cars, human beings were constantly exposed to alternating heat and cold. These days, many people even sleep in heated rooms instead of in a cold room with an open window, carry out their morning toilets in overheated bathrooms, have breakfast in a kitchen which has been heated through the night, and then get into cars already pre-warmed by an independent vehicle heater. At work, they have to spend hours in overheated, or air-conditioned offices, only to go home in the evening to complain of a lack of natural defences and the sniffles which have already set in again. I am telling you these thoughts simply as a means of calling your attention to the fact that we often don't reflect consciously on our behaviour. I find it very interesting that pregnancy provides us an opportunity to think about our habits. It's fascinating what functions children already carry out before they are even born. Again and again, I find parents telling me: "If it hadn't been for our child and your thought-provoking words, we probably still wouldn't have really thought about our own health and the way we live." I have great sympathy for these parents, since I went through exactly the same thing with my own children and a wonderful older colleague who once wagged her finger at me, saying: "You young midwives and mothers, just wait and see where your thoughts and actions will take you. For every little ache and pain you have to take a pill, instead of just using cold water and putting some faith in your body." To this day, I am grateful to Thea for this remark, because it really got me thinking.

Herbal Medicine

Midwive's Tea Rosemary, a blend of one part each of common broom and rosemary leaves and two parts of hawthorn blossoms has proven very effective. As always, you should drink the tea for several days at least, and then stop drinking it when your condition has improved.

Homoeopathic Remedies

Homoeopathy can be very helpful here as well, but it is essential to carry out treatment on the basis of a thorough anamnesis since usually not much can be achieved with time-tested remedies. Possible choices are: *Veratrum album, Arnica, Natrium Muriaticum, Gelsemium.*

Aroma Therapy

I have had excellent success treating low blood pressure with *rosemary oil*: one, or at the very most two, drops of rosemary on a washcloth in the morning and used for washing or showering often already suffices to stabilize your blood pressure within just a few days. Many women prefer to make themselves a body oil containing rosemary and administering it to the skin in an upward (!) direction. At home, you can use your aroma lamp, the same rule applying here as in the case of high blood pressure: always think about the people who are being subjected to co-treatment. Used to counteract low blood pressure, rosemary is a helpful oil which heightens stamina and boosts our faith in our own strength. Because this faith has often dwindled in pregnant women who already have a difficult time getting to their feet in the morning, are still tired at noon and sink into bed weaker than ever in the evening. In such a condition, you easily begin to wonder: "How am I going to manage everything when the baby is here?" Incidentally, rosemary is a desert plant; in other words, it grows in an environment in which there are virtually no nutrients left, just sand! But it can subsist on the few drops of water that fall from the sky, stand upright and grow. In my opinion, it is surely also possible in our own lives to mobilize our last remaining reserves of energy, arouse our wills and motivation and find our staying power with rosemary oil. Give it a try; maybe even just the refreshing *rosemary hydrolat* will help. By the way, both the oil and the hydrolat are a great tip for midwives who have to work a night shift or are just tired and out of energy, or for colleagues who would love to go home after ten hours on duty but the next expectant mother in labour is knocking at the delivery suite door. Rosemary also has a very nice side effect: it arouses hidden appetites. Mothers whose children were sickly or poor eaters have confirmed this time and again: the problem children developed an appetite and gained strength quickly ...

... another case, for example, was the grandmother who lived with the family and was already being treated for high blood pressure and then, for initially inexplicable reasons, found that she had abnormally high blood pressure levels. But interestingly, she didn't have any of the unpleasant side effects which otherwise accompanied this condition. After her daughter had used up her stock of rosemary oil in the aroma lamp, everything soon returned to normal.

Yes, essential oils have been proved to have an effect and really should be used only when indicated, and never thoughtlessly. All naturopathic remedies help when their administration is sensible, but should definitely not be used when there are *contraindications*. For this reason, I would like to impress the following upon expectant mothers: it is better to ask one time too many than one time too few! And for all of my fellow midwives who are just beginning to gather experience: take essential oils seriously, and keep careful records of how the pregnant women react to them – and learn as much as you can about the topic.

Rosemary is thus a substance to be used within a strictly defined area of health problems, and please note: it *can* be used in cases of low blood pressure – but only rosemary of the cineole type. It *cannot* be used in cases of normal or high blood pressure. Because of these prohibitions, many books state that rosemary should not be used at all during pregnancy. It is my hope, however, that my readers – expectant mothers and midwives alike – will live up to the faith I am placing in them and really take these recommendations seriously. If you dislike the smell of rosemary, you might want to try the *Original D® Aroma Blend Kräuterkorb/Basket of Herbs D®*. But please be aware that this mixture also contains peppermint. So please use it only if there are not the slightest signs of increased uterine activity, and only in cases of extremely low blood pressure.

The Breech Position

Normally, children turn themselves around so that their heads are pointing towards the birth canal in about the thirty-second week of pregnancy; i.e. they are then lying in the womb "on their heads".

There are some children, however, who are still upright in the uterine cavity, bright as a button, in the thirty-fifth week. At the antnatal appointment, a so-called breech position is then diagnosed. The medical records always include a documentation of the presenting part, which will then be a breech presentation instead of a cephalic (head-down) presentation. Naturally, it is very important for all midwives and obstetricians involved to know of this circumstance beforehand, and not suddenly be surprised when they see the baby's behind. This condition is not abnormal, to say nothing of pathological. It is merely a variation on the "cephalic presentation".

Assessment Methods

With the help of an *ultrasound examination*, it is very easy to determine the child's position without a doubt in any given week of pregnancy. We midwives, however, and a few scattered doctors, try to ascertain the fetal presentation manually, from the outside. All midwives learn a method for doing so, the so-called *"Leopold's manoeuvres"*, during their training, in order to be able to determine the child's position in the uterus.

The advantage of this method is that it enables us to judge the fetal position without technology and electricity, while also providing an opportunity to establish good physical contact to the mother. During childbirth she will also be attended to by a midwife's hands and not by machines. In the context of this external examination, we can demonstrate to the mother where her baby's back, bottom, head, legs and arms can be felt (and at the same time, she can also try to feel these body parts herself). The child's growth naturally makes this examination increasingly easier towards the end of pregnancy. Until the year 1975, it was frequently the only method of determining the child's position, for it was not until then that ultrasound devices came into use even in the smaller obstetrics hospitals. And it was only many years later that these expensive apparatuses became common in doctors' practices, and since then they have undergone constant further development. Naturally, the obstetrics wards quickly became familiar with ultrasound devices, especially since technology very quickly arouses the enthusiasm of men in particular. To this day, ultrasound is the most reliable means of clearing up immediately any doubts as to the fetal position.

During the ultrasound examination carried out routinely within the framework of the antenatal check-up, the mother can see on the screen what position her child happens to be making itself comfortable in at that particular moment. This is of course a very special experience, but feeling and seeing are two different forms of sensory perception. It is undoubtedly interesting to see pictures of the unborn child. But to feel and touch one's own baby inside one, to know that this is where its behind, its legs, etc. are, is actually much more unforgettable. Mothers get to know their children better by touching them than by looking at ultrasound pictures. There is always something very special about showing mothers and fathers how to touch their babies. Especially the expectant fathers are overjoyed when – during the antenatal class or at the antenatal check-up – they are allowed to feel it themselves, with their own hands: here is the back, there is the head, here are the child's arms and legs. To see "my" child is certainly impressive, but to touch "my" child means: to grasp the reality that it is really there, there in my own paternal hands and not on the screen of a machine. Again and again, I experience that fathers have enormous respect for – even a certain shyness with regard to – his partner's pregnant womb, and hardly dare to touch the child properly. I believe this circumstance is connected to the high-tech means of surveillance – after all, it has often been observed that technology evokes respect, even a certain feeling of awe in us. But it is a false sense of respect when the woman's abdomen appears fragile in the eyes of the father and is handled with the same excessive care as is often the case with electronic devices – fearfully, as though something might break. Many women confirm that they can't understand why their partners always touch them so gingerly. The expectant fathers are grateful when I show them how clearly they can feel and touch the child. For the women, this proper, firm grip is much more pleasant and natural; it even gives them a sense of safety. If the man's grip is too tight, of course, it can happen that the expectant mother has to point out to her husband that it is her tummy and he should be a bit more cautious. A happy medium is always best. If parents are vocal about their desires, sensations, feelings and expectations, this happy medium can surely be found.

Spontaneous Vaginal Delivery or Caesarean Section

A great number of high-risk vaginal breech deliveries have undoubtedly been avoided thanks to ultrasound examinations. But many midwives are concerned about the fact that scarcely any *spontaneous vaginal breech deliveries* are allowed any longer these days, and can accordingly no longer be learned. In the past few years, fortunately, we note a cautious trend at various university hospitals for allowing first-time mothers to deliver their children vaginally, despite the breech position. In the case of women who have already given birth at least once in the past, the trend towards caesareans has fortunately not been confirmed. Many women have surely defended themselves and insisted on spontaneous delivery if possible.

It is well worth your while to find out what hospital in your vicinity will offer you, as parents, support in delivering the child spontaneously. Just like the birth of a child in the cephalic (head-down) position, vaginal breech delivery can take place entirely normally and without problems, or – again as in the case of a head-first birth – there can also be a delayed expulsion or pushing phase. As at any birth, the obstetrics team has to pay careful attention and take the appropriate measures in the case of emergency. Due to the fact that a doctor must be in attendance if there are complications during a vaginal breech delivery, it is always advisable to plan a hospital delivery. Moreover, the necessary obstetrical manoeuvres require a certain amount of experience, so you should try to choose the doctor or hospital accordingly well in advance of the due date – and ask about the rate of spontaneous vaginal breech deliveries at that hospital. Unfortunately, the latter are a rarity, and often a combination of worry and inexperience is the chief factor in deciding to end the delivery with a caesarean section. Recent studies carried out in Dublin prove that vaginal delivery is safe for the breech position. With quite some interest and pleasure, I read that, in this context, artificially induced labour and oxytocin infusions are taboo for these doctors, and that they attribute the low complication rate shown in the study to these strict standards.

It is my wish that everyone involved will aspire towards the best and safest solution for the mother and child. Naturally, however, I would advise all women to do everything in their power to avoid a caesarean. People are fortunately becoming increasingly aware of the fact that a caesarean section is absolutely the wrong way of overcoming fear. Sadly, for many years, women told their girlfriends: "Have a caesarean; they'll give you a general anaesthetic and when you wake up, everything will be over." And as a matter of fact, for years it was no problem to convince doctors to carry out this type of delivery, especially in the case of older women having their first child. Today, even more unfortunately, the opposite is more likely to happen: doctors urge women to have a caesarean even though they know that a general anaesthetic and caesarean section should really only be carried out in an emergency. Please take into account that a caesarean is always a major surgical intervention, of which the risks are far greater than those of spontaneous delivery, even if caesareans are undertaken these days as a matter of course, and thus perhaps trivialized. Sometimes I am even tempted to accuse the hospital directors of supporting caesareans because they bring in more money and because they make deliveries schedulable.

Natural Support for Turning a Baby from a Breech to a Cephalic Position

Time and Rest

Women are often already alarmed and come for a consultation when their babies are in the breech position in the thirtieth week of pregnancy. At this point in time, we midwives console the women by telling them that the child still has several weeks in which to turn around. I try to convince them that they can calmly wait a number of weeks: the child will turn around when it is good and ready. If the expectant mother had not been made aware of the breech position by way of an ultrasound examination, she wouldn't even know to worry at this point in time.

In any case, in the antenatal course I use a doll to demonstrate to the women how much space the baby still has. In her thoughts, she should regularly remind the child to turn its head downwards, and imagine the child making this somersault in her tummy.

It is also important for me to point out to the parents that it makes no sense to have excessive numbers of ultrasound examinations carried out, since they will do nothing to change the situation. On the contrary, they only represent unnecessary stress for the unborn baby since, after all, the latter is exposed to a volume of one hundred decibels! So my advice to you is, be patient. Give your child the chance to turn around on its own for as long as possible. I just think it's a shame when labour is induced two weeks before the due date – maybe the baby would have turned around three days later, as was the case with Mrs. W. ...

... she wanted to know whether it was really necessary to carry out the caesarean already two weeks before the due date. Her doctor had told her to come into the hospital on Thursday in order to carry out the planned operation on Friday. I could well understand her and, as concerned as I was for her

safety and that of her child, I couldn't determine any indication for premature intervention. I sup-
ported her in her desire to wait and recommended that she negotiate with the doctor and ask him to
wait. On Monday Mrs. W. asked for another appointment. She had had a restless night, the child had
been very lively and her belly had repeatedly gotten as hard as stone, so that she suspected labour
pains were already taking place. Now she was worried that perhaps it had been the wrong decision to
wait. But when I felt her belly, I was able to comfort her: "In my opinion, the baby has turned around;
I can feel the head at the bottom, and the fetal heartbeat is now clearly to be heard below the navel. I
would suggest that you go to your doctor and let him carry out an ultrasound, which he is sure to want
to do. I am certain it was worth your while to wait!" That afternoon, Mrs. W. rang me up: "You're
right, the doctor who is substituting for my gynaecologist confirmed it with ultrasound: my child has
now got its head pointing downwards and, just as you said, the cervix has opened slightly; maybe la-
bour will get under way tomorrow."

Patience and faith in the child really are worth the effort – and that's something that
proves true in situations later on in life as well. I have no doubt that our children
could already show and teach us quite a bit before they're even born – if only we parents and health professionals didn't think on such a short-term basis and weren't so
easily worried.

The Emotional Background of the Breech Position

When a woman comes to consult with me because of a breech position, one question
that should be raised is whether or not she can imagine why her baby might have assumed this sitting position instead of standing on its head in her womb as the medical
textbooks prescribe. Maybe it has some reason for this behaviour. In the talk that
ensues, the following often comes about: with its "sit-in", the child has managed to
get the parents thinking about the coming childbirth and the new situation of becoming parents. Frequently it becomes clear that the parents have taken the pregnancy
too much for granted until now, or have paid too little joint attention to what will be
a major change and new situation in their lives. Again and again, I notice that it does
the expectant mothers good to have talks like these. For many, it is a new but very
pleasant way of looking at the situation from the child's point of view or involving the
child in the current events, rather than just accepting a worrisome diagnosis. Now
suddenly the concern is no longer with doing something or being worried, but with
learning to interact with the child and what it is trying to communicate. Just such a
talk alone already helps many mothers. Parents have confirmed to me that when
questions of upbringing have arisen later on, they have often remembered my advice
to consider the child's perspective on the situation.

In these breech position cases, I also always ask how the coming child's two grandmothers had their children. With great regularity, the answer is something like: "Yes,
my mother-in-law had my husband in breech position!" Usually everyone present
reacts to this statement by laughing, and we realize that maybe even now the unborn
child has something in common with its father. Above all, the parents should think

seriously about the type of delivery and very consciously ask the grandmother about the events surrounding that breech position delivery.

Indian Bridge – All-Fours Position – Vena Cava Syndrome

During the antenatal class, sometime after the thirty-third to thirty-fourth week of pregnancy, the women learn to use the so-called *Indian Bridge*. This is an exercise where the mother lies on the floor with her abdomen in as high a position as possible while her knees are bent and her calves hang down as far as possible, creating a pronounced lordosis or hollow back. This will be uncomfortable for the child, and it may try to assume a different position of its own accord. Every woman should decide for herself how long she can endure this exercise. Often the directions for carrying it out tell you that the pregnant woman has to stay in this position for a specified length of time, but such recommendations can only have been made by people who have never been pregnant. This extremely inclined dorsal position frequently causes severe shortage of breath, since the baby slides all the way up to the ribcage, interfering with the function of the mother's lungs in two ways: proper breathing is prevented on the one hand by the child itself, and on the other hand by the dorsal position, which is inadvisable for a woman during pregnancy anyway. In many cases, the Indian Bridge can lead to the *Vena Cava syndrome*. This is triggered by the large uterus, which presses against the inferior vena cava (the large vein that drains blood from the lower body), blocking the return flow of blood to the heart. The mother gets dizzy and faint and has to turn on her side immediately. As a matter of fact, pregnant women are advised in general always to lie on their sides in order to avoid this syndrome. And all expectant mothers should exercise great care in doing the Indian Bridge, breathe slowly and intentionally into their tummies for as long as they can as they maintain the position. It is advisable to change from the Bridge to the *All-Fours Position*, in order to recover and breathe deeply, for in this position the lungs have all the space they need. You can assume the latter position for as long as you like, and remain with your child in your thoughts. The "all-fours" also leaves the child plenty of scope for movement and therefore might also facilitate its decision to do a somersault. If the Indian Bridge position makes you feel nauseated because the child presses against your stomach so hard, an alternative is the knee-elbow position for about twenty minutes. What is important here is that the abdomen is higher than the shoulder girdle so that the baby can slide out of the small pelvis.

⑤ Aroma Therapy

For the Indian Bridge exercise, I recommend that women involve their partners by having the latter support their abdomens. While she carries out the exercise, he can treat her to a gently abdominal massage with the *Original 𝒟® Aroma Blend Purzelbaum/Somersault 𝒟®*, containing the essential oils lavender, rose, yarrow, ylang-ylang and cedar. It is most sensible, of course, to massage in the right direction, in the "somersault direction", which the midwife will show the couple.

☙ Other Methods

Many a woman also finds it very pleasant when her partner massages her feet instead of her tummy. I would recommend proceeding very cautiously, however, because only trained persons should work with pregnant women by way of the foot reflex zones. I have often heard from expectant mothers that they had been to see a masseur who had gotten the child to turn around by means of *foot reflexology* or *acupressure*. But I would like to remind you once again that you should be sure the treatment is carried out by a competent person. As long as this is the case, these two types of treatment are very helpful means of turning a child in the breech position "upside down".

An equally helpful method is *acupuncture* carried out according to Penzel, or the *craniosacral therapy* successfully employed by many of my colleagues.

And many midwives also advise encouraging the child to turn with the help of a *torch (flashlight)*. The beam of light has to be moved very slowly over the mother's tummy in "somersault direction" several times in succession. For the mother, this is in any case a painless and pleasant way of literally lighting the child's way – for the beam of light penetrates the layers of muscle through to the child. Within the framework of a manual external examination, the midwife will show the mother the side of her belly on which to shine the torch.

☙ Homoeopathic Remedies

I am frequently confronted with the question as to whether it isn't possible to turn the child with the help of a couple of "globuli". It isn't as easy as all that, since homoeopathy is not capable of directly moving something. The midwife must make the effort to find a substance which will help the mother in this situation, i.e. which encourages the self-activation of the uterus and the child. In other words, a *homoeopathic medication* can serve as a means of support, but cannot get a child to move if that child isn't able to move, regardless of the reason. High potencies of the following substances can be prescribed by midwives and doctors with knowledge of homoeopathy: *Pulsatilla, Sepia* and *Tuberculinum*. I myself never cease to be amazed at what can be set in motion with the help of homoeopathy!

☙ Moxibustion

Sometimes women are sent by their doctors with the remark, "Go and see a midwife; they have a method. I don't think much of the things they do on the whole, but this method does help." What they are referring to is the *moxibustion method*. In the "Erdenlicht" midwife's practice in Kempten, my fellow midwives have been administering "moxa" for several years, and can achieve a correction of the child's position in fifty to seventy percent of all cases. This therapy is very similar to acupuncture, but instead of needles it employs mugwort cigarettes. By applying warmth to a certain point on the woman's little toe, the entire bladder meridian is warmed. This has a positive effect on the uterine muscles and the pelvis minor, and supports pregnancy in its normality. And as we know, it is normal for the child to lie head downwards in the uterus at the end of pregnancy.

Uschi's child hadn't heard of this normality yet, though, because …

… she came into the practice saying, "Just imagine, my baby is in breech position, and I only have less than four weeks until the due date. So I guess I can forget about having a normal delivery. Tell me, do I just have to accept this fact or is there something you can do?" I began by comforting her, telling her that it was by no means too late and she could keep dreaming, because things always turned out differently from the way we dreamed them anyway. After this typical remark of mine, which she already knew inside out, I said "I'd like to do a manual examination in order to get an impression of how much space it's still got and how much it can move in your womb." I also explained to Uschi that I can't "do" anything, but that, at best, with the help of the moxa, could support the child. When I examined her by means of the so-called "Leopold manoeuvres" in order to determine the child's position in the womb, I was able to comfort the worried mother. I told her that it was certainly worth a try with moxas. The examination made it clear that the child still had plenty of space and, what is more, had readily followed the movements of my hands. As a matter of fact, I almost had the feeling: just a little more courage on my part and one last turn, and the somersault will have been achieved. But in such cases my training looms over me and keeps me from taking such action. Without a medical background, and without control by means of ultrasound, the risk of carrying out this turn with my hands appears too great for the child. In many hospitals, doctors have now reverted to trying to turn children manually, where the process can be followed on the screen and an anaesthetic is always on hand. Uschi and I made an appointment for the following day at a time when her husband could also come so that he could learn the treatment and be able to carry it out on his own at home during the next few days. It's not at all difficult for the expectant mother's girlfriend or partner to work with the mugwort cigarettes if he or she has received proper instruction from the midwife.

The following day we had our meeting in the home of the young expectant parents. As I had directed, they had the lovely scent of lavender emanating from the aroma lamp to make Uschi relax and feel good. Peter had already been hard at work turning very firm, fat mugwort cigarettes, and we could begin with our treatment as soon as Uschi had made herself comfortable on the sofa. By candlelight, with Peter at the little toe on the right, I on the left, we commenced literally to heat Uschi up – the point was to be heated to the point of reddening. I asked Uschi to concentrate with all her might on her child and treat it to plenty of abdominal respiration. It took her no more than a few minutes to become accustomed to the heat and she told us that she had a pleasant sensation of warmth all over her feet. After another three minutes she could feel the warmth rising up her calves. Soon she said with great pleasure: "Just look at that little 'buzzel' [Allgaeu dialect for baby], wide awake and dancing around." And in fact, we could clearly see Uschi's belly bulging and the child moving beneath the abdominal wall. We were very happy about this because it was a very positive sign that the baby was reacting to the therapy. A few days later, after which the parents had "moxed" regularly, Uschi rang me up and I already suspected what she was going to tell me from the happy tone of her voice: "I was at the doctor's today, Inge; the baby is lying head downwards, isn't that terrific? Now hopefully everything can go the normal way." Yes, that was one of the first of my many positive experiences with moxa.

I'd also like to tell you about a very interesting experience I had treating a mother of twins with moxa…

… Evi came into the practice with her husband on a Friday afternoon in quite a sad state. I had been her attending midwife for several weeks already. She was now in the twenty-ninth week of pregnancy and her abdominal girth had increased substantially. Evi had just gotten home from a stay in the hospital a few days previously. There she had had a cervical cerclage carried out. Due to the twin pregnancy, her cervix was subjected to considerable stress and therefore had to be sewn shut. She also had to take a tocolytic (contraction inhibitor). Now for several days she had been suffering from congestion of the kidneys. She came with a beseeching expression on her face and I knew immediately that she had kidney pains again. And, yes, that was in fact the reason for the visit, but the expectant parents also wanted to tell me that the twins were still in the breech position. "Tell us, Inge, what in the world should we do; do you have any advice for us? You have some strange method", the worried father asked. I told them about moxas and explained that I didn't expect it to help in the case of twins, but it certainly would do no harm to try; on the contrary, if nothing else, moxibustion would support the function of the kidneys. When they agreed to try I was really encouraged, and we eagerly set about "smoking her toes". Already during the first ten minutes, Evi felt so much better that I was amazed. She relaxed, her facial features softened and at the end of the treatment she said she could endure the pain much better now, which seemed incredible to me. The next morning she called me and cheerfully reported to me that for days she hadn't been able to urinate as well as she had the previous night. Her husband – a doctor, incidentally – told me: "You know, Evi was on the toilet half the night. If I hadn't experienced it myself I never would have believed it possible." I was just as happy and amazed as they were. It's just terrific what the ancient Chinese already knew!

The two children could not be persuaded to turn themselves into the cephalic position, however, though that wasn't something we had really dared hope would happen. But the strain had been taken off the kidneys, and that was more than was to be expected.

Success is on the horizon particularly when the child moves actively during the moxing procedure. It is surely enjoying its parents' mental attention and will have all the more pleasure in doing a somersault.

Reasons for the Breech Position

Very many breech babies adamantly refuse to change positions, no matter what anybody does. After a caesarean, the reason often becomes obvious: it was literally impossible for the child to turn around because the maternal pelvis was too narrow for a normal delivery. Sometimes umbilical cord complications can also lead the unborn baby to stay in its sitting position. Children always know themselves what's best for them. For the mother, it is important to know after the delivery that she has done everything in her power to help the child turn. The nagging question as to whether one did too little during pregnancy can often lead to emotional disturbances, which in turn can put great strain on the relationships between the mother, child and partner.

Partnership/Parenthood

The relationship between the expectant parents usually becomes very intense during the final three months, and this is the time to resolve any conflicts that might be causing discord between you. Take as much time as possible to talk to each other about your feelings – and to listen to each other. One very nice exercise is to sit opposite one another, all four of your hands on the child you are awaiting. Look into each other's eyes without talking, then both of you close your eyes and try to concentrate on the child. After several minutes, each of you tell the other what feelings came up in you during that "meditation". Don't interrupt each other; give one another the opportunity to communicate your feelings, needs and expectations with regard to this parenthood. Make an effort to be good listeners and develop a sense of your partner's needs. This way you will experience parenthood as a team. For the coming birth and the initial months following, these are important prerequisites. The level of emotional intensity may be something new for you, but during pregnancy, childbirth and the postnatal period it represents a natural form of protection for the mother and child. For pregnant women, it is very important that the expectant father also talk about his sensations, feelings and expectations regarding parenthood, because it confronts him with thoughts about becoming a father. Women often tend to expect their partners to show understanding for their situations as mothers-to-be, but never put themselves into the place of the father-to-be. I often have the feeling that women expect too much of their partners.

For the expectant father, this is a good way of allowing himself to express his feelings and learning to talk about them – and of experiencing that he doesn't always have to be the man whose supposed responsibility it is to understand the unfamiliar feelings of an expectant mother. It is usually not possible for him to have more than a vague notion of what is going on inside the woman's heart and mind and what it means to be subjected to fluctuations in feelings brought about hormonally. Many men are likewise confronted with a very out-of-the-ordinary situation during their partner's pregnancy. They often find themselves confronted with new professional challenges related to the prospect of having to support the family on their own. In my opinion, society still pays much too little attention to these pressures and the stress of becoming a father. A father will often tell me that the questions asked by the people around him show concern but also depress him a bit: "How is your wife? Is the baby healthy and growing?" Many men would be happy if people also asked about their feelings as expectant fathers. Men also think about this change and the new responsibilities that the role of father will bring.

For men and women, becoming parents means undergoing change. Both of them will realize that the time they now spend together talking about how they imagine their duties and responsibilities as parents are the hours they will later need to cope with the baby's evening restlessness. In the partner classes I always recommend: take at least one weekend and rehearse being parents. In other words, the expectant mother sits in an armchair or on the sofa with her legs propped up six to eight times in twenty-four hours for as much as an hour and "nurses". Because that's how long and how often a newborn demands attention and care, i.e. needs to be breastfed, changed, carried and loved. This "baby care routine" will initially take you one to one-and-a-half hours or even longer, before your child finally gets back to sleep for two hours. For the mother, simply caring for the baby is therefore a full-time job. What this means for the father is that he should be mentally prepared for this temporary neglect, the fate of every initiate to fatherhood. Among other things, he will now have to take care of the mother and the child for awhile – an unaccustomed task. The help of the father in the household is nothing unusual anymore. But in the final weeks before and the initial weeks after the birth of the child, men are increasingly taking over completely on the shopping and cooking, to the extent permitted by their professional lives. On a rehearsal weekend of the kind mentioned above, both partners can practice taking on these new roles which, for the woman, include giving up certain daily and household habits and leaving them to her partner.

As Anita once related to me...

... *"Inge, you know, the evenings with you were so good. It's only now that we realize how necessary it was for us to attune ourselves to this child. It's only now that my husband has become truly aware of the fact that he will soon be a father. He even sometimes cancels a date with his buddies, and he no longer insists on watching the news like he used to. And we're having talks the way we did at the beginning of our relationship, after that kind of communication had fallen more and more by the wayside. And I'm in the process of learning to leave certain household tasks to him, and am beginning to accept that he goes about things differently."*

In these sessions on the subject of parenthood, men often ask: "Is there anything positive to be said about the first few weeks of being a parent?"

It is then that I realize that, as hard as I try to tell them something about everyday life as young parents, I can't convey much of the "happy young parents" image that beams out at us from brochures and book covers. In reality, a few days after the initial joy, everyday life is dominated by stress, lack of sleep and worry, and parents-to-be should take their expectations down a notch or two.

There is no doubt in my mind that all of this is much less of a problem and can be coped with all the better when expectant parents truly accept that their situation is very special and very out-of-the-ordinary: the birth of the child really will bring about a major change in family life. For me as a midwife, it is important to confront the parents with facts and not romanticize about everyday life during the first few weeks. Naturally, even at the beginning, parenthood is associated with many pleasant and happy moments and hours, but they will not always dominate.

Sexuality

The physical relationship between partners can be experienced in extremely different ways, ways as different as people themselves – along with their experiences and feelings – can be. What is important is that the same "rules" that apply to most other areas of life also hold true for sexuality: everything that is fun and makes you happy is allowed. If the woman's body sends her signals such as lack of desire, lasting stomach pains after intercourse or the like, then it is important that they be interpreted correctly. There is no evidence that sexual intercourse is harmful for the child at any time and should therefore be prohibited. Naturally, an orgasm is likewise harmless; as a matter of fact, there are certain advantages to it: it helps to improve the tonicity of the uterine muscles and prepare the body for labour. Many women report that pregnancy is one of the best phases of sexual experience, and that it was during pregnancy that they first learned what it meant just to allow things to take their course. Maybe this is the nicest way of learning to "let go" in the manner required for childbirth, for the latter is also a kind of orgasmic dissolution/release. Here again, it is very important for both partners to talk about their feelings. It is important to know that the baby is well protected and is happy about this affectionate embrace. If carried out in the right position, everyone – the child, the woman and the man – can experience joy in the togetherness of intercourse. Many parents report that they are glad to have broken some of their old sexual habits, and that the pregnancy – with the help of lots of cushions – has inspired them to find other fun and gratifying possibilities and variations.

On the other hand, it is not at all unusual for women to have no desire for physical love during pregnancy. In order to make clear that it is not a deeply rooted problem, however, you should by all means talk to one another. There are also men who no longer want to sleep with their wives because they are worried about the child. Unfortunately, his lack of desire often leads to the fear that he might find her misshapen body repulsive. Again, what is important here is to talk to one another, and to obtain the advice of people with experience in these matters.

I am frequently asked whether it's true that pregnant women should not have intercourse in the final weeks. This is an unjustified statement which I cannot endorse. Once again, I would like to emphasize: every couple can decide for themselves whether they want to make love, when, how and how often. Your body tells you of its own accord what will do it good, by signalling desire or the lack thereof. It is true, however, that – due to her enormous girth, shortness of breath and similar discomforts – some women lose their sexual desire towards the end of pregnancy. Intercourse can also trigger minor contraction activity, i.e. the abdomen reacts immediately afterwards with a tightening of the muscles. This tightening is entirely normal and should not prevent you from enjoying the relaxation following the orgasm. The triggering of labour pains through the prostaglandin content of the semen (prostaglandin is a hormone which stimulates contractions) is extremely rare. This can only happen when the due date has been reached or exceeded, i.e. when the woman's body has begun to produce the kind of hormones that stimulate labour. And at that point in time it is desirable for labour to begin. Only when the body is ready for labour does it react to the prostaglandin. This hormonal substance is also produced by certain cells in the cervix, and makes the latter soft and pliable.

Sometimes women have a trace of spotting after sexual intercourse, which comes from small injuries to cervical vessels caused by the contact during coitus. Usually this is no cause for concern, but you should talk to your midwife or doctor about it.

A Baby Sister or Brother

If you already have one or more children, you should prepare them for the new addition to the family during the final weeks of pregnancy, if not sooner. Try to involve your children, introduce them to their infant sibling, let them put their ear to your tummy, feel it and try to guess the baby's position in the womb. It makes a child happy to know that the baby inside already hears his or her voice and will surely recognize it again after the birth. Bigger children sometimes like to sing songs to their baby brother or sister in utero, give it a good-night kiss and include it in the going-to-bed ceremony. I rather doubt that children can imagine the appearance of the baby on the basis of ultrasound images. Let your child rely on its own powers of imagination instead, and get him or her a good picture book on the subject – your local bookshop will surely be able to recommend one.

Make sure you give your children enough time to adjust to the coming change. Don't expect them to be wild about the idea from the start. Upon being told the "happy news", a five-year-old boy made it unequivocally clear that "No babies are coming to live in my house!" Today, this boy loves his sister dearly. Gisela's ten-year-old daughter reacted by saying: "I'd rather have a puppy!" But she adored the new baby from the very beginning. So be aware that your "big" child won't always be very happy about the news. I have the impression that children know instinctively – perhaps better than we adults – what an addition to the family means.

It is well worth your while to get children accustomed to the fact that Daddy is just as good at reading a good-night story as Mummy, and to acquaint older children with other trusted adults. During pregnancy, a problem can arise from one day to the next and you have to go to the hospital for a little while. In such a case it is very helpful already to have rehearsed such a separation from your child. After all, when the labour pains begin, the child will have to be taken to Grandma, a neighbour or close friend. But it is equally important not to confront children with the advent of a sibling too soon and talk about it constantly, since forty weeks are an incomprehensibly long time for a child. The process of waiting for the baby sister or brother is strenuous and exciting enough at the end of pregnancy.

Preparing the Baby's Room

A nice way of preparing for parenthood is to get the baby's room ready. If you already have older children, this is also a good opportunity to get them used to the idea of a new member of the family. The children learn that the baby will not exist only in Mummy's tummy, soon be present in the children's or parents' bedroom as well. For those children who still sleep in their parents' bed, the preparations for the new baby often involve getting the older child accustomed to sleeping on its own. But don't wait to begin this "weaning" process until shortly before the due date, because this is often very difficult for children to understand: not only does the "big" child – often no more than a toddler itself – have to give up space in its own room, but it is also not allowed into Mummy's bed anymore. Approach these changes in the life of the older child with caution, and be aware that the newborn might be content to sleep in its cradle from the beginning. In a pinch, you'll be able to sleep quite alright as a four-some in the parents' bed.

The Changing Table

When making preparations for your first child, your first priority should be to make sure that the changing table is practical and well thought-out. This table is going to be your "workplace" during the next few months, even years, if a second child follows close on the heels of the first. The changing table should have a healthy working height, i.e. at least 95 centimetres. If it is too low or too high, you are sure to develop back problems before long. The changing surface can never be too large, but should in any case have high sides to keep the risk of the baby's falling off as low as possible. It is a big help if either the table is large enough to place a bowl of water on it or there is running water in the room. Many parents install a quartz radiator over the changing table, but make sure you place it high enough – your child will grow fast and you shouldn't expose your head to direct heat either. I find quartz radiators very practical, because then you don't have to heat the entire room all day. The heat is at your disposal when you need it, and is very pleasant to have on days when the central heating has been turned off and above all at night. Particularly in the early phase, it is important that the baby is warm enough and doesn't catch a chill while it is being changed. Under the radiator, changing is a joy for the child and its parents alike. But please don't use an infrared radiator, because the area it heats is too restricted and it is difficult to place in such a way that neither the child's nor the parents' eyes are exposed to the light. Infrared lamps have wonderful therapeutic qualities, but they should not be used to provide warmth.

I would like to recommend to all parents that they purchase only the most basic furnishings for the baby's room. In the course of the coming months, any number of presents and loans will make their way into your house. What is more, once you are parents you will notice that you view these things differently than before the baby was born. For the newborn, the most important thing is to have a little bed with a hot-water bottle and a soft sheepskin in a place that is well-protected from draughts. Too much furniture and baby clothing are inadvisable, because the fumes emitted by the solvents represent a danger and the risk of the baby's developing allergies is very great. When choosing the interior, make sure that the furniture is environmentally friendly and free of formaldehydes. Consult with an expert, look for suitable litera-ture on the subject and ask experienced parents. People also often ask us midwives when we pay them house calls. Unfortunately, however, in many cases it's too late by then – when I come for my first postnatal call I can tell by smelling that there is new furniture in the room. When the children are restless, I have often had to advise the parents not to change the baby or let it sleep in the polluted room.

For this reason, I would like to recommend to all parents that they begin thinking about the subject of the baby room furnishings well in advance of the due date. Many women think they'll be able to take care of all that when they go on maternity leave. But I would advise you against doing that, because who knows what surprises the pregnancy will bring with it? Many a child has thwarted its parents' plans by forcing the mother to spend most of the final weeks resting on the sofa or even by being born prematurely. And anyway, in those last weeks it really isn't very pleasant shopping for furniture in department stores or moving furniture around at home, wallpapering and painting the walls.

Baby Care

Aside from the antenatal classes, there are also special infant care classes. There you not only practice changing a baby, but all kinds of other useful things besides. The various kinds of nappies/diapers are introduced, methods of using cloth nappies are tried out. And everyday problems are discussed, with a focus on everything from the nappy bucket to the laundry detergent, from the bassinette to the carry sling, giving the baby a bath and lots more.

Cloth Nappies

Here a few remarks on the pros and cons of cloth nappies: decide early on what you want "your" nappy method to be, because once the baby is born, it will be difficult to break the habit of using the convenient disposable plastic nappies. If you've already stocked up on the practical cloth nappy panties or the pleasant fluffy cotton nappies, it will be a matter of course to nappy the baby with them. The advertising slogan "Nothing is too expensive for my child!" can also be interpreted to mean: nappy your baby in cloth! The time spent washing, drying, hanging up, folding and changing your baby with cloth nappies – part of the everyday working life of a young mother or househusband – is in fact of inestimable value. During the time it takes for other parents to drive into town for a quick shopping spree, get caught in traffic, not find the brand of disposables they want, and then come home stressed out, you could be sitting on the balcony or in the garden with your baby and peacefully folding the cloth nappies. A few years later, every time you clean the windows with the rags made from the cloth nappies, you'll be reminded of your child. You will find any number of further uses for those nappies, for cleaning, for leg compresses when a member of the family is sick, etc.

Baby Clothing

To an ever greater extent, pure fashion considerations determine the range of available baby articles. So when you're shopping, don't forget to ask yourself: is this offer good for my child or for the company making the offer? Don't buy too many small playsuits or rompers, because sometimes they're too small for your baby from the start. And also take into account that, as experience shows, you'll get a number of cute little playsuits as presents. Grandmas, aunts, girlfriends – everyone loves to buy baby clothes. Unfortunately, baby articles have come to constitute a huge branch of the fashion industry. When shopping, make sure that particularly the undergarments are made of pure cotton, wool or silk. At the risk of sounding old-fashioned: white clothing is really preferable, because dyed cloth can be dangerous for your baby's sensitive skin. Believe it or not, medical journals contain reports on allergies and respiratory difficulties in newborns dressed in colourful undergarments.

And another piece of advice from an Allgaeu grandmother: back in the old days, children were all swaddled and dressed in the same things their parents and grandparents – i.e. several generations – had worn, and on a chest of drawers in the kitchen, because there the mother always had the stove going and could get warm water from the oven, while simultaneously keeping an eye on the older brothers and sisters and watching that the soup didn't boil over. What I am trying to say is that there's a lot we can do even today – without spending a great deal of money – to show a child that it is loved and part of the family. A child doesn't need the most modern and most expensive furniture or clothing to be happy and content.

Home Birth/Independent Birth Centre

In the last three months of pregnancy, the contact between the midwife and the parents planning for the birth at home or in an independent birth centre becomes very intense. Women go to their antenatal classes regularly, and their partners take part in the information session/s.

Information Sessions/Tuning In to Childbirth

It is ideal when the midwives' practice offers opportunities for the exchange of experience between parents who would like to deliver outside the hospital. For us midwives, it is important to attune the parents to the baby which is on its way. Particularly fathers who already have children appreciate these opportunities, because at home they usually don't have much energy left over for the unborn baby. We are always happy when they tell us at the end: "That was nice; now I'm conscious of the fact that I'm going to be a father again soon – my wife was right when she urged me to come along. At home it wouldn't have been the case, but here at the midwives' practice I have become much more aware of the coming birth of the new baby."

The sessions are used to learn about the contractions as well as the breathing exercises that can be employed to cope with those contractions. Parents who have their first child at home or at an independent birth centre receive a lot of information as well as encouragement from experienced fathers. I'll never forget, for example, how suspensefully Oliver could relate his experience of the force of labour pains. He described something that had happened to him once on holiday. He was sitting on a beach and trying to avoid a storm tide that kept coming closer and closer, the turbulent seas making the stony shores roar. In this situation of vulnerability, with no place to retreat to – since the beach was closed off at the back by a high, insurmountable cliff – he thought of his son's birth. When retold in the first-person by a real live father, these experiences are often more impressive than any descriptions of waves or labour pains I might come up with.

During these evening sessions, we practice how accompanying persons should hold, support and massage the woman in labour. We midwives attach great importance to talking about the course of childbirth: using pictures to explain what happens in each individual phase of labour. Naturally, we also try out and practice various birthing positions. It gives the mother a sense of confidence to be corrected or told she is doing it right by the midwife, because she has the security of knowing she can be reminded of what she has practiced later on, when she is in labour. When we do a "dry run" of the expulsion phase, it is possible to point out her strengths and weaknesses to her. The training session provides the man the opportunity of becoming aware of his position and function during the birth of the child, and he recognizes that his help could well play an important role in the baby's being born quickly and soundly. It gives all of us a means of attuning ourselves to one another, verbally and mentally. Naturally, we tell the expectant parents over and over again that we have to be flexible while labour is in progress, and that we may have to forget everything we've learned. And I never tire of saying: "First of all, things won't always happen, second of all, the way you expect, but, third of all, sooner or later entirely of their own accord!" – an expression other midwives, and even doctors, have also meanwhile adopted. All expectant home-birth parents must become aware that a home delivery cannot be planned in detail beforehand. Many parents have found themselves confronted with this truth. Suddenly everything happened so fast that there was no time to set up the aroma lamp, play the favourite CD, light a candle or enjoy a relaxing bath in a cosy atmosphere. For children often already reveal a will of their own during their birth, and do things much differently from what the parents expect. In the independent birth centre, it is frequently also a very special challenge to conjure up a good atmosphere at the drop of a hat. It is very helpful to have a midwife-in-training in the background to take care of such matters while the midwife and the father attend to the birthing mother. There are even children who don't even wait around until the parents have driven to the birth centre, but decide they'd rather be born right there at home, when the midwife – having perhaps been intuitively summoned by the parents to pay a call – correctly judges the situation and considers the drive too time-consuming.

Another important function of the group sessions is to provide a forum for the fathers to voice their fears and worries about these matters, for example: "What if I don't get home in time?" "What if the baby is born in the car?" "What if I run out of petrol?" "What if there's a storm or a whole lot of snow?" Etcetera. For me it is very helpful to experience the men communicating to one another, because naturally my perspective on the birth of a child is different from that of a father.

Home Assessment

Of course it's not always possible for expectant parents to participate in these information sessions, in which case we talk about everything at the parents' home within the framework of a house call. These house calls are extremely important for the midwife and the parents alike. They create a basis of trust, and any preparatory measures which are still unclear can be discussed all the better at the "scene of the action". When the time comes for the birth to happen, the midwife already knows exactly where the parents live and will be waiting for her. It increases her confidence to know the way, and be able to assess dangerous curves and slippery spots or difficult inclines in the wintertime. In the case of well-travelled routes, she can find out from the parents about alternative routes and which roads are safer and faster. Here in the Allgaeu, the fathers are relieved when they see that the midwife drives a car that is equipped for snowy conditions. How many times have I been told: "Thank goodness you have a good car. I thought I might have to come and fetch you with the tractor, the way my father did when I was born."

Preparation List for the Home Birth

Together, when they meet at home or at one of the information evenings, the parents and midwife go through the preparation list for the home birth. For this purpose I have drawn up a checklist. Other midwives are sure to have other wishes or suggestions for the parents. So with regard to the following list, I can only speak for myself.

My intention in including it here is to give home birth parents information and midwives embarking on home obstetrics a collection of ideas and reminders. The nice thing about our profession is the individuality it allows – and that applies as much to us midwives as it does to the expectant parents who decide in favour of home birth.

My pointers on preparing for a prospective home birth are as follows:
- write out a list of important telephone numbers, including that of the emergency medical service, the hospital, the attending physician (in the practice and at home), the paediatrician you are planning to consult

In the birthing room
- an easily accessible bed with a pillow, a light blanket, possibly some cushions or an (adjustable) head support
- enough space in front of the bed to allow for a birthing stool
- a stable chair with a cushion at the back as a support for the father if the birth is to be carried out on a birthing stool
- a table or other surface to put things on (can be the changing table)
- an additional source of heat (radiator, fan heater, etc.) in order to maintain an ideal room temperature (approx. 25 °C/77 °F)
- a floor lamp, clip-on lamp or a good torch/flashlight
- a clock or watch which keeps precise time for recording the time of birth
- possibly an aroma lamp with essential oils appropriate for the birth situation and a candle to create a pleasant atmosphere

At the changing table
- a heat lamp or other good source of heat (see above)
- everything you will need for the baby, including a cap, a cloth to wrap the baby in and a swaddling band, a wool blanket, baby bathtub, soap, baby comb, towel and washcloth
- good-quality baby oil consisting of cold-pressed plant oil (almond, jojoba, olive oil)
- a baby bottle and slow-flow bottle teat (nipple), fennel or cornsilk tea and dextrose

Keep on hand for the delivery
- the medical records of the pregnancy – whatever equivalent you have to the "Mutterpass" booklet described on p. ■
- a hospital suitcase with a suit of clothes for the baby and one for the mother – enough for a one-day stay in the hospital
- nappy/diaper inserts
- a soft covering for the floor in front of the bed to protect the knees when kneeling and for warmth in cases of hard, cold floors (e.g. camping mat, sleeping bag, old mattress protector)

- two sheets of waterproof material (plastic tarp or oilskin tablecloth) – one for the bed and one for the floor in front of the bed (dimensions approx. 1.5 m × 1.5 m)
- one or two bed sheets (on top of the sheets of waterproof material)
- four to five medium-sized (soft) towels, ideally in shades of red, pink, etc.
- 1–2 large wastebaskets or refuse bags in order to separate paper and residual waste
- a bucket, large plastic bowl or plastic bag for the placenta
- 1–2 hot-water bottles
- a sickle-shaped cushion filled with spelt or styrofoam pellets (a cushion especially designed to provide support to pregnant women, women in labour and during breastfeeding) or other large cushion
- a teapot warmer and a bowl in which cotton or tissue paper can be kept damp and warm to prevent the perineum from tearing
- a small bowl for the *Dammmassageöl/Perineum Massage Oil* $\mathcal{D}$®
- a thermos bottle containing extremely strong, hot coffee, also for the protection of the perineum (let the midwife decide whether and when to use it) and a somewhat larger bowl to pour the coffee into later in order to dip a piece of cotton, a nappy or a washcloth into it and apply it to the perineum

In the bathroom:
- approx. 1 kg of salt, if the woman in labour likes to take baths – Salt makes the water buoyant, stabilizes the circulation and serves as an emulsifier for essential oils
- for the midwife: hand brush, towel, dishtowel

Deposit in a visible and easily accessible spot in the freezer:
- ice cubes and cold packs
- arnica ice cubes and calendula ice cubes (made of 125 ml water and 1 tsp of the respective herbal extract)

For the postnatal period:
- the usual postnatal period garments (nightgowns, large panties)
- fever thermometer
- a means of taking a sitz bath (large plastic bowl, bidet insert)
- sitting ring in case the perineum is badly torn
- wheat germ, linseed or other means of maintaining regular bowel movements
- plenty of milk curds (quark) in the refrigerator for when the milk "comes in"

There's always a lot to explain and discuss in connection with this preparation list. As I already mentioned, other midwives will have other habits. So a list like the one above can never replace a talk with the midwife in attendance. A meeting is really the only suitable opportunity for explaining why you need the baby comb, the teapot warmer, the coffee, the placenta bucket, the ice cubes, etc.

In view of all these items and bits and pieces of information on the previous pages, you will surely have noticed that a home birth has to be well considered and requires careful preparation. You will understand that it is accordingly necessary to make contact with the midwife as early on as possible, to allow plenty of time for these discussion and preparation appointments. In addition to these preliminary measures, regular contact must naturally also be maintained with regard to the child and how the pregnancy is going. Up until the very last minute, the plans for a home birth can be thwarted due to some risk that arises (or on account of fear or a negative premonition) – and the trip to the hospital can become necessary after all.

Early Discharge from the Hospital

Parents often come for consultation and explain that they actually would like to experience a home birth but have several concerns in that connection, which they would like to discuss with the midwife. In these cases, the best solution often proves to be planning for early discharge. Naturally, many parents come for advice on this compromise solution to begin with, already having decided that it is the best alternative for their needs. Incidentally, in several European countries it is par for the course for parents to go home with their newborns within twenty-four hours of the delivery. In Germany, the possibility of introducing this system is discussed again and again by the powers that be.

For the parents, an out-patient birth means: the child is born in the hospital, the mother leaves the hospital with her newborn within twenty-four hours and spends the postnatal phase at home, where she is attended to by a midwife within the framework of regular house calls.

The reasons for parents to decide in favour of this option are usually the same as those for home birth: on the one hand the mothers don't want to leave their babies to be cared for by the hospital staff following the birth, to say nothing of being separated from them spatially. (Unfortunately there are still maternity wards in which the mothers cannot have their babies with them around the clock.) On the other hand, women are very well informed about what it can mean for a child to be separated from its mother. Such an intimate, forty-week-long bond should not be severed so abruptly. Separation causes both the mother and the newborn pain. A lot of research has been done into the long-term consequences of such separation. Even Sigmund Freud already talked about the postnatal bonding between mother and child and about the emotional traumas of persons who were separated. A mother's heart "bleeds for her child" – I didn't really understand this expression until I became a mother myself: she undergoes genuine pain. Again and again, it has been obvious to me that newborns who are integrated into the family from the first day on are much calmer and well-adjusted. Naturally, there are also the exceptions that prove the rule.

Fathers complain that it's horrible for them to have to drive home alone after the birth, and leave the mother and child behind in the hospital. Both parents have a longing for intimacy and a lot to tell each other, or want to rest from the strains of labour together. But the everyday hospital routine does not allow for such intimacy. The Dad has to drive home, the mum stays behind, the baby is taken to the baby room. Expectant fathers not only want to be involved in the pregnancy, and participate actively in labour, they also want to be the child's father from the very beginning ...

... one man related how, after the birth of his first child in the hospital, he felt like the odd one out. The mother was surrounded by other visitors, the baby either sleeping in its bassinette or in the arms of one of the visitors. His job was to have a pad of paper and pen ready to write down everything he should get for tomorrow or the next day or for when the mother and child came home. Instead of spending a happy hour with his newborn son, he was on the road to run some errands, rushing home to take care of the household, water the plants, have a bite to eat at his mother's house. When he came back in the evening to visit his wife and child, he had to wait for ages in the corridor because the doctor was busy doing something in the room, and then he had to leave again right away because the "new arrival" in the neighbouring bed wasn't feeling well.

I hear hordes of stories like this one. The present-day father doesn't want to wait several days to have contact with his child, he wants contact from the very beginning. During a consultation, Werner told me with a laugh: "You know, I'm going to make sure that doesn't happen to me again, that my wife comes home on the sixth day and already has a huge head-start as regards coping with the baby. It was so frustrating to be told constantly, 'Sweetheart, I learned to do that differently, look, this is how I've been doing it the past few days ...!'"

Another reason for an early discharge is the presence of an older sister or brother in the family. The parents want the two children to be together from the beginning and to avoid confronting their older child with "Mummy's not home now because of the baby." Parents want to prevent feelings of jealousy to the extent possible, and be a "real family" as soon as they can. I do, however, urge parents to prepare the older child for the eventuality that the mum might have to stay in the hospital for a day or two.

In spite of our well-equipped obstetrics wards and our medical knowledge, it can and does happen that there are problems during labour and cause for concern. Neither an unproblematic pregnancy, good and careful preparation for childbirth, a healthy and natural attitude towards labour, friendly, personal care or family-oriented facilities in the delivery room can guarantee that the birth will go smoothly. Despite all the means of monitoring offered by our highly technologized world, childbirth can – in rare cases – represent a danger for the mother and the child. Moreover, it is never possible to predict how the mother and baby will fare in the first few hours following delivery.

Parents should accordingly never promise their "big" kids that they will be able to greet the baby as soon as it has been born. Explain to your child over and over again that it will have to be patient – maybe even more patient than when it's waiting for St. Nick – until the baby comes home. Remember that children don't forget promises as quickly as adults do.

Preliminary Information Meeting with the Parents

Naturally, both the parents and the midwives require certain information in advance of an early discharge from the hospital. The expectant parents almost always bring a list of questions with them to their consultation with the midwife. Together, on the basis of that list and the information list the midwife has drawn up, they talk about everything important. One of the most fundamental matters is the due date. In the period around that date, the parents should be able to reach the midwife – in other words, she should not have any holidays or absences planned during that phase. If she does, the parents should know who will be substituting for her.

The presence of the father at these meetings is absolutely essential, because his behaviour later on in the hospital will be decisive. If the new father makes the impression of being worried, afraid or overwhelmed with the situation, the midwives and doctors at the hospital will have to recommend to the parents that the mother and child be admitted and stay on as in-patients. Naturally, the hospital personnel can only assume that his lack of confidence will continue at home and therefore the mother and baby are in better hands in the hospital ward. For this reason, the father should be involved in the preliminary meetings so that he knows how to prepare for an early discharge from the hospital.

In the hospital it is initially advisable to be cautious with the question as to leaving and going home. There are still many hospitals which advise against an early discharge. If you actually do encounter a doctor or midwife who thinks that going home so soon is essentially negligent or dangerous, then they are purely and simply inexperienced. We self-employed midwives attend to a constantly rising number of parents who want to spend the early postnatal period at home, and I myself have never once encountered any problems in this context. Never once has a mother or a newborn had to be taken back to the hospital within the early postnatal period. I should add, however, that the often-cited dangers are avoided for the very reason that the expectant parents have informed themselves during the pregnancy and arranged for daily house calls by a midwife as well as for a doctor who would be willing to come as well if necessary. When the father immediately makes the impression on the maternity unit personnel that everything is well prepared and well arranged, they nearly always consent to letting the parents leave the hospital a few hours after delivery.

Midwives can also provide information on the practices common at the local hospitals. Particularly if this is not the case, however, I would advise all parents to take advantage of the information events offered by the hospitals in their area in order to obtain the relevant information.

Conditions for/Thoughts about Going Home

At the consultations, midwives inform the parents as to the conditions under which early discharge from the hospital is possible. Naturally, the labour has to have been normal, and the baby has to be healthy and "mature" (as opposed to any degree of prematurity). In general, the parents can assume that there is nothing standing in the way of going home if the mother would otherwise now be admitted to the postnatal ward and the baby to the newborn nursery or "baby room". From this point in time onward, the child is no longer under the midwife's constant control, and the mother likewise doesn't require continual surveillance. All examinations have been concluded, now there is time to rest and recover. At this point in time, the parents can safely take responsibility for the situation, because at a maternity ward the doctor and the nurse do not stand in readiness outside the door of the patient's room, but have to be called with a bell or buzzer if there is a problem. And in some cases, it can take ages for them to come. Even in a case of emergency, quite a bit of time elapses in a postnatal ward until medical help is provided. The same applies to the newborns. The baby room nurses always have several babies to attend to at once, are on their way back and forth to the mothers' rooms while a newborn baby is back in the nursery, unattended. At home, however, the new parents won't take their eyes off their baby at all during the first few days. At night, most newborns sleep in their parents' arms, or at least in a bassinette next to the parents' bed, whereas in the hospital, the night nurse has to feed and change several babies at once and take them to their mothers. Of course she has quite a lot of routine, but parents usually have a very intimate connection with their child and a sure instinct for its needs. What is more, almost all women are a bit wound up and wide awake the first night after delivery. The reason for this is the increased secretion of endorphin brought about by labour. This hormone can be described as the body's natural pain reliever. Our bodies thus have a wonderful solution for the protection of the newborn, helping the mother to be alert to and heedful of her baby's needs right away. This hormone function lasts several days, only decreasing on the third day of the postnatal period, when the child is usually well provided-for with milk and has overcome its initial adjustment problems.

Shortly after Delivery: The Situation in the Hospital

As a way of determining whether everything is normal and the family can set out for home, I advise the father to ask repeatedly whether everything is really alright with his wife and the newborn. This is because the hospital personnel will always respond to worried-sounding questions on the part of the father in a manner that corresponds to the actual situation. For example, he could ask: "Is this bleeding really normal?" If he asks, "What do you think – we'd like to go home now", the doctor is likely to enumerate a number of possible risks, but entirely omit to assess the momentary condition of the newly delivered mother. Relatively few hospitals are against an early discharge anymore these days. But unfortunately, statistics – the degree to which their rooms are used to capacity and the financial losses for the hospital if they aren't – also play an important role in their decision. So simply ask very directly about the mother's and child's momentary condition. "Is everything really alright with my child and my wife?" In the great majority of cases, the answer will be "Believe me, they're both fine. We'll be taking them to the maternity ward in just a little while." Then you can answer: "OK, we're going home now." I know that some of my colleagues are of the opinion that parents should tell the midwife on duty about their intention to leave the hospital soon after the birth right from the start. But as I mentioned above, there are various attitudes on this issue, at least here in Germany. The best is for you to ask your own midwife about details during a preliminary meeting.

But to return to the hospital situation, when it has been confirmed to the father that everything is alright, he can drive home with the newborn and the new mother, even if he has not announced it in advance. Naturally, he will first make contact to the midwife entrusted with the postnatal care to be sure that she can come for a call the same day. In many hospitals this is the only – surely well-meaning – condition for allowing the parents to leave. The hospital personnel is thus reassured that the necessary medical care of the mother and child by a midwife is guaranteed.

If a woman has had an episiotomy – a surgical incision of the perineum during childbirth to facilitate delivery –, she will have to decide for herself whether or not to go home. When I am asked, "Does an episiotomy prevent an early discharge?" my answer is: "Every woman has to endure the pain, no matter where she is, and get herself in and out of a sitz bath on her own. Perhaps her wound will be attended to more individually at home, but it must heal on its own, whether she is at home or at hospital. Neither the doctor's rounds in the hospital nor the midwife's house calls can work wonders."

Back Home: The Father as "Childbed" Manager

Once you are back home, the father will be the one to care and provide for the woman and the newborn infant. He is the chief contact person for the midwife, the doctor, the concerned or caring grandmother, the visitor, the neighbours. The woman in the postnatal phase will communicate all of her joy, her fears, worries and maternal feelings to her partner first. For the man, this means: he is the father from the first moment of the child's life. This is a wonderful challenge for every man, the consequences of which should not be underestimated.

Ewald, who attended to his wife during the postnatal period at home, referred to himself as the "childbed manager" – a fitting designation, if there ever was one.

The fathers always attach great importance to changing their children's nappies themselves so that the mother can stay in bed. Often this is absolutely necessary, because circulation problems can make it hard for the new mother to stand. And due to the pressure it is subjected to, a perineal wound always hurts more when the woman is standing than when she is lying down.

Most fathers do everything they can to anticipate their wife's every need and desire, simply to be with her and process the experience of the birth jointly. During the first few days, the new parents want to change and breastfeed the baby, feed it tea and put it down to sleep together. The father almost always wants to be present when the midwife comes to call, so as not to forget any questions, not miss any information, not overlook any of the professional manoeuvres the midwife uses in handling the child. The presence of the midwife is an important daily question-and-answer session for the parents.

During the postnatal period, it is moreover the job of the father to manage the household – do the shopping, cooking, cleaning and laundry, in addition to directing the flow of visitors or sometimes even turn visitors away, take care of the bigger children or at least take them to Grandma or a friend and fetch them again later; watch out for the mailman and the vegetable man, take care of official matters, since the child has to be registered with the civil registry office, the health insurance scheme and the employment office, and the application for the child benefit allowance has to be filled out.

I have often been asked by fathers why there isn't a single, central birth registration institute. I usually respond: "Those are the father's labour pains: to have to sit outside municipal offices and not know how long he's going to have to wait."

Questions for Thought: Planning the Postnatal Period at Home

As is obvious from my various observations above about the postnatal period, it is important to plan this phase well if you want to spend it at home. In this context, ask yourself the following questions:

- Who will run the household?
- Who will take care of the older children?
- Does the father or the person entrusted with that responsibility have experience with children?
- How did you organize the postnatal period after the births of your other children?
- Is your doctor prepared to pay a house call if it should prove necessary?
- Do you know what paediatrician will be attending to the baby? Is this person prepared to make a house call to carry out the routine examinations necessary during the first ten days?
- Is it clear to you that you will be solely responsible for your child for at least twenty-three hours a day, that you will have to decide on your own: is it hungry, does it need to be changed, can it sleep, should we wake it?
- And are you aware that so-called infant jaundice can develop to the point where the child has to be admitted to the hospital?

These questions will also be discussed with the home birth and independent birthing centre parents. Parents almost always remark: "Why do you think we want to spend the postnatal period at home? For that very reason: so we can decide for ourselves when it has to be fed, so we can allow the child to find its own rhythm. What we want, purely and simply, is to be responsible for our child from the first minute on."

A Midwife's Experiences with the Postnatal Period in the Home

During my first years of self-employment as a midwife, I was often amazed at the degree of self-confidence and conviction possessed by parents who had decided in favour of early discharge from the hospital. It was they who contributed decisively to my breaking out of my hospital routine and overcoming the excessive anxiety that went along with it.

I will always remember the postnatal period of one of the first "early-discharge mothers" I had the good fortune to care for:

… Mrs. R. was expecting her third child and asked me if I would look after her in the capacity of mid-wife. When I paid my first preliminary house call, I realized that hers was a family of doctors. The paediatrician, whom I knew well, was the grandfather of the expected baby. I felt quite queasy, but Mrs. F. made a self-assured impression and told me about her negative experiences with her first birth in a hospital. She never wanted to go through anything like that again. It was just awful the way they handle newborns in the hospital, she said, and she was certainly going to come home as soon as pos-sible after childbirth this time. If she already couldn't give birth at home, with two "medicine men" in the family, then at least she wanted to go home immediately afterward. I could understand her point of view very well and confirm that it was certainly unpleasant for a newborn to be awakened during its sleeping phase and left alone in the infants' nursery during what was perhaps its most active phase, separated from the mother. When I expressed my concern about infant jaundice and the stress of spending the postnatal period at home, the father – who had just joined us – answered: "Little do you know! When my wife gets something into her head, she goes through with it. Our Grandpa will carry out the necessary examinations with regard to infant jaundice." Soon Mrs. F. had her baby, a girl, and went home with it two hours after childbirth, against the objections of the doctors – back then (1984) it was often still inconceivable to get up from the maternity bed and go home. When I arrived a few hours later for my first house call, the new mother lay in a room she had prepared specifically for this purpose, held her daughter in her arms, beamed at me and said: "I think the hospital staff are glad I went home because after refusing to let them open the amniotic sac we also didn't allow them to attach an electrode to our baby's head and I already had a reputation as an obstreperous mother. They're probably happy not to have to put up with me in the ward." The first day of the postnatal period went smoothly and I looked forward to visiting the two nice "ladies" again the next day. But then came the big scare: on day two, little Lisa was already as yellow as a quince. The levels were in the danger zone, and I therefore agreed with the mother that the baby should be exposed to sunlight. So now little Lisa was allowed to lie in the children's room in the sun which, fortunately, was shining. I was a bit shaken by this jaundice, but the mother, father and grandfather all consoled me (things have changed since

then: now I'm the one who consoles the parents). Her condition gradually improved and Lisa developed an increasing appetite and we thought everything was alright. But we were wrong! Lisa had contracted an eye infection. Mrs. F. asked me: "Do you know of any herbal remedy? My father-in-law always prescribes antibiotic eye drops immediately. He knows I have a different opinion on these matters, but you know how that is." I gave the newborn eyebright drops and advised the mother to repeat the procedure frequently. Two days later, our problems increased when Mrs. F. developed retention of the lochia – retention of the vaginal discharge following childbirth. We analyzed the situation together and came to the conclusion that her condition was surely psychosomatic: first the excitement about the jaundice, then with the baby's eyes, and now Grandpa was planning to vaccinate her the following day. And on the previous evening she had reached the typical postnatal-period low, when mothers often spend the day crying, and now she had decided to stay in bed for at least another few days. We came to the realization that a lot had accumulated – not just the vaginal discharge. By means of massage, gymnastics, rest and a hot-water bottle on the tummy, the discharge began to flow again that evening. In the end, everything was fine, and on the tenth day I visited Mrs. F. for the last time. I had learned quite a lot just caring for this one mother and child: that doctors are only human, that the dangers of jaundice are only half as great as my fears made them out to be, that with herbs, time and attention, many a postnatal problem can be overcome wonderfully at home.

Quite a while later, I think it was two years, I was once again called upon to attend to Mrs. F. during the postnatal period. In the meantime I had gained quite a bit more experience and had our own third child. My talks with this woman – herself a psychologist – during her postnatal phase gave me a great number of valuable insights for my further career. I will always remember her as a true friend.

In this book I would once again like to thank all mothers who have helped me with their convictions and openness during the period of my attendance – helped me to gain experience and develop understanding for other mothers in the course of my career. Nobody can learn from a textbook how to work with women during the postnatal period, but only by communicating with mothers. And I am entirely convinced that the women who went home shortly after birth many years ago contributed not only to my having reached the level of knowledge I possess today, but also to the following conviction: there is nothing nicer than spending the postnatal phase at home, surrounded by the family. In the course of those years, I learned that the critical and worrisome situations described in the textbooks can usually be dealt with very well at home and without medicine.

It is not my intention to try to convince parents dogmatically to have their babies on an early-discharge basis, for this is a decision every couple has to make on their own. But it would be dishonest of me to report on my experiences with the postnatal period in a negative way, because to this very day I have never had a single unpleasant experience. Below I will describe the postnatal period from all angles, I will tell you about the stressful and worrisome aspects as well as the lovely hours with the newborn at home in your own bed. The feeling of holding your child in your arms right there where it was perhaps conceived some forty weeks earlier in the parents' embrace is simply indescribable; parents have to experience it for themselves.

THE LAST SIX WEEKS – PREPARATIONS FOR CHILDBIRTH

When a woman has reached the thirty-fourth week of pregnancy, she can breathe a sigh of relief. The critical weeks in which labour would have been premature are over and she enters the final spurt: the child has developed to a point of near maturity, is still growing and putting on a bit of fat. It should gradually betake itself into the head-down position. It is now, at the latest, that most breech babies decide to do a somersault.

Employed women enjoy their maternity leave and make final preparations. Mothers who already have children at home should gradually begin to clear out the bassinette and make it serviceable for its original purpose again. It's time to wash the baby clothes and stow them in the changing table along with a sufficient number of nappies.

I advise pregnant women to make it a habit of cooking double portions in the last weeks of pregnancy so they can freeze half. In the weeks following childbirth, when the father isn't doing the cooking anymore and the Grandma has left for home again, you will be glad to have these reserves in the freezer. A pleasant and practical form of security, because it will be a long time before you can lead your housewife's and your mother's existence to equal degrees.

A major housecleaning is almost always on the agenda several weeks before childbirth. In the months after the birth, you won't have time. In this period, many fathers report: "My wife is starting to clean, cook in advance and get rid of things, she's 'building her nest'. Looks like I'll be a father again soon." There is undoubtedly a great amount of truth in the claim that cleaning and preparations for childbirth are closely related. Many women are familiar with the same phenomenon a few days before they begin menstruating. During pregnancy, the same urge is felt, but several weeks earlier instead of only several days. Symbolically, there are many similarities between bleeding, birthing and cleaning: the uterus discharges the unneeded mucous membranes and begins to generate new ones. So why not make a clean sweep in the home as well?

Many women experience the culmination of their urge to tidy and clean shortly before childbirth. I would like to advise all mothers and fathers to take a "spell" of this kind seriously and be prepared when the first signs of labour set in within twenty-four hours.

Moodiness and Pulsatilla

During the last few weeks of pregnancy, many women say they experience great fluctuations of mood, but often only when asked specifically if this is the case. Almost all women are familiar with the problem, but are somewhat shy about admitting it. Many pregnant women still think they have to play the role of the blissful mother-to-be. In my opinion, this topic should always be brought up during the antenatal class. When it is, a sheepish look makes the rounds and it is apparent that the women find it a difficult subject to talk about. But when the midwife tells them about any number of comparable cases, the expectant mothers are very quick to confess that they are all too familiar with this moodiness: the ecstasy at the thought of the baby, the despair brought on by the fear of becoming a mother!

Hormonally influenced fluctuations of mood also frequently occur before a woman begins menstruating. Then the people around her know: aha, she's about to have her period. At the end of pregnancy this translates as "Oh, well, you know, she's pregnant." During pregnancy, partners are usually understanding about this side effect. But sometimes the fathers do say things like: "I no longer have the slightest idea what to say. If I say I'd rather stay home and not go bowling she accuses me of not letting her out of my sight. But if I do go out, she says I don't pay her enough attention. And either way, she's miserable. I'd like to see the guy who can get it just right!"

One thing is certain: shortly before the process of childbirth gets under way, a woman feels like, no matter what she does, she can't escape the impending labour. She feels vulnerable and, often, misunderstood. The older children experience Mummy as being irritable and moody. The mothers themselves suffer greatly from this state. They say that they experience huge fluctuations in their basic mood. When they wake up, they look forward to the new baby, later on in the morning their eyes suddenly fill with tears when they discover the hospital suitcase while vacuum cleaning. Around noon the whole world seems bright and sunny, and in the evening when her husband gets home, one critical word is enough to get her tears running again.

It is the female hormones which are the cause of all these ills, because shortly before labour there is a strong increase in the pregnancy hormones. But knowing this doesn't help much. When women consult a midwife about this condition, they usually ask: "Tell me, is it normal that I'm sometimes so temperamental? Is there anything you can recommend to me?" With an understanding smile, I respond: "I certainly can: Pulsatilla!" This homoeopathic medication is one of the most suitable remedies for this problem. Also called pasqueflower, it is known to counteract precisely this kind of fluctuation in hormone-related situations. What is more, it is the homoeopathic remedy most frequently employed during pregnancy. Following the administration of a high potency (see p. 441), or of a lower potency over several days, you will find that your can cope with yourself and your situation again. You'll find your inner balance and be able to face birth with confidence. Many therapists advise every pregnant woman to take Pulsatilla four weeks before the due date. I must advise against this, however, because homoeopathy is an individual form of treatment and should always be prescribed according to individual need. After all, there are also pregnant women who are quite even-tempered and stable. A large proportion of pregnant women develop the Pulsatilla symptoms, but not all of them.

Consult a midwife who has experience in homoeopathy as to whether or not you should take Pulsatilla. You will find more information on the so-called "pharmaco-logical picture" of Pulsatilla on page 171 f.

"Very Pregnant"

In this advanced stage of pregnancy, in addition to all the cleaning and preparations, the woman needs and seeks rest. She likes to take a break in the rocking chair and commune with the child inside her. Because an intimate friendship has developed between the mother and the baby, they have become a unified whole. A pregnant woman often knows exactly when the unborn infant has its waking and sleeping phases. Outsiders often have the impression that the two of them know each other well; they talk to and are considerate of one another.

The expectant mother becomes increasingly aware of the fact that these weeks of twosomeness may be coming to an end very soon. Pregnancy is literally at its peak; a circumstance felt clearly by the mother, and seen clearly by everyone else. The child reaches all the way up to her ribcage, the belly is high and protrudes more and more. The woman's posture is upright, her upper body held high. The baby is taking up her entire middle, as is clearly reflected in the mother's posture and the form of her belly.

The Expectant Father/The Partner Relationship

It is also very obvious to the father that his wife will be having the baby very soon. During this phase, pregnant women often say: "My husband has started reacting to my slightest move or remark. He's constantly asking me if everything is OK, and how I'm feeling."

This attentiveness contributes to an intensification of the partner relationship. During the final six weeks, the fathers like to come along to the midwife's practice, to the antenatal check-ups; they ask what labour and the postnatal period will be like. The closer the due date, the more important it is for many men to be reachable at all times and in constant contact with their wives. It is touching to see how affectionate and gentle the two partners are with one another during this period. And surely it is one of the things that helps a woman endure these often rather uncomfortable final weeks with patience. In one of my couples' courses, Dietmar told us:

... I try to put myself in her shoes: when the baby, with its sharp little heels and bony elbows moves inside my wife's tummy and she wants to lie down, and has to hoist an extra fifteen kilograms over to the other side every time she wants to turn over she. I just can't imagine it, no matter how hard I try. But what I can do is prop her up on all sides with plenty of cushions so that both of them, my wife and the baby, are as comfortable as possible.

This pampering and spoiling undoubtedly does every woman a lot of good in the final weeks of pregnancy and contributes to the intensification of intimacy in the partnership. The expectant parents learn to be close to one another and to the child, to be there for one another and respond to the needs of the respective other. In the partner relationship, the final weeks of pregnancy are nearly always a time of affection and tenderness. Sexual love will often recede into the background during this phase, but the emotional bond becomes stronger. As always in life, there are the exceptions, and there are partners who continue to feel sexual desire for one another right up until the day before the birth. But disinclination towards and abstinence from sexuality are just as common. As already mentioned in the previous chapters, it is up to each individual couple to decide on the role sexuality will play during these weeks. It is not imperative nor is it taboo. In the final days before the due date, it can happen that the prostaglandin hormone in the man's semen triggers contractions in the woman. This can only happen, however, when the female hormone system already signals a readiness for childbirth. On these days it can only be of advantage to sleep with one another as a means of inducing labour by natural means. But again, I would like to emphasize that the couple should decide this for themselves, and that both partners can have reasons for wanting to abstain from sexual love.

Going Swimming

Now and then, you still hear the old dictate: "During the final six weeks, a pregnant woman should not have sexual intercourse and should not go swimming."

There are many women who enjoy both and wouldn't want to go without a regular swim in the public swimming pool right up until the due date. I am certain that the supposed danger of infection is not greater than in connection with a vaginal examination. Pregnant women feel good in water – the backaches many of them suffer from are relieved through the exercise and the circulation is boosted. Gisela told me that she was sure the baby inside her liked it when she went swimming, because it always responded with lively pedalling movements itself.

Choosing the Independent Birthing Centre or Maternity Unit

In these final weeks before childbirth, if not before, the parents choose the birth centre or maternity hospital. As mentioned above, it can already be too late to register with a birth centre. If you know the midwives from the antenatal class or check-ups – i.e. have already developed a trusting relationship with them – but were only recently able to decide in favour of giving birth in a birthing centre, the midwives may be able to make an exception if they are not already booked up for the period in question. There still may be time to plan for giving birth at home or in an independent birth centre. Exceptions are also made when parents have to move on short notice and a midwife in the new place of residence is prepared to consider taking you on at this late stage of pregnancy. Naturally, she will want to meet with you and get to know you before making her decision.

In any case, it will put your mind at ease to know the streets, traffic lights and intersections between your home and the place of birth. Are road construction or other obstacles to be expected? It certainly doesn't hurt to look for alternative routes. Another thing you can do is time the drive: for the woman in labour it can be extremely reassuring to hear: "Just ten more minutes; we're already halfway there." Are there plenty of parking spaces near the hospital, can the father drive right up to the entrance, is there perhaps a different entrance for the maternity ward? Where do the parents have to ring when they come at night? It is of great advantage if you have already acquainted yourself with the route through the building from the entrance to the maternity ward, if you know what stairs and what elevators to use and whether there are opportunities to breathe your way through a contraction, leaning on a railing or a windowsill. It is very soothing to be greeted by a hospital midwife during a preliminary visit and hear about they run things in her department. You will become familiar with the atmosphere and can discuss your personal questions with a midwife or perhaps a doctor. Many hospitals offer information sessions. In my opinion it is important that you find out as early as possible what examinations are carried out routinely in the respective maternity ward. Later, when labour is in progress, is not the time to discuss the sense and necessity of being shaven, having an enema, an infusion, a routine episiotomy, early clamping and cutting of the umbilical cord, "skin to skin" and countless other measures. Whatever questions you may have, discuss them at the maternity hospital of your choice in advance if at all possible. One of your main objectives is to bring a sense of trust along when you arrive at the hospital for labour, your contractions already in progress – a sense of trust that will last throughout labour. One reason why labour is not the time or place for discussion is that it keeps the birthing woman from relaxing and devoting herself entirely to the 'labour of labour'. It is no wonder if labour comes to a standstill on account of what seems to be mere 'trivialities'. It may sound strange, but it becomes plausible when we think about the effects of our hormones: the contraction hormone oxytocin works best when the woman is relaxed, when she is happy, because our bodies also produce this hormone during sex. But as soon as a woman's attention is diverted, the body produces adrenaline, our escape and activity hormone, which in turn reduces the labour hormone as well as the endorphin, a substance that makes you feel happy and reduces the sensation of pain. The woman therefore has to be able to concentrate entirely on the physical work of labour and simply allow the birth process to take its course, and should not have to worry about external matters. Just compare it with the act of lovemaking: when the place and atmosphere are right, two people making love are happy and feel like they're in seventh heaven. But if someone were to come into the room in the midst of it and ask if the room should be lighter or darker, the music softer or louder or tell you that you can now move to another room, or wanted to record personal data, the lovemaking would come to a screeching halt! And the same thing applies to labour: if the woman feels good, if the atmosphere is right, if she gets the attention she needs, she produces plenty of serotonin – the hormone that is released when you eat chocolate or get an affectionate abdominal massage and that brings about a sense of relaxation and happiness – and she can let go.

Information obtained in advance thus enables you to choose an obstetrics hospital that corresponds to your wishes and expectations and helps you gain a sense of trust in the staff, all of which contributes to a good atmosphere during labour. This atmosphere, in turn, is the prerequisite for a smooth birthing process.

Psychologists are becoming increasingly aware of the effect the hours of labour have on the child's life. I often witness parents going to all kinds of trouble to give their baby a pleasant nest for when it gets home. But little is undertaken to shape the hours of childbirth itself, and the responsibility for greeting the infant is simply delegated to strangers. I would like for parents to think about the fact that, for the baby, being born is probably something like arriving at a longed-for holiday destination. You'll often hear people talking about how disappointing and discouraging it was, how unkind and impersonal, the way they were greeted by the hotel staff with no accommodation of their needs. What is the good of an expensive room if the people attending to you are impersonal? For the birth of a human being, the feelings and experiences are surely a great deal more formative and inextinguishable when the first impression is a technologized, cold, loud, glaringly bright environment. During the final weeks of pregnancy, I would like to urge you to think about whether you would prefer a safety-oriented, possibly very technical environment or a maternity unit which takes natural aspects into account. Another thing you may want to think about is whether the hospitals you are considering will provide you support in breastfeeding your child. In Germany there is even a rating – "stillfreundliches Krankenhaus" (breastfeeding-friendly hospital) – for maternity hospitals. This may not be the case in your country, but if expectant parents make it a point of asking about this aspect, maybe things will begin to change to the benefit of the newborns.

However much you plan and anticipate, however, it is essential that you be flexible, because there are children who are in a great hurry to see the light of day. To be on the safe side, in addition to the maternity hospital of your choice, find out where the hospitals nearest you are located and how to get there. Be inwardly prepared for possibly having to give up your chosen hospital and maybe just being happy to reach the nearest hospital in time, according to the motto:

> *First of all, things won't always happen*
> *second of all the way parents expect but,*
> *third of all then and there where IT wants them to!*

Gerda was compelled to experience this wisdom first-hand …

… she wanted to drive to the hospital of her choice, which was many kilometres away from where she lived. She didn't trust the obstetrics methods of the local hospital. She had been so shocked by certain remarks made by a doctor during a lecture there that she was prepared to do anything conceivable not to have to give birth there. One evening she rang me up in a state of great excitement: "Inge, what should I do, I've been having contractions for hours, and we were already at the hospital, but the mid-wife there said they were just false pains. Just a minute … [I heard her trying to breathe through a contraction with a great amount of difficulty.] Now I'm afraid to drive all the way back there for noth-ing. Could you examine me?" "Of course I can. But your contractions don't sound like false labour anymore to me; don't you think it would make more sense to drive back to I. City? Unfortunately, I can't get away right at the moment; you'd have to come to my practice", I replied. "No, I'm afraid to go all the way back to I. This is the way the contractions were this morning, and like I said, the midwife there said these weren't genuine labour pains. I want you to examine me. We'll be glad to come to your practice." A short time later, the woman, her husband and their older son arrived. It was immediately obvious to me that the birthing woman was concentrating hard on trying to get through her contrac-tions, but that she was extremely tense. After I examined her I was all the more worried. The cervix still wasn't dilated to any appreciable degree, so I gave her a suitable homoeopathic remedy and tried to help her relax. When I talked to the father, he confirmed my opinion that the hospital of their choice was much too far away. It was clear to me: she was tense because she was afraid that the midwife in the hospital might be dissatisfied with what she had accomplished in the course of the day. We decided that the father would take the older boy to his grandmother's while the birthing woman remained in my care. We would see how things were going when her husband returned. In this pleasant atmosphere the woman felt more secure, she relaxed and the cervix got softer. But it was clear that she wouldn't be able to endure such strong contractions for several hours to come. So I advised the two of them to go to the local hospital and have an epidural in the hopes of soon delivering a healthy baby. At first it was extremely difficult for her to accept this sudden change of plans, because that was exactly what she didn't want – a large hospital, medication during labour. But that's the way it is with children: first of all not, second of all the way mothers expect …

When Everything Happens Differently

It is very disillusioning and almost cruel for women when everything happens differ-ently at the birth of their child. For this reason, I advise all parents, particularly ex-pectant mothers: don't get bent on anything, not on a particular place of birth, not on a particular birth method, and certainly not on a certain course of events. In my ex-perience this is particularly difficult for women having their first child: to go into la-bour as openly and unprepossessed as possible. I can understand them very well, but I nevertheless advise them to take the trouble to acquaint themselves with the various possibilities. Later on, in your life with your child, you will undoubtedly often experi-ence that everything happens much differently from the way you thought they would. It's the hardest for women who were adamantly against having a caesarean section and it turns out that such an operation is ultimately the only solution for the mother and child. Again and again, we midwives observe that women are not open to information on caesareans during pregnancy; they purposely don't pay attention when this topic comes up in the course and skip the respective chapter in the book, only to voice the soft accusation later on: "I wish you had told me more about all the things a caesarean can confront you with." I have a lot of sympathy for these women, before it happens and after it happens. First of all, there is the fact that it lies in the nature of the matter that a woman should enter the phase of pregnancy and childbirth with a sense of faith and confidence, because she will constantly be encountering uncertainties, and for this reason she puts on a protective outer shell. And I can likewise understand the disappointment that comes later, because a caesarean is not so easy to accept and cope with. **I highly recommend the book by Theresia de Jong and Gabriele Kemmler *Kaiserschnitt – wie Narben an Bauch und Seele heilen können* as an aid to helping you come to terms with the experience of a caesarean in the course of time.** We midwives do make an effort to talk to the woman about the birth when we are making our postnatal house calls, but often her thoughts and feelings about it only surface much later on. This is what happened once after a lecture I gave:

… I already noticed one of the women in the audience while I was holding the lecture. She sat there, wrapped in thought, tears filling her eyes now and then. At the end she spoke up, saying: "It's good to listen to you and what you say makes a lot of sense, particularly about natural birth, but you know, when a caesarean does turn out to be necessary, the world is suddenly totally different. That's what happened to me, I just don't think it's right that you – like my midwife at the time as well – said so little about it." I made an effort to quote a few lines from my book and show her understanding. I said it was certainly justified from her point of view to doubt my words, but as I had said at the start: first of all, it doesn't happen …and I had mentioned that a birth could turn into an emergency situation, but was always a very personal and intimate experience that defied generalization.

After the lecture, a colleague came up to me and told me she was at her wit's end; she had tried so hard to help this woman and had had the impression that everything was alright during the postnatal period. And anyway she could remember only too well that in that particular antenatal class there had even been four women who had already undergone caesareans, and they had reported on their experiences often – too often, she had thought at the time – and now this woman's reaction … My fellow midwife could also remember that the woman had only been prepared to talk about an entirely normal home birth and turned a deaf ear on other information. Yes, her child showed her that you can't always plan your route in advance, and realizations of this kind truly are difficult to digest. Just like the colleague who experienced that a woman can't come to terms with a negative birth experience during the postnatal period but often takes years before she can more or less make her peace with it, and even then, certain aspects can remain unresolved.

Packing for the Hospital

One of the preparations to be carried out in the final weeks is packing a bag for the hospital. I can only advise every woman to do this as early as possible, preferably six weeks before the baby is expected. It is a very tense situation when, for example, the child suddenly announces itself three weeks before the due date and nothing has been packed. Fathers don't like rummaging around in their wives' things, and they end up bringing the wrong nightgown along. Spare yourself and your husband unnecessary tension.

When you pack, take into account that very few hospitals have huge closets, and take a travel bag with you rather than a cumbersome suitcase. These are the things you should take along:

For the *birth:*
- *A comfortable, short, favourite nightgown or men's shirt.* Many hospitals offer a white hospital nightgown for use doing labour; decide for yourself and talk to the midwife if you'd rather wear your own, simply because it's more personal. And also, it is a nice memory every time you take it out of your closet later on. If you wear a hospital nightgown you can tie it in the front so that the baby can be laid on your breast immediately after birth.
- *Well-worn slippers*, since in the final weeks your feet are often swollen. For the postnatal period, slippers with a somewhat higher heel are suitable, because they help to take the strain off the perineum in case an incision turned out to be necessary.
- Warm *socks*, because cold feet are the worst thing for labour. They keep the birthing woman from relaxing and make the labour pains all the more painful.
- A *bathrobe*, which is easy to close.
- For your partner or the person accompanying you, *comfortable clothing* (T-shirt, jogging pants, slippers).
- If you have long *hair*, a *slide (barrette)* or elastic to tie your hair back.
- A jar of *salt* mixed with *lavender oil* for the bathtub. As a bath supplement, lavender is ideal for relaxing and feeling good. Many midwives report on positive experiences with lavender baths. The women relax, the cervix softens, the labour pains become regular; even the excited father calms down. The *Original $\mathcal{D}^®$ Aroma Blends Entspannungsbad/Relaxation Bath $\mathcal{D}^®$* and *Verwöhnbad/Spoil-Yourself Bath $\mathcal{D}^®$* are excellent alternatives. Take along whatever you like best. In many hospitals, these good oils are already in stock on a regular basis – you can ask beforehand whether the aroma blends are available there or you should bring one yourself. Some hospitals may not purchase them for reasons of cost.
- *Geburtsöl/Childbirth Oil $\mathcal{D}^®$* for massages to alleviate the contractions, and *Dammmassageöl/Perineum Massage Oil $\mathcal{D}^®$* for the delivery.
- *Rose hydrolat* to refresh yourself with, since the scent of roses is most suitable for the birth process.

- Perhaps refreshing *mints or candies*, to help moisten the mucous membranes of the mouth.
- A discman or MP3 player with your favourite *relaxation music*.
- A thermos bottle full of *raspberry leaf tea*, which provides good support to the activity of labour.
- A *little something* for the father to eat, in case labour takes awhile. Many hospitals still don't allow birthing women to eat. But if you are moved to the maternity ward at night, after the delivery, you are likely to be hungry, and you won't have to wait until breakfast.
- Your *family register*, and marriage or birth certificate.
- Whatever *documents* you may need from your health insurance scheme, particularly if you are privately insured.
- The referral from your gynaecologist, if necessary.
- The *medical records of your pregnancy* (the equivalent to the German *Mutterpass*)! Tack a note to the outside of your bag with a reminder of these records, because it can be extremely maddening to leave without them and for your husband to have to rush back home to fetch them. This has often led to a father's not being present at the birth of his child – he had to rummage around too long looking for the Mutterpass, and the baby was already born by the time he returned.
- An *aroma lamp* and your favourite oil. The most suitable is *Entbindungsduft/Childbirth Aroma D®*, which is available as a ready-to-use blend, which saves you from having to buy the expensive oils individually. It consists of: benzoin Siam, grapefruit, jasmine, linaloe wood, mandarin, rose, sandalwood and ylang-ylang. But simply the scent of lavender extra can also be very pleasant. Perhaps the midwives will already have all these aromas on hand and you can choose what appeals to you most that day. But remember, an aroma you are familiar with triggers pleasant memories, which are important for relaxing. If you love *Rosengarten/Rose Garden D®*, for example, then take it along. You will find more detailed information on essential oils in the chapter on "Childbirth" as well as in my books *Aroma Therapy from Pregnancy to Breastfeeding* and *Time-Tested Aroma Blends*.

For the *postnatal period*, you should pack:
- About four comfortable nightgowns or pyjama tops which button down the front and are washable in hot water.
- Take plenty of *nightwear* along which should not be too warm, since you will sweat often in the period following childbirth, and the rooms in the hospital are moreover heated on account of the babies.
- About eight pairs of large, warm, hot-water-washable *cotton underpants*. During the first few days you will need large sanitary pads or nappy inserts for the uterine discharge, so the underpants should be large enough to accommodate them. And even if it sounds old-fashioned, it really is necessary to keep the uterus warm in order to avoid extreme afterpains.

- To be on the safe side, approx. twenty *maternity pads* to use as sanitary pads, since many hospitals only have ordinary sanitary pads on hand. During the first few days of the postnatal period, the latter absorb far too little and can also subject the perineal wound to unpleasant pressure.
- A light *bed or jogging jacket* for when your room is being aired.
- Leggings or jogging trousers in case you'd like to take a walk in the hospital. Particularly women who have given birth for the second time or more should be very careful not to be exposed to a draught in the hospital corridors, and not to get a chill, because that would only increase your afterpains. You can take a wool scarf or woollen kidney warmer along for use on the first few days following childbirth.
- Several *towels* and *washcloths*, especially a bath towel, because most women in the postnatal period like to shower twice a day. The readjustment of the hormone system causes them to sweat profusely and they constantly feel the need to freshen up.
- Your usual *toiletries* (toothbrush, toothpaste, soap, shampoo), the *Original $\mathcal{D}^®$ Aroma Blend Wochenbettbauchmassageöl/Childbed Abdominal Massage Oil $\mathcal{D}^®$* and your *cosmetics*.
- A *blow-dryer*, because freshly washed hair contributes decisively to a feeling of well-being. The legend that women in the postnatal period shouldn't wash their hair is most likely to be attributed to the fact that women used to catch colds and develop fevers when their hair was wet. And it is true that a woman who has just given birth is especially vulnerable, because her immune system is very much weakened by the birth process.
- At least two *nursing bras*, which should be two sizes too big, because the chest measurement increases considerably when the milk comes in.
- *Nursing pads* made of wool or wild silk, since these natural textiles keep your nipples from getting sore and are very absorbent, antibacterial and pleasant to wear.
- The *Original $\mathcal{D}^®$ Aroma Blend Stillöl/Nursing Oil $\mathcal{D}^®$* and *Stilltee/Nursing Tea*; here again, ask what they have in stock in the hospital.
- If you are convinced of the effects of essential oils, I would recommend that you take *Sitzbad/Sitz Bath $\mathcal{D}^®$* on a Dead Sea Salt basis with you. But ask beforehand whether the hospital has it on hand.
- Your *address book and small change*, so that you can call all of your loved ones. Remember that you are prohibited from using your cell phone in the hospital.
- A pad of paper or journal for writing down your memories of the birth and your first impressions of your child.

The "Wrong" Aromas for the Hospital Bag

I would already like to call your attention to the fact that you should be careful with *perfume* during the postnatal period. Perhaps you will wonder what this information is doing here in the chapter on "Pregnancy", but experience has taught me that it is better to think about these matters now than when you are actually in the postnatal period. Because then your hospital bag is already in use and it is your husband who will have to go shopping rather than sitting at your bedside or changing the baby's nappies.

Take care not to change the natural scent of your own body with foreign aromas, natural or synthetic. They irritate the newborn baby, whose sense of smell is already very well-developed in the first ten days of life. It is entirely natural for women to sweat a lot during childbirth: when the baby is laid on our breast, it is confronted with this individual odour immediately and is therefore capable of recognizing its own mother right away – and from then on – by the way she smells. But if you use lots of scented shower gels or perfume, your smell will remain strange to your child and it will have trouble recognizing and accepting its mother. What is more, the use of synthetic aromas – which make their way into the baby's body by way of its nose – places an unnecessary burden on the child's organism. It is not yet been determined, incidentally, what effect synthetic substances have in our bodies, and whether they are ever eliminated. A press release dating from the summer of 1994 confirmed what had already long been known in the field of aroma therapy: artificially produced essential oils are not harmless. Traces of musk oil compounds were found in a great number of breast milk samples. This oil has come to be used only as synthetic oil and is an ingredient in many perfumes and laundry detergents. With the investigations cited, experts proved that, first of all, essential oils find their way into the breast milk and, second of all, they really do remain in the human body. What is more, synthetic musk oil is suspected of containing chemical compounds which represent a health hazard.

It makes me very happy to know that babies possess a means of protecting themselves from such synthetic aromas. When I worked in the hospital, I regularly witnessed newborns refusing the breast when their mothers were lying in bed freshly perfumed – the same babies who had drunk with relish early that very morning. In the morning, the mothers are often awakened to nurse their babies and haven't had a shower yet – they just smell like mum.

So when you pack, please consider carefully what cosmetics you really want to take along. And when you are shopping and making preparations for the baby you should also take this matter into account. Please do not use any fabric softeners for laundering the baby clothing, because they also contain synthetic aromas, which often cause irritations of the skin in newborns. In many families, the birth of a child leads to the parents finally making more conscious decisions regarding the purchase and use of laundry products. The other members of the family will often complain at first about the roughness of the freshly washed laundry when you stop using fabric softeners, but within a very short time even the adults will notice that their pimples and impurities of the skin have disappeared. If the baby's things are too rough, it helps to add a few drops of lavender oil to the last rinse cycle or/and a cup of vinegar, or have recourse to the old-fashioned method: the iron.

Preparations for the Drive Home

The following *clothing for the baby and yourself for the drive home* should be assembled and waiting at home so that your partner can bring it to the hospital the day you are discharged. In the hospital you probably won't have enough space for it.

For the mother:
- Roomy, comfortable clothing suitable for the time of year. Remember that, even though you have given birth to the child, your abdominal girth is still much larger than it was before pregnancy. As a nursing mother, your chest measurement will also be a great deal larger than usual. Really, your maternity clothing will fit you the best, but almost all mothers are happy not to have to use it anymore, at least for the time being.
- A sitting ring which you can put on the passenger seat so that the perineal wound, if you have one, won't cause you too much pain. If you don't know where to buy one, you can fashion one yourself by rolling up a large towel or small blanket, starting at one corner, and then forming a ring with it. Or you can use your older children's swim ring – or borrow one from your neighbour's children –, but only blow it up slightly.

For the baby:
- A baby carry-bag, which you should by all means line with a sheepskin, has proven an excellent means of transport. According to traffic regulations, it has to be strapped onto the back seat of the car with a seatbelt. Actually, I should probably recommend a baby car seat to you at this point, but have a hard time reconciling these seats with my midwife's conscience, since many models do not provide enough warmth or protect the child from draughts. If you do use such a seat, make all the more sure that your baby is well-covered.
- A hot-water bottle or warm cherry stone cushion, which should be placed in the carry-bag – despite the sheepskin lining – in the winter or colder months of the year. Incidentally, a thick wool cushion fulfils the same purpose.
- A set of baby clothing including a jacket, shirt and bodysuit, preferably in two sizes, since you can't possibly know how large your child will be at birth.
- A cap, a woollen jacket and knitted wool or cotton booties.
- A wool or cotton blanket which can be tucked in underneath the carry-bag cushion.

- If you have decided in favour of cloth nappies, take one or two of them with you. Don't forget to take a pair of nappy pants along. No matter what you might hear, newborns can be nappied in cloth despite the remainder of the umbilical cord. It saddens me when health-care professionals tell mothers that they shouldn't use cloth nappies before the stump of the umbilical cord has fallen off and the navel has healed. In those cases I ask myself how people could possibly have survived before the invention of disposable nappies. Don't allow yourself to be talked out of the best nappy type – the cloth nappy – before you have even left the hospital.
- You don't need anything for the care of the umbilical cord. Before you leave the hospital, the navel will be attended to by a baby nurse, and at home this care will be taken over by the midwife in attendance, who will place the necessary utensils at your disposal. The costs are generally covered by the health insurance scheme.
- Assemble all of the clothing and accessories for the drive home in one place or, even better, pack them in a small travel bag so that your partner doesn't leave half of it at home in all the excitement.

If you are planning an early discharge after birth or the home birth has to be moved to the hospital, then of course you will have to take all of this clothing for mother and baby with you when you drive to the hospital. I recommend that you then leave them in your car. After the birth of the child, when it is clear whether you really can leave the hospital a few hours later, you'll have plenty of time to fetch everything from the car. In these cases it has proven very helpful to have a wool blanket in the car so that the new Mum doesn't freeze. A second hot-water bottle is also a very pleasant thing to have.

Birthing outside the Hospital

Final Preparatory Meetings/The Possible Transfer to the Hospital

When the midwife visits the parents who are planning childbirth at home or at an independent birth centre, her chief concern in the last weeks of pregnancy is to discuss the final preparations. She talks to the parents about the eventuality that the birthing woman may have to be moved to the hospital in the middle of labour. In the lines below, I will make repeated reference to the failure of home births and births in independent birthing centres, which might give my readers the impression that it is a frequent occurrence. But before I start, I would like to reassure all parents: in Germany, extra-clinical obstetrics record a hospital admission rate of 10 percent, and within that percentage, the proportion of cases in home obstetrics is lower than in independent birth centres. Even if this is an encouragingly low number, it is nevertheless important to talk about this situation in all detail in order to avoid any unnecessary problems if an emergency really does arise.

It is important to think about what hospital is nearest you and offers the best facilities for an emergency birth situation. The parents have almost always informed themselves in advance and know what measures are taken on a routine basis. The birthing woman and expectant father usually cope well when what began as a home or independent-birth-centre birth suddenly becomes a hospital birth. They are just as happy as the midwife is that, in an emergency, there are possibilities such as block anaesthesia, ventouse deliveries or, in acute cases, caesarean sections. We all know that a caesarean is sometimes the only means for the baby and the mother to get through the birth healthy and alive. For the "labour support team", what this means is that the natural birth has turned into a natural event of such forcefulness that it will only end well under the protection of medicine.

The move to a hospital in the midst of labour is often just as difficult for the midwife as it is for the parents, and unfortunately we are not always greeted in the friendliest of manners. The number of critics is decreasing gradually as far as I can tell, but there are still fellow midwives and doctors who refer to us professionals working in home birth and birthing centre settings as "potential murderers". This is very unfortunate for all of us, since I am sure that home birth parents are particularly well informed as to the responsibility they are taking upon themselves, the risks and the consequences for mother and child. The kinds of people who consider giving birth at home are very aware of the fact that children can be born with handicaps. It is par for the course for everyone involved to talk openly about acute and emergency situations, about disablement and death. Parents often ask me: "Inge, tell us, are parents who are planning a hospital birth also this well informed?" Midwives who attend my seminars and are interested in information on conducting home births are often surprised at how frankly we talk about possible birth-related risks. They are amazed when parents who visit the hospital tell them that they are well aware that a child can be born disabled or sick. As a matter of fact, it is for that very reason that they plan to give birth outside the hospital, so that – if worse came to worst – the child could die in their arms and not hooked up to all kinds of machines. When I began conducting home births I also found it very remarkable that parents could cope with suffering much better than I could. Many of the families I attended helped me get to the point where I am today – i.e. where I am able to talk about these subjects as a matter of course.

As far as the move to the hospital goes, I am sorry to say that those very parents who initially fought tooth and nail against even discussing the topic of a hospital birth are often the ones who are forced to experience it. Sometimes I even have the impression that their children have the task of showing their parents that giving birth in a hospital can represent a good and necessary aid when the means of home birth have been exhausted. For me personally, it would be wonderful if both sides – obstetrics in the hospital and outside of it – would communicate more and learn to accept one another. "Both are integral parts of our society and have an equal right to existence." – That sentence was uttered by a doctor who had bitterly opposed home birth until he learned from me about the in-depth preparatory meetings we carry out. In many places there really is good cooperation and the transfer to the hospital goes smoothly. I am very happy about the fact that this book has also contributed to an increase in discussions between hospitals and self-employed midwives on this subject. Even if there are still large discrepancies, I would like to encourage all of my colleagues not to grow tired of making contact from "inside to outside" and vice versa and exchange views and experiences with one another. Moreover, with their honesty and openness, parents who have experienced such a situation can also help to eliminate misconceptions and one-sided points of view.

If you are planning a home birth, it is likewise very important for the expectant mother to prepare a hospital bag with the necessary items for a possible stay at hospital. During a home birth, we have to be prepared to drive to the nearest hospital at the drop of a hat. Women who have already delivered several children at home are often amazed to hear this. But they have to be aware that there is no guarantee that the birth will be normal just because it has been so in the past. It can and does happen that women who have already given birth to one or more children have to move to the hospital in mid-labour.

One very clear memory I have of such a situation was the case of Eva's birth ...

... we, the expectant father and I, had already been supporting the birthing woman in her labour efforts for several hours. The doctor we had called confirmed my suspicion that it would be too difficult for a home birth; the child would not manage its way to the light of day without technical assistance. Our decision to drive to the hospital was firm and, as arranged, I wanted to fetch the hospital bag, but I couldn't find it. The mother hadn't prepared one. The result was unnecessary delay and tension. I could not conceal my anger about the fact that the parents had not followed my instructions. At the birth of Eva's brother, two years later, the first thing the expectant mother showed me when I arrived was the hospital bag, all packed and ready to go. Thankfully, we didn't need it that time; the mother was able to give birth at home.

One of the nicest jobs awaiting a mother after the home birth has been carried to completion at home is the unpacking of the unused hospital bag!

No Home Birth After All?

It can happen that, in the final weeks of pregnancy, parents who had been planning a home birth suddenly have a change of heart. I myself have not experienced such a change among the parents I have attended to. On the other hand, sometimes I myself have been the one who noticed that the demands of a home birth were possibly over their heads.

Sometimes I simply had an uneasy feeling, usually without any specific medical justification. In cases like this, the midwife talks to the parents again about what is means to give birth at home. A joint attempt is made to figure out what is causing this intuition on the part of the midwife; the due date, antenatal check-up results and our feelings are carefully examined once again. After talks of this kind, it often becomes clear that it would be better to prepare for birth in a hospital with early discharge. As far as home birth goes, the "game rules" say that everyone involved is allowed to change his or her mind. Whether it is the parents, the doctor or the midwife who announces misgivings or feelings of uncertainty, these should always be accepted by the others. This joint decision-making process is undoubtedly the most important basis for the good success of home births.

Fortunately, only in about ten percent of my home birth cases was it necessary to come to a joint decision of this kind – brought about when a risk became apparent shortly before the due date or after labour had started.

Antenatal Care

At the antenatal check-ups, which are now generally carried out every two weeks, the question often arises as to when the Braxton-Hicks contractions – the primary purpose of which is to help the baby to engage with the mother's pelvis – set in.

Braxton-Hicks Contractions

Since it is very difficult to explain what a pregnant woman feels in moments such as these, I would like to cite a few cases I witnessed.

I remember Andrea quite well …

… *"I only have less than four weeks left until the due date – can I expect Braxton-Hicks contractions to begin now?" I asked her whether she still had the feeling that the baby was pressing up against the bottom of her ribcage and giving her breathing trouble. A. replied, "No, actually I don't. On the contrary, I can breathe better now and there's space in my stomach for more food again. But now I have to get up at night more frequently. Tell me, Inge, does this mean the baby has already dropped?" I could only confirm this suspicion. "Well, yes, the way it looks, you've just ascertained that that's the case, and when I look at your tummy, that's the way it looks. Last week at the antenatal class it seemed to me to be much higher. You're apparently one of the type who don't feel the contractions which help the baby to 'drop' downwards or have them while they're sleeping." At this the expectant mother stopped to think and then said, "Or – wait a minute – two days ago I had a constant ache in my lower back and that evening I didn't know how I should lie, either my belly was hard or my groin ached or my back ached. Were those the Braxton-Hicks?" I told her yes, that was surely the case.*

Many women really don't feel the Braxton-Hicks contractions – the ones which cause the baby to "drop" or "lighten" – clearly as such. Particularly those who are pregnant for the first time have difficulty identifying these contractions correctly. To confuse matters even more, these contractions can express themselves in various ways. Either the pains occur throughout a day in rhythmic progression or are experienced merely as a hardening of the abdomen at brief intervals in the course of an evening. Many women say that they had strong pains in the small of the back repeatedly for several days. Another may not notice any change at all, and is surprised when the examining obstetrician or midwife tells her that the forward end of the baby has dropped snugly into her so-called pelvis minor. After all, the purpose of Braxton-Hicks contractions is to establish contact with the birth canal. There are also children who don't drop down into the pelvis until shortly before, even during labour. Midwives and obstetricians generally only observe this last-mentioned phenomenon in women who have given birth before.

Braxton-Hicks Contractions/"Lightening" Contractions in Multiparas

… Simone came to the antenatal class one Monday and wanted to talk to me briefly alone. As had been the case with her first two children, we had agreed to plan for a home birth, circumstances allowing. She was now quite worried about the fact that she had been having such strong and regular pains that weekend – at ten-minute intervals – that she had almost rung me up. "Don't be ridiculous, Simone, you can't have the baby at home this early; if this is true labour, you'll have to go to the hospital. Remember, we arranged that you can have it at home anytime after the middle of the month at the earliest, and today is only the third", was my spontaneous reaction. "Did you have any other signs of birth? Mucus discharge or bleeding?" I asked her. She shrugged her shoulders in response: "No, that's just the point, but they were real labour pains; after all, after two births I can remember what contractions feel like. And anyway, I told you that I've constantly had the feeling that this child would be born early. Inge, could you please examine me?" The examination confirmed my suspicions: Simone's cervix was not at all ready for birth; the baby's head hadn't even made contact with the pelvis. On my examination glove was a tiny bit of sticky, milky mucus. This also was not a sign of imminent birth. Simone had merely been having false labour. I explained the results of my examination and my assumption to her: "Simone, I think your uterus is practising – and trying to get across to the baby that it should gradually be making friends with the birth canal. But the baby apparently isn't interested, and is still moving freely above the entrance to the pelvis. You were having regular Braxton-Hicks contractions. These will not lead to the birth of the baby. And what's more, I can't find anything to confirm your fear or hope (?) that this baby will be born early. On the contrary, the results of the examination lead me to suspect that you'll have no trouble making the due date. Let me examine you again in a week and then maybe I can tell you more about when I think the birth will commence." One week passed, and then another, and Simone's cervix remained unchanged, although she kept having regular Braxton-Hicks contractions. In the end the child was born ten days past the due date.

I could tell you similar stories about many other multiparas (women who have already given birth one or more times in the past). The expectant mothers are often disappointed that they have misjudged the situation and been thrown off balance by these premonitory contractions. But in my opinion, they are quite useful: they serve to draw the woman's attention to the child and make clear to her that this child is entirely different from the ones she has given birth to in the past. The expectant mothers gain an awareness of the fact that they can't rely on past experience, that they have to attune themselves to this birth as if it was the first time, and to the fact that labour and delivery might take place in an entirely different manner. When we talk, the pregnant woman and I both come to the conclusion that there will never be any such thing as routine when it comes to giving birth. The worry that the child will be born prematurely actually almost always reveals itself to be a secret hope: not to have to endure the final unpleasant weeks of pregnancy at least once. Because the more children you have, the more burdensome the final weeks are. The body has to mobilize an enormous amount of strength to carry a child to the full term.

Premonitory Contractions

These contractions serve to maintain good circulation in the uterus, and the abdominal muscles tighten frequently as an aid in supporting the weight. The uterus "practices" until labour begins, and shows the child the way to the birth canal. With these exercises, the cervix is also prepared for labour. At the antenatal check-up, it is usually ascertained that "the cervix is effaced, in mid position and admits one finger". In multiparas, the cervix often opens as much as four centimetres. This is no cause for worry, because no child is born without true labour pains. So if it is your third or fourth pregnancy, don't be all too concerned if you are told this is the case. I often get calls from these mothers, who are worried that their child will be born while they are out and about, or several weeks too early. As in the case of Dorothea …

… we had arranged an appointment to talk through everything concerning the home birth again. Dorothea was expecting her third baby. The first child had been born in the hospital, right on the due date, with an early discharge home,. The second had been born at home a little less than three weeks early, but the labour had been quite a bit more difficult than the first time around. The third pregnancy had now progressed to the thirty-third week. My external examinations told me that this baby was still very small and that we could by no means plan for a home birth before the end of the thirty-eighth week of pregnancy. The mother was a bit puzzled that I was laying out such clear conditions because, in the case of the second child, the midwife in attendance hadn't been concerned when labour commenced three weeks early. But for me there was no doubt: this baby was too small and the risk too great if it was born early. For the mother it was now clear that she would have to rest a lot, because she had been having increased Braxton-Hicks contractions for weeks. She wanted to do everything in her power to be able to have the child at home. The vaginal examination confirmed my misgivings: the cervix was open 'two fingers' wide, not yet pointing in the correct direction for birth, though, but quite decidedly towards the sacrum. The baby's head was already trying to make contact with the pelvis. I explained to her that if she rested a lot lying down and regularly did the all-fours position, she could surely stick it out for several weeks yet. But nevertheless it wouldn't hurt for her partner and her to take a practice drive to the hospital and talk to a midwife there. I advised the expectant mother to try to get used to the idea that maybe everything would turn out differently from the way she had imagined. Nine days later, Dorothea rang me up in the evening and said, "I've been having strong contrac-

tions all day already. They're sill irregular, but clearly perceivable. And I also have the feeling that the baby's head is pressing downward hard. I'm afraid I should have taken your warning more seriously and rested more. What should I do?" I advised her to wrap a compress containing Toko-Öl/Toko Oil 𝒟® around her abdomen and simultaneously carry out the all-fours position. Her husband should take care of the older children so that she could really rest. If there was no improvement, she should ring me up again. She didn't call again until the following day – The oil had caused her abdomen to relax, the pressure had lightened and the "wild contractions" had stopped. She also told me that she had applied to the health insurance scheme for help in the household and was planning to pay a visit to the hospital with her husband as soon as possible. It had apparently become clear to the expectant father in view of these increased Braxton-Hicks contractions that it would be better to follow my advice after all.

Dorothea didn't have her peace and quiet for long, however. Ten days later – she had now reached the thirty-seventh week – I got a call at 10 o'clock in the evening: "Inge, my wife is having contractions regularly every ten minutes; what should we do?" "If the contractions continue, you'll have to drive to the hospital, but I'll be happy to come by first", I offered. "No, you don't have to drive all that way. It's alright; we'll pack our bag", the expectant father announced. The next morning the phone rang, and a laughing Dorothea told me that she was home and slept wonderfully all night and everything had calmed down again after she had gently rubbed the oil into her abdomen again. Several days later, after our antenatal class session, we tried to figure out what kept causing this "wild" contraction activity. I asked her if she had taken any medication which might have triggered contractions, and she remembered that she had taken a combination drug that past weekend. She thought she was coming down with the flu and had been trying to boost her immune system. When I read the package insert, I found what I was looking for: the medicine contained thuja, a plant extract known to have a contraction-stimulating effect. This medication is a good means of activating the natural antibodies and perhaps thus preventing the flu, but in sensitive pregnant women it can bring about contractions. This was the case with Dorothea, because she had been taking only natural medicines for years and her body was accordingly sensitized.

But the story doesn't stop there. I made another house call thirteen days before the due date and wanted to take the opportunity to examine Dorothea again. She claimed her premonitory contractions had now decreased to a minimum. At the antenatal examinations carried out by the doctor, he had consistently determined that the state of the cervix was unchanged. The entire situation was calm and relaxed. From my external examination it was clear to me that the baby had grown and gained a good amount of weight. During the vaginal examination I had a slight shock: her cervix was already six centimetres open but still not fully effaced, and the baby's head was fixed in the entrance to the pelvis! I told her to let me know as soon as the contractions started because it was sure to be a fast birth. I wasn't worried, because I know that a child cannot be born without good, strong contractions. Three days later the father rang up and asked me to come for the birth. After labour lasting a single hour, Dorothea gave birth to a daughter weighing 2,860 g nine days before the due date.

My reason for relating this story is to tell all women and young midwives once again that no child is born without strong labour pains, no matter how frequently Braxton-Hicks contractions, false labour or "wild" contractions have set in. Every woman worries now and then that the child could suddenly just be there. And every home birth midwife is afraid that the child will be born before she arrives on the scene. But we all have to recall, again and again, that in order to give birth a woman has to have contractions, and you feel contractions. There are children who take a long time to be born and children who "slip out" very quickly. But no human being can be born without labour pains.

Problems during the Final Weeks

One of the most frequent results of the antenatal appointments during the last six weeks is a vaginal infection – most frequently thrush (a fungal infection), Chlamydia or a Group B streptococcus infection. A herpes virus infection can also occur during pregnancy.

Unfortunately, an increasing number of women are confronted with these vaginal disorders. If you have discomfort in the form of redness, itching, burning and increased flaky, greyish-white discharge, take it seriously and have yourself examined to find out what is causing it. But you don't have to be inordinately worried. If women had to have a sterile vagina for childbirth, evolution would have arranged for it in one way or another. And by all means, don't forget: fear weakens your immune system!

Vaginal Thrush

At the first sign of vaginal thrush, treatment should be undertaken. The longer the infection has been in your system – sometimes it has been chronically present for years – the more difficult and tedious naturopathic treatment of it will be. Vaginal thrush, a yeast infection in the area of the vagina, is unfortunately relatively common during pregnancy. The vaginal pH changes during pregnancy and is more susceptible to the candida, the genus of yeast causing the infection. Stress, anaemia, treatment with antibiotics in the recent past or the intake of too much sugar are often associated with the contraction of canker. It is very important to get rid of it entirely before childbirth, because the baby can become infected during labour, i.e. develop the candida infection in the mouth or nappy zone. For newborns, the treatment is very bothersome, painful and tedious.

The medications prescribed by doctors, antimycotics or antifungal agents, often bring about only a temporary improvement, particularly when treatment has already been carried out frequently. These medications are often used for too short a time, and the fungus is not completely eliminated. The spores then merely lie dormant and flare up again immediately during the slightest stress situation.

Every woman should know that yeast can only grow in a moist, dark environment and thrives best when her diet contains a large proportion of sugar and refined flour products. Accordingly, you should see to it that you keep the area around the vagina as dry, light and airy as possible by wearing breathable cotton under- and outerwear. You should drastically decrease your intake of sugar; ideally eliminate it from your diet entirely. But many women don't get rid of their yeast infection even if they abstain from sugar. Natural healers thus consider the cause to lie in general acidosis (an abnormal increase in the acidity of the body's fluids) and, above all, stress.

Means of Prevention

In order to heal this condition by natural means or prevent yeast or other infections, a number of fundamental measures are necessary.

- Wash with cold water and preferably with your hand as opposed to a washcloth, so that the spores don't accumulate in the laundry. Or you can use a washcloth made of raw silk, which has an antibacterial effect.
- Use alkaline soaps, but no vaginal lotions, sprays or other scented vaginal products.
- Wear underpants made of cotton or silk.
- No synthetic clothing such as nylon stockings or tight synthetic leggings. Skin-tight trousers should also be avoided.
- If possible, allow plenty of air and light to circulate in the genital area; i.e. don't wear underpants when you are at home.
- During pregnancy, see to it that you get plenty of rest and relaxation; avoid all stress.
- When you go to a public swimming pool, wear a tampon which has been soaked in olive oil – this provides ideal protection against a yeast infection because the spores literally slide off.
- Regular pelvic floor exercises promote circulation and strengthen the immune system.
- In general, all abnormal sexual practices should be refused or discontinued, since they are often the cause for the spreading of germs.

Naturopathic Treatment

There are of course various naturopathic means of treating an acute vaginal yeast infection.

The use of yoghurt containing live active cultures and dextrorotary *lactic acid* is very helpful. Before you go to bed at night, spread a teaspoon of yoghurt on the walls of the vagina or on the vulvae, depending on where the infection is, and – very important – wash if off thoroughly with the shower head in the morning, or rinse your vagina out with a douche bag. If you begin with the treatment as soon as you feel itchy, it often suffices as a means of preventing the yeast from spreading. If you missed this early stage or contracted the infection quite some time ago, it is very effective to treat it with *garlic*. Take a clove of garlic and run a string through it, insert it into the vagina and leave it for at least twelve hours; then insert a fresh clove for another twelve hours, etc. Again, with this treatment you may well succeed in doing in the yeast spores for good.

In order to avoid a burning sensation of the vaginal mucus membranes – which are particularly sensitive during pregnancy – I advise you to wrap the garlic clove in a tampon or a finger bandage, tied firmly shut with a piece of string. This garlic treatment can naturally be repeated as often as necessary. The regular consumption of garlic is also helpful. I never cease to be amazed when I once again find confirmation of the fact that women who eat lots of garlic never suffer from yeast infections.

⑥ Aroma Therapy

The *Original 𝒟® Aroma Blend Rose-Teebaum-Essenz/Rose-Tea-Tree Essence 𝒟®* , consisting of the essential oils lavender extra, manuka, rose and tea tree, has likewise proven its value. Women who have treated themselves naturopathically for a long time, and whose bodies accordingly respond well to natural remedies, are usually successful when they administer *Rose-Teebaum-Hydrolat/Rose-Tea-Tree Hydrolat 𝒟®* immediately at the first signs of infection. The treatment is most successful when the intimate zone is sprayed quite regularly or vaginal douches are carried out – in cases where vagina is infected (then the hydrolat is diluted with sterilized water at a ratio of 1:1). As soon as the itchiness has decreased, it suffices to carry out three applications a day until the infection is completely healed.

I have a great many memories about yeast infections in stock, e.g. the one about Marion …

…"Inge, just think I have a yeast infection again. What should I do – I've already used the vaginal suppositories the doctor prescribed me two weeks ago and now the whole thing is starting all over again. Do you know of any essential oils I can use?" My advice was to take a sitz bath every morning and every evening containing: one tablespoon of Dead Sea Salt mixed with five drops of Rose-Teebaum-Essenz/Rose-Tea-Tree Essence 𝒟® and a clove of garlic with slits cut into it. Already a week later she reported to me: "Super, Inge, I'm rid of the infection."

Many women have managed to cure their thrush infection without using garlic. When non-pregnant women ask me for advice, I recommend treating the vagina with yoghurt and the above-named essential oils rather than sitz baths. A tampon soaked in St.-John's wort oil or, even better, evening primrose oil and a few drops of *Rose-Teebaum-Essenz/Rose-Tea-Tree Essence 𝒟®* also helps. This therapy almost always leads to the desired results.

During pregnancy, however, I would generally recommend beginning the treatment with sitz baths since, due to the heightened sensitivity, they usually suffice. The mucus membranes are protected from the danger of irritation and the vaginal pH soon restabilizes.

⟳ Homoeopathic Remedies

Homoeopathy likewise has various remedies in store, whose administration, however, should only be carried out on the advice of a doctor or midwife with experience in homoeopathy. The two most common substances are *Sepia* and *Kreosotum*. In the case of a chronic infection, one of the major miasmatic remedies such as *Psorinum*, *Luesinum* or *Medorrhinum* should naturally be taken into consideration.

Other Forms of Vaginal Infections

Group B streptococcal Infection

Infections of the vagina with the Group B streptococcus have become very worrisome for pregnant women, because they have heard that this malady can lead to a problematic infection in the newborn. Their fears are unjustified, however, because actually the danger of an infection only arises when the pathogen finds a way of reaching the child. Often these examinations are carried out too early – at a point of time irrelevant for childbirth because by then the Group B streptococci can already have disappeared again of their own accord. Even doctors don't always agree on whether this examination is necessary during pregnancy. From the scientific-medical point of view, however, the search for Group B streptococci is indicated if there are signs of an impending premature delivery before the end of the thirty-seventh week or if the mother's temperature rises above 38 °C/100 °F during labour. If the pathogens are found in this situation, treatment with antibiotics is essential and the newborn must be attended to by a paediatrician.

In order to prevent the baby from being infected, it would be very sensible to desist from artificially puncturing the amniotic sac, because the latter protects the baby and prevents any and all contact with the mother's mucus membranes. Moreover, every vaginal examination should also be carefully considered, because it can lead to a spread of the pathogens farther up into the vagina. It is not only I that sometimes have the impression that these "modern" illnesses are brought about more by overly cautious precautions and excessive control than by anything the mother does, because insufficient intimate hygiene has become extremely rare these days. Presumably this is another case of medicine being able to control and examine all kinds of things, but not knowing exactly how to cope with the results.

Herpes genitalis

An acute herpes genitalis infection rarely occurs but represents a grave danger to the child's life during birth. The delivery must be carried out by caesarean in any case. In the weeks preceding childbirth, vaginal herpes should always be taken seriously and treated accordingly.

(◉) Aroma Therapy

In aroma therapy, treatment with a combination of *lemon balm hydrolat* and *lemon balm 10% in jojoba wax* has led to excellent results. First the hydrolat is sprayed onto the infected area, and then the oil is applied to it.

Bleeding

I often receive phone calls from worried women in the final stage of pregnancy due to *bleeding*. What they usually tell me is something like: "What should I do? I've had slight bleeding constantly since this morning."

Fresh Red Blood

The first thing I ask in these cases is whether the bleeding is as strong as, stronger than or lighter than menstruation, and what it looks like: bright red, fresh blood or dark, old blood. I have never received the answer "as strong as menstruation and bright red, fresh blood". During the antenatal class and from their gynaecologists, women learn that the latter is a sign of grave danger and, in the rare cases when women have this type of bleeding, they always go to the hospital immediately. The fact that red is a sign of alarm is fortunately known all over the world, and no matter when it occurs during pregnancy, expectant parents should react as follows:

In the case of strong, bright red bleeding, as strong as menstruation or stronger, go to the nearest hospital immediately!!

This is unfortunately almost always a sign of premature detachment of the placenta, in which case medical assistance in the form of an emergency caesarean must be provided without delay. Women who experience this are naturally very shocked and require a lot of attention and understanding for this sudden change in their situation. In such cases, everyone involved is always grateful that we have such an outstandingly well-functioning emergency rescue system and hospital management that the babies can usually be born alive. Unfortunately, however, it can happen that, due to the major loss of blood, the baby will not be sufficiently provided for and will not survive the birth. I know that such facts are horrible, brutal, and cruel, but that is one of nature's many faces. Due to the fact that most of the women who undergo this have already either had bleeding during early pregnancy or the low position of the placenta is diagnosed within the framework of an ultrasound examination, they are usually prepared to a certain extent and know that they have to go to the hospital immediately. In these cases, we owe a great deal to ultrasound technology, because it gives the expectant mother the opportunity to explain to her neighbours, boss, colleagues, etc. that – if bleeding should occur – she will immediately place her older children in the neighbour's care or leave her place of work in order to reach the hospital as soon as possible. The same applies to the expectant father, who can likewise take immediate action without having to go into big explanations. After this ultrasound diagnosis, many women are completely distraught and see themselves and their babies buried at the cemetery. This panic is understandable but, as described above, usually the situation calms down because, as mentioned, in Germany all hospitals can be reached within the necessary span of time. What is more, this extreme mislocation of the placenta and its detachment really happen very rarely. Usually the initial diagnosis states that the placenta is in an abnormally low position and partially covering the cervix. I would greatly prefer it if such statements weren't made at all, because – particularly in early pregnancy – there's a good chance that everything will change of its own accord. But the woman should be – and wants to be – informed about every medical finding, and indications such as these are also possible.

I would, however, like to address the topic of warning blood again. If it should happen that the low position of the placenta is overlooked during the ultrasound or the woman has not wanted an ultrasound examination up until this point in time, the organism nevertheless calls attention to the situation. After all, this condition already existed before the days of ultrasound diagnostics, and midwives and obstetricians also knew what to do back then. Here I would like to quote my so highly respected older colleague again, who once said: "My goodness, do you spring chickens really think we were that stupid? We kept our eyes and ears open and really studied the textbook, and we were able to identify risk situations. All you have to do is listen carefully. When you listen to the fetal heartbeat, you also hear where the afterbirth is." For me that was a whole new insight, but from that point on I really began learning and listening to where the so-called wind noise was. Thanks to our excellent fetal heartbeat devices; I soon managed to confirm the doctor's findings: the placenta is here. As a matter of fact, it can even be determined with the ear trumpet. It's a shame that today we think only technology can convey such knowledge, and that the old midwives weren't able to pass on their wisdom – or our generation no longer listened to what they had to tell us. Because this age-old knowledge shows that a great effort has always been made in the interest of the mothers' and children's well-being, so that the mothers could go through the process of becoming mothers calmly and well-informed. On the other hand, as the historian Barbara Duden says: "There has always been fear!" And fear is justified, can be voiced, and must be taken seriously. As an expectant mother, I urge you to keep looking for an open ear until you have the feeling someone understands you and you can be calm and confident even after such an unsettling diagnosis as placenta praevia – i.e. when the cervix is wholly or partially covered by the placenta (praevia = in front of the way). That's what midwives are for.

Dark Blood – Consequences of Vaginal Examinations

The women who ring me up to report on bleeding, however, usually tell me that it is light, initially bright red, but then "old" and dark red. As in the case of Mrs. A. ...

... when I asked her about the results of her medical examination, she said: "Nothing special, I was at the doctor's and since then I've been bleeding. And I also have constant back pains, as well as a steady ache in the groin. The doctor says childbirth could begin any minute. But these aren't labour pains, when I had my last child it was totally different. What should I do? What does this blood mean, without real contractions?" Before giving Mrs. A. any advice, I thought about whether she had already exceeded the due date and, if so, by how long, and I asked her again, just to be certain. And anyway, I wanted to know what the results of the examination had been and whether the examination had hurt. "Yes, that's the strange thing; the due date isn't until the day after tomorrow. But he said the cervix was already in the condition it should be in for labour and three centimetres wide open. But I bet you the doctor stretched it at least a centimetre – it hurt so much I thought his fingers would be coming up through my throat and out my mouth! All he said was, I shouldn't be afraid, he was just trying to stimulate and stretch the cervix a little so that labour might begin a bit sooner. Before I could even answer, he had already started and since then everything hurts. But maybe I made a mistake, because the first thing I said to him when I said hello was that there was nothing I was longing for more than true contractions, I was finding it very difficult to wait this time around." With her answer, Mrs. A. had already realized herself what had caused her discomfort and bleeding. The examination had turned into a major intervention, which had injured some small vessels of the cervix and caused the bleeding, which was, however, harmless. The stretching of the cervix had irritated the uterus to such an extent that pain in the groin and the small of the back had come about, because so-called wild contractions had been triggered. My advice to Mrs. A. was: "Try to relax, take a warm lavender or lemon balm bath and then go to bed; maybe the uterus will calm down, or true labour pains might get under way in a few hours." Mrs. A. later told me she had had the pains the rest of the evening, but had felt calmer and cooler after the bath. It wasn't until four days later that she started having real contractions.

My reason for relating this story to you is to point out that for you as an expectant mother it is always important to be patient – and not lead the gynaecologist to undertake such massive interventions by making impatient remarks. On the one hand, his action might really trigger labour. On the other hand, however, often all the women get out of it are unnecessary aches and pains. Unfortunately there are still obstetricians around who have recourse to these somewhat insensitive methods in order to get the contractions going. I advise all women who have experienced such a situation to talk to their doctors about it, so that they will more careful the next time. A vaginal examination does not have to be painful. But I often have the feeling that many women lack the courage to talk about feelings and experiences like these.

Natural Methods of Preparation for Childbirth

One of the questions asked most frequently in the antenatal class and during a consultation with a midwife is: what means are there of preparing myself for childbirth as well as possible with natural methods?

Naturally, I am very happy when a woman asks this question. It means that she knows that good childbirth depends a great deal on her as a woman and mother, on her behaviour and her body. Such a woman does not want to surrender the responsibility for a good birth entirely to the personnel attending to her, and she doesn't want to blame the child later on for not being able to find its way out. At the same time, however, it is also very important to me to make women in general as well as all of my fellow midwives understand that even the best preparations, the most suitable homoeopathic medicines and the most appropriate essential oils cannot enlarge a maternal pelvis, and cannot make an unborn child lighter or smaller. Even the best preparatory measures will not be able to prevent an obstetric emergency. Natural methods of preparation serve to let us expect that labour will take its normal course and will last a normal amount of time, and to get the mother's body in the best possible physical shape so that it can perform optimally and does not represent an obstacle to the child. In order to achieve this, I have been recommending the following measures for many years:

☉ Raspberry Leaf Tea

Beginning with the end of the thirty-fourth week of pregnancy I recommend the regular consumption of *raspberry leaf tea,* either two to three cups a day in addition to the *Schwangerschaftstee/Pregnancy Tea* blend, or tea made from half a teaspoon of the blend and half a teaspoon of raspberry leaves. It has not yet been scientifically determined how or why raspberry leaves effect pregnant women. But there are a great many midwives who swear by raspberry leaf tea, and that is proof enough. We midwives are convinced that this herb loosens the muscles of the pelvis minor quite substantially. It is known that raspberry leaves have a detoxifying and purifying effect on the smooth muscles of the intestines. This means that the metabolic process is stimulated by way of the intestine and the purification contributes to the maintenance of health in the entire body. A healthy body, in turn, is capable of carrying out labour within a normal time span. Moreover, regular bowel movements mean good intestinal peristalsis – wavelike muscular contractions – and since the intestine runs directly along the wall of the uterus, the muscles of the latter are constantly stimulated into action. This is undoubtedly the reason why raspberry leaves are thought to have a labour-inducing effect. Many women say that they have a rash on their tummies or thighs after they start drinking raspberry leaf tea. In that case I recommend reducing the amount per day and drinking plenty of other fluids, preferably water. The rash is a sign that a detoxification process has commenced, but that the liver and kidneys cannot cope with the elimination process and the skin is being used as an excretory organ. Rashes and itchiness don't always have to be designated as allergies – we have to learn to understand the skin as a possible vehicle of excretion and not suppress that function. It is an entirely normal and healthy process for toxic substances to make their way out through the skin when the body no longer stores them internally. The rash usually subsides after a while.

⑤ Linseed

It is likewise advisable to take one tablespoon of coarsely ground linseed per day from the thirty-fourth week of pregnancy onward. According to the vernacular, at least in German, linseed is said to make the children "flutschen" – i.e. slip out. Linseed has a positive effect on the mucus membranes. The reaction of the intestinal mucus membranes to linseed is the most well-known example. Many pregnant women confirm the mucus-stimulating effect in the area of the vaginal mucus membranes. The regular consumption of freshly ground linseed does in fact lead to increased vaginal mucus production, and the benefits for childbirth are sure to be obvious to all. The likewise well-known bowel-movement-regulating property of linseed undoubtedly has the same effect on the muscles of the uterus as raspberry leaves – in other words, due to increased peristalsis the uterine muscles are also stimulated. When you take coarsely ground linseed, make sure to drink plenty of fluid, since otherwise the opposite can happen, i.e. constipation. Moreover, it is also important to know that the consumption of only one tablespoon does not have a laxative effect, but merely serves to regulate the activity of the intestines.

⑤ Perineal Massage

It seems to me that the most important preparatory measure for childbirth is the regular massage of the perineum with the *Original D® Aroma Blend Dammmassageöl/ Perineum Massage Oil D®*, a blend of St.-John's wort oil and wheat germ oil supplemented by the essential oils of clary sage and rose.

I have been recommending the massage of the perineum to every pregnant woman since the late 1970s, and it has since become an entirely self-evident piece of advice throughout the world of obstetrics. I am convinced that this measure has enabled very, very many women to give birth without having an episiotomy – surgical incision of the perineum – to facilitate childbirth. The massage of the perineum is intended as a means of making the latter soft and elastic so that the baby's head can pass through it without the mother's having to be injured by an episiotomy. Naturally, small tears in the perineum cannot always be avoided, but they heal much faster and less problematically than an episiotomy, as I have witnessed again and again since I began working in independent midwifery. Moreover, in the meantime, studies have been carried out by midwives which support this observation with numbers. A study by Gisèle Steffen provides proof that women with perineal tears suffer less discomfort during the postnatal period and the months following childbirth. These women accordingly make far less use of pain relievers in the postnatal phase. Another aspect is that very many women have the feeling their intimate zone has been gravely violated by an episiotomy. For years afterward, this incision represents an emotional injury and damage to their femininity. This intervention should therefore always be well considered beforehand, and never carried out unscrupulously. Unfortunately, it wasn't until I gained personal experience with childbirth that it became clear to me what it means to have an episiotomy or remain uninjured.

And it was not until I began accompanying home births that I truly understood the responsibility I, as an obstetrician, was really taking on with regard to the protection of the perineum. To this day, all of my protective measures have been successful. This borderline situation – to cut or not to cut? – represents a huge stress factor and a complex challenge. But for us midwives, no effort should be too great in the interest of keeping the perineum of a woman uninjured. In addition to the oil and the determination to convince the woman of the importance of the matter, we also require the deep conviction that a woman is capable of giving birth without an episiotomy. It may take a few contractions longer; the stretching of the perineum progresses more cautiously; thanks to the oil on a warm, moist washcloth the woman can endure the stretching pains quite well; she breathes regularly so that the child is well supplied with oxygen. Without a labour-inducing infusion, the intervals between the contractions are pleasantly long, a factor which also works to the benefit of the child; the woman can recover and gather strength for the next contraction and the perineal tissue has time to adjust to the stretching. Every midwife must keep all of these considerations in mind with inner conviction every time she assists a woman in giving birth. And even if someone is standing there, surgical scissors in hand, she is called upon not to lose her patience and her confidence and not allow herself to be dissuaded from the cooperation between a midwife and a woman in labour which has proven so effective in the course of many millennia. If the perineum then tears, the pain it causes is nowhere near as great, because a tear is a natural injury and the tissue always tears at the weakest point. Injuries to the blood vessels are extremely rare. When the perineum is cut, on the other hand, vessels are severed, often causing effusions, which can impede the healing process and cause additional pain.

All midwives and obstetricians know that we cannot do without this surgical intervention entirely. Fortunately, between 1990 and the present, the episiotomy rate has decreased from approximately 90 percent to an average of 45 percent; 20 percent would – in my opinion – be very positive. In a report issued by the World Health Organization in 1988, it is estimated that this target for the reduction in the episiotomy rate may well be scientifically justified.

In order to help us reach this goal, it is necessary for you as an expectant mother to contribute by taking to heart the following pointers for how to carry out a perineal massage so that your perineum remains uninjured when you give birth: about six weeks before the due date, begin energetically massaging and stretching the perineum – i.e. the tissue between the back wall of the vagina and the anus, with *Dammmassageöl/Perineum Massage Oil ᴅ°* , so as to make it soft, resilient and elastic. In addition, insert first one, later two or three fingers approximately three centimetres deep into the vagina, take hold of the perineum between your thumb and forefinger and massage it with a U-shaped movement, exerting slight pressure in the direction of the intestines. If you carry out this massage every day for about two to three minutes you will soon notice that, with the use of the oil, the perineum is becoming soft and supple. In the final days before childbirth, it is worth the additional effort to apply oil to the labia and massage them gently as well, because it does happen now and then that the perineum remains intact but the labia are slightly injured. Try to pull the vulvae apart for about twenty seconds to the point where you feel a prickling or slight burning sensation – the same you will feel when the baby's head passes through. For the perineal massage you should only use as much oil as your skin can absorb; otherwise dab off the remaining oil with toilet paper or a towel when you are finished. Naturally, your partner can also take over on carrying out the massage. Perhaps he will regard this task as a means of doing his part to protect the perineum from injury during the birth. Many women are worried, however, that the massage might turn into lovemaking; that is something you must decide for yourself; at any rate, sexual intercourse is harmless. For the partner, it can be a good exercise to treat the perineum without ulterior motives, because during childbirth it is often difficult for men to adjust to the medical objectiveness of the events in the genital zone – which are otherwise so intimate and full of feeling.

Your midwife may well massage the perineum and labia during labour, but don't assume that every midwife has *Dammmassageöl/Perineum Massage Oil D*® at her disposal: you can, however, take a bottle of it with you and offer it to her. In any case, the midwife in attendance will make an effort to protect your perineum because that is one of our professional duties. And incidentally, most of my colleagues are very pleased when you, as an expectant mother, are aware of this duty, and they see it as a welcome challenge if you attach importance to giving birth without a surgical incision.

Technology has not remained at a standstill in this context: a gynaecologist developed a device known as the EPI-NO. It consists of an inflatable balloon with a manual pump which the woman can insert into the vagina regularly during the final weeks of pregnancy, pumping it up to increasingly larger circumferences until she reaches that of the baby's head, about 10 centimetres. The woman can thus become accustomed to the stretching pain and the tissue becomes elastic. This device is the subject of a lot of controversy among midwives and expectant mothers. Some think it's great, others disgusting; some regard it to be a sensible means of preparation, others fear that it can cause an overexpansion of the pelvic floor before childbirth. I myself also have a hard time recommending an apparatus when a woman or couple can achieve the same results with their hands, sensitively and individually. Particularly the idea of getting used to the stretching pain seems a bit strange to me: after all, the baby doesn't keep sticking its head out and retracting it again during childbirth but, when the time has come, purposively leaves the birth canal with one final thrust.

The History of the Dammmassageöl/Perineum Massage Oil

It was with the development of the *Dammmassageöl/Perineum Massage Oil D*® that my success with the use of essential oils in the context of midwifery began. When I used it for the first time during the birth of Frederik, the effects were amazing. His mother had already given birth to a child several years earlier, but had had a major episiotomy which had been causing her pain for many years. Her greatest wish was to give birth without an episiotomy this time, something that was difficult to promise her in view of the old, fleshy scar. But to my astonishment, due to the use of the oil, the child was born without even the slightest tear to the perineum.

Within a very short time, I learned that children who were considerably bigger and heavier than their older siblings – who had been born with the help of a supposedly absolutely necessary episiotomy – could be born easily without a perineal wound. For me it was soon clear that the success was to be attributed to the essential oils, because I had always recommended perineal massages. But often the mothers confessed to me that they had felt very unsure about treating themselves "down there". I realized that many women have an almost insurmountable feeling of shame. They very simply have inhibitions about handling their genitals. But when I started recommending the *Dammmassageöl/Perineum Massage Oil* $\mathcal{D}^{®}$ I had developed, a product containing clary sage and rose, this threshold suddenly disappeared. The pregnant women I attended to all began talking about their experiences with perineal massage. The number of women who gave birth with intact perinea – even in hospitals – grew from month to month.

For me there was no doubt: this was the effect of the essential oils. Today I am grateful to my pharmacist, who allowed himself to be talked into manufacturing this blend for interested mothers and selling it at a realistic price. Due to the fact that the essential oil of the Turkish rose is quite expensive and the price has tripled since my first experiments in the 1980s, I couldn't expect mothers to pay such enormous sums for a little bottle of rose oil if they really only needed one to two drops for a perineal massage oil blend. It seemed to me rather unreasonable to recommend such costly products which very few mothers could have afforded or would have been prepared to buy. Moreover, it was also important to me that only flawless, high-quality essences be employed in the obstetrical context. Due to the fact that I was not in a position to test the quality myself, I was dependent on the professional know-how and competence of a pharmacist. These considerations paved the way to the Bahnhof-Apotheke pharmacy in Kempten, which I knew as being naturopathically oriented, well-informed and highly experienced with pharmaceutical practice. Since that time, with my involvement and quality control, the pharmacy works only with high-quality oils. Throughout Germany it is the only pharmacy which tests oils in its own laboratory, using the techniques of gas chromatography and mass spectrometry. This proved necessary because the oil suppliers only carry out random inspections of their products. As a result, a great number of mothers, midwives, hospitals and pharmacies throughout the country can be supplied with manually filled essential oils of the very highest quality, and they can rely entirely on the complete flawlessness of these oils.

As a "layperson" it is sometimes very difficult to know what oils are unadulterated and thus can be used without hesitation. Unfortunately, due to the rising costs of pure oils, trade with synthetic oils and oils diluted with inferior essences is being carried out all over the world. I would like to take this opportunity to point out once again that the success of aroma therapy depends to a great extent on the quality of the oils, i.e. on the individual components, which vary, in turn, depending on the cultivation, climate and distillation conditions. My experience is based only on the compositions of my own blends using oils from suppliers I have chosen myself. If you use essential oils from other sources, you may well find that your results and experiences will differ considerably from mine.

Composition and Description of the Essential Oils

I would like to explain to you why I have chosen the following fatty and essential oils for my *Dammmassageöl/Perineum Massage Oil* $\mathcal{D}$® blend.

- *St.-John's wort oil* has a strong nerve-strengthening effect and can be used when sensitive nerve ends are to be treated.
- *Wheat germ oil* has a very high vitamin E content and therefore improves the elasticity of the tissue and supports the muscle and gland function.
- *Evening primrose oil* is the most valuable vegetable oil there is, since it is rich in unsaturated fatty acids and moreover has an influence on the female hormone system, particularly on the oestrogen.
- The essential oil of the organically cultivated *rose* is surely the best and most valuable oil when it comes to treating the vaginal zone. This oil has strong antiseptic and antispasmodic qualities. Rose oil was already used in obstetrics during antiquity. As early as 1629, the midwife Marie Louise Bourgois reported on using rose oil for women in labour. I would like to point out that with rose oil it is more important than ever to take quality and purity into consideration. Since it is one of the most expensive oils – approximately five thousand kilograms of rose blossoms are required to extract one litre of essence – it is unfortunately often offered on the market as synthetic or diluted oil.
- I use the essential oil of *clary sage* because it likewise has a strongly antiseptic, antispasmodic and pain-relieving effect and, due to the sclareol it contains, also possesses hormone-like qualities. When purchasing this oil for the pharmacy, we therefore always attach great importance to the presence of this substance. On the psychological level, clary sage helps primarily in transcending one's own limits and sticking things out – precisely the demands made on a woman by childbirth. For weeks beforehand, people prophecy to the expectant mother: "You'll come through fine. All you have to do is overcome your inhibitions and let go, let the child out."

All women know that, at the end of the second stage (expulsion phase) of labour, the "only" obstacle is the perineum. It is precisely this image, the dilation of the vagina for the baby's head, that seems inconceivable to many women, and surely to men as well. Already well before labour, by employing the qualities of clary sage, the woman gains the ability to overcome her own inhibitions and massage her perineum. During labour, the essential oil helps everyone present, because it affects the attending obstetricians by way of the sense of smell, and the confidence that this child can pass through the perineum increases. I would like to point out to midwives that they should use

Dammmassageöl/Perineum Massage Oil 𝒟* sparingly, because it is highly concentrated and particularly clary sage possesses a substantial hypotonic (antihypertensive) and anaesthetizing effect. And in general, essential oils are highly potent and costly and should therefore be used sparingly.

🌀 Herbal Medicine

Beginning in the thirty-eighth week of pregnancy, steam sitz baths with *hayflowers* (flores graminis) are very suitable as a means of preparing for childbirth. They help to make the tissue softer and more elastic. This is highly advisable especially for primiparas (first-time mothers), since their pelvic floor muscles are generally still very firm. For so-called multiparas (women who have given birth before), this treatment is recommended in cases where a major episiotomy was necessary during past deliveries. An old midwife tradition is hayflower treatment in cases where the labour pains are irregular or too weak, either in the form of a dry, hot sack of hayflowers or as a hot bath. Even in the form of tea, hayflowers have an antispasmodic and contraction-regulating effect. Women who suffer from hay fever should remember, however, that a steam bath with these flowers can trigger an allergic reaction.

I recommend taking a hayflower steam sitz bath once a week from the thirty-eighth week of pregnancy onward. Once she has reached the due date, an expectant mother can take a steam sitz bath as often as she likes. Applying this measure when labour gets under way is ideal for making the pelvic floor soft and resilient. Women who have varicose veins in the area of the vulvae should be careful, however, because these veins can cause her quite a lot of pain after the bath.

Many women have no idea how such a bath is carried out and ask me: "What in the world to you mean by a 'steam sitz bath?'" It's as simple as can be: take a small fireproof pot, put a handful of hayflowers from the pharmacy into it and then pour boiling water over it. Place the pot in your bidet or toilet and sit on it for as long as it emits steam.

Renate reported to me …

… "Inge, if I'm not mistaken, this hayflower steam not only softens the tissue but also wakes sleeping children. When I sit over the steam in the evening, I can't get to sleep anymore afterwards because the baby in my womb is moving so energetically. In future I'm going to take my steam bath in the morning."

🌀 Homoeopathic Remedies

The most frequent question posed by expectant mothers is: "What homoeopathic remedies can I take in preparation for childbirth? I read that pregnant women should take *Pulsatilla* and *Caulophyllum* four weeks before the due date. [These substances are supposed to ensure that the woman will give birth within a relatively normal period of time and with so-called effective contractions.] What's your opinion?"

My answer is: "Yes, it is possible to use these substances to prepare a pregnant woman for birth homoeopathically if she is not in a state of inner harmony. But only those pregnant women who really need it – who have problems or discomfort of a physical or emotional nature – should take a homoeopathic remedy." It is complete nonsense to give all expectant mothers one and the same remedy. This would mean that all women are the same. But as we all know, that is not the case, and since homoeopathy is an individual form of therapy, it is incorrect to assume that Pulsatilla and Caulophyllum are required by all pregnant women. Therefore, you should by all means talk to a health-care professional with experience in homoeopathic treatment to learn whether it is advisable for you to take any of these remedies in preparation for childbirth, and if so, which ones.

The Pharmacological Picture of Pulsatilla

Pulsatilla, or pasque flower, can be taken by women who recognize themselves in the description of the so-called pharmacological picture, i.e. if the following symptoms occur. Please be advised that not all of them have to be distinctly present.

The guiding symptoms of Pulsatilla are:
- changeability in every respect – mood, pain, habits – like the weather in April
- crying fits at the slightest little thing, consolation helps quickly
- the woman looks fantastic
- major fluctuations of mood, particularly in hormonally affected situations (also see p. ■f.)
- problems with stases such as oedema or varicose veins, primarily on the right side of the body
- bodily discharge (eye secretion, sniffles, vaginal discharge) is mild and yellow
- has difficulties letting go
- has an aversion to fatty foods, fruit and ice cream
- always feels better in the fresh air, by an open window

In fact, the tendency to be weepy occurs most frequently in the final four weeks of pregnancy, the 'bloom' of the Pulsatilla candidate. She doesn't want this phase to end; she knows she will have to let go of her baby soon, but it is difficult for her. Naturally, it can happen that you already discover these symptoms in yourself several weeks earlier; then the time has come to take Pulsatilla. By taking this substance, you will regain your inner centre, your inner balance. Homoeopathic remedies help to restore harmony in the human being.

Here I would like to tell you about one of my numerous experiences with Pulsatilla …

… Mrs. S. was pregnant with her third child and still had seven weeks to go until her due date. "So tell me, how are you?" I asked her when she came to my practice. Apparently it was the perfect moment to ask her that, because her eyes immediately filled with tears and she told me: "I don't know myself. I often feel like a stranger to myself. I get upset at the slightest triviality; I scold the children for nothing. My husband is already saying he doesn't know what he should do at all anymore, because I cry no

matter what he does. And it's true – you see? I'm crying right this minute. You know, I'm already feel-
ing a bit afraid of the birth. What if it takes as long as it did with the other children?" I was totally
astonished at this outbreak because I knew her to be the ideal mother, always even-tempered and radi-
ant. I knew that the whole family was looking forward to the baby. In view of this unexpected loss of
inner balance, I asked her: "Don't you think it would be advisable to take Pulsatilla?" "Yes, please, I
wonder why I didn't think of asking you that. I should have known you'd have some 'globuli' for me." I
advised her to take Pulsatilla twice a day for a while. If things didn't improve, she should call me. After
two weeks of successful administration, Mrs. S. stopped taking this homoeopathic medication and then
took it again for three days shortly before the due date when the same symptoms cropped up again.
The birth of her daughter went very fast and she was happy to have experienced such a good birth.
There is no doubt in my mind that the Pulsatilla helped.

The Pharmacological Picture of Caulophyllum

Caulophyllum thalictroides, blue cohosh, is a time-tested herbal medicine of the Native Americans. As a homoeopathically potentiated substance, it can be administered:

- when the cervix is found to be unripe on the due date, i.e. long, rigid and tightly closed (but only when there is no doubt about the correctness of the due date)
- when the labour pains are too weak and ineffective
- when the water breaks but no contractions ensue.

I can report on good experience with Caulophyllum for women whose cervix is scarred as the result of a cerclage (a sutured cervix) or other gynaecological interventions carried out in the past. With the help of this substance, the first stage of labour – during which the cervix dilates – can be kept to a reasonable duration. I also recommend it for women who have undergone extremely long labour in the past: they should take it shortly before the due date – but not weeks before, as is frequently directed! The most positive Caulophyllum results are attained in cases of prelabour rupture of the membranes. This medical term refers to the condition in which the water breaks but no contractions set in. In view of the fact that there are still a great number of obstetricians who immediately want to administer a contraction-stimulating infusion, their patients often ring up the midwife's practice or come by on short notice. These mothers want to avoid such forcible obstetric measures if at all possible, and seek advice from their midwives. If the unborn child is still faring well and the examination results are good, the expectant mother should take Caulophyllum in a low potency at fifteen-minute intervals. By the time the parents have reached the maternity hospital, the labour pains are usually regular and the oxytocic agent can be avoided, at least for the time being.

It is not unusual for a woman to ask: "If I take Pulsatilla and Caulophyllum, can I have normal childbirth this time? Last time I had to have a caesarean because the baby was too big and my pelvis supposedly too small." In such cases, I always have to point out very clearly that homoeopathy can't work wonders. There are no pills that can make a baby smaller or a pelvis larger. On the other hand, it is certainly advisable to check the correctness of the diagnosis "relative disproportion". It does happen that the prognosis "caesarean" is refuted by Nature herself, as was the case with Manuela …

… her first child had been delivered by caesarean section at a weight of just under three kilograms on account of "relative disproportion". Her second child was a proud four kilograms heavy. The parents had just managed to reach the hospital in time for its birth because the baby had pushed its way through the supposedly "abnormally narrow" pelvis at lightning speed. The mother had been treated with Pulsatilla in a high potency, and she was now able to cope with letting go, an issue that had been causing her problems for quite a while already.

Postterm Pregnancy/"Going Overdue"

As soon as expectant mothers are past the due date, concerns come up that the baby might be postterm. Very many women allow themselves to be unnerved because suddenly friends, neighbours, relatives are asking almost daily: "Well, have the contractions started yet? It's getting to be about time that baby was born. Aren't you worried about it? What did the doctor say? You know when I was pregnant, they induced labour on the due date so as not to endanger the baby." These and similar questions and comments are very upsetting for a pregnant woman. She often literally feels under pressure to perform, because everybody seems to be expecting her to come up with contractions on command. But this pressure makes her increasingly tense and it becomes more and more difficult for her to let go. Naturally there are cases in which expectant mothers stay calm and confident and receive support and consolation from those around them. Every woman should be so lucky. On the other hand, it doesn't help the mother at all to hear the famous sentence: "No baby ever stayed inside; sooner or later yours will come out too." By a few days after the due date (at the latest), many pregnant women regret ever having told their friends and acquaintances the exact date at all, because that is when they understand my advice, which is the following: consider carefully who you inform about the due date. It is extremely nerve-wracking when the telephone no longer stops ringing and everyone constantly asks whether the baby has been born yet. Tell them some date a few weeks later, because in the age of ultrasound, everyone will believe you if you say the due date has been revised.

The gynaecologists are most commonly the ones who put the pregnant woman under pressure. That is certainly not intended; it happens as a result of the frequent antenatal check-ups, which should be carried out, already before the due date under certain circumstances, and afterwards under all circumstances. In many cases the women are supposed to come in every two days, often even every day. They are even given appointments on Saturdays and Sundays. Mrs. H. was puzzled: "Strange – first I was supposed to come in every two days for a control, and now that my doctor is going on vacation suddenly it suffices if I go to his substitute after the weekend." There's not much I can say in response to such stories, but they do make you wonder.

There are obstetricians who don't ask the pregnant woman to come in again until a week after the due date and only begin with intensive supervision after ten days. No matter what the situation, every woman influences the situation greatly with her own behaviour. When she appears uncertain and frightened and constantly asks questions, the doctor will naturally have to give her appointments at short intervals. An expectant mother who demonstrates that she is patient and capable of waiting calmly will not be asked to come in for an examination so often.

Intensive Monitoring Methods

A number of very different methods are employed for the purpose of intensive monitoring if there is suspicion of a postterm pregnancy:

- a *vaginal examination* in order to determine the progress of the cervix's ripening and to make sure the child's position is as it should be.
- a *CTG check-up (cardiotocography)* in order to record the child's condition and any contractions that might be occurring. It is important to determine whether the fetal heartbeat remains stable during a contraction.
- an *ultrasound examination* in order to check the fetal heart rate, the amount of amniotic fluid and the placenta function. At this point in time, a Doppler ultrasound scan may be indicated, since it is capable of testing the flow of blood in the umbilical cord and the baby's vessels.
- an *amnioscopy (examination of the amniotic fluid)*: With the aid of a tube and a light source, the colour of the amniotic fluid is determined. This examination can only be carried out painlessly if the cervix is already partially open. Ask whether this is the case if your doctor wants to carry out this procedure, because otherwise it is sure to be extremely painful. Moreover, it causes a strong irritation of the uterine muscles and you will have to endure unnecessary abdominal pains or even ineffective 'wild' contractions. Unfortunately, many women ring me up in tears because they have been taken completely by surprise with this examination method. They complain of pain and can no longer tell whether they are having contractions or merely pains which are the result of the examination.

If the cervix is already open, however, this is an entirely painless means of examination. The endeavour is made to determine whether the baby is still well provided-for on the basis of the colour of the amniotic fluid. Clear fluid and visible vernix caseosa (a waxy white protective substance covering the skin of the fetus) mean that the baby is clearly not postterm and still has some leeway until it has to be born. If the fluid has already become slightly greenish, it is time to undertake labour-inducing measures. There are many doctors who no longer carry out this examination because it doesn't really tell them much. One reason for this is that only the amniotic fluid in the lower section of the uterus can be assessed. Due to the fact that the baby's head is nestled firmly in the birth canal, the amniotic fluid may no longer be circulating sufficiently. As a result, the fluid in the upper section may already have turned green while that in the lower section is still clear. Moreover, there is a great danger of causing the water to break by carrying out this procedure. It happens again and again that the amniotic sac is damaged during the examination, and labour thus inadvertently induced. For the woman, this means that she has to be taken to the hospital immediately.

- a *hormone test:* This is a blood test which must be carried out more than once because every placenta exhibits different hormone values. If the values are determined repeatedly, a curve can provide insight into whether the baby's nutrient and oxygen supply is still sufficient. This is a relatively expensive laboratory method and is carried out less and less frequently, because cost plays an increasing role in the medical care of pregnant women as elsewhere.

- an *oxytocin challenge test (OCT)*, generally carried out only in the hospital. There are, however, a few gynaecologists who conduct it in their practices. The expectant mother is given an infusion containing a labour-inducing hormone, namely oxytocin. This hormone is usually produced in the woman's pituitary gland and it triggers contractions. The OCT is another method of checking whether the placenta is still providing for the baby properly. In the place of an infusion, a nasal spray might be used, but the latter method, in my opinion, does not allow the dosage to be controlled – to the point where I regard it as irresponsible.

When Should Intensive Monitoring Begin?

As regards the question as to whether a baby is already postterm or whether everyone can just be patient and wait, I'm always amazed at how stubbornly everyone suddenly adheres to this estimated due date. Apparently the only place you can read that the due date is not the be-all-and-end-all, but merely a point of reference, is the midwife's textbook. Only four in every hundred children are actually born on this day. It has already been known for ages that very many deliveries take place within ten days before or after the calculated date. Exceeding the due date by ten days is therefore completely unobjectionable, and the word "postterm" applies only after ten days.

Naturally, it is necessary to keep an eye on the unborn child. I would like to point out to all expectant parents, however, that there is not a single means of keeping the baby in the womb under surveillance for twenty-four hours a day. What I mean to say is that parents should take their own responsibility, their confidence in the child and faith in nature as their orientation. The child will let us know when it needs to be born because it is no longer receiving sufficient nutrients and oxygen in the uterus. Parents should be receptive in this situation, but also have faith. Women were born to give birth and to preserve our species, and not to let the unborn child die. This, namely, is the accusation with which many women are faced: "Do you want your child to be born dead?" But I also know that, despite the very best means of surveillance, it will unfortunately sometimes happen that a baby dies in the womb. This was the fate of some very close friends of mine. It is very difficult to understand these oc-currences in life; they hurt and make us sad. But death is as much a part of the world as life. It was the experience of that death which taught me to communicate any un-easy feelings I have to the parents immediately. At that time – many years ago – I wasn't capable of that; I was very nervous when I didn't hear anything from the par-ents, because they had promised to let me know immediately when the child had been born. Even though I wasn't the midwife in attendance, I was extremely worried and went to see the parents. We decided that labour should be induced in the hospi-tal the following day, even though a home birth had been planned. It was too late; the little girl was dead. Even today it makes me sad and my tears flow when I think about it, but that's how life is. Nothing is predictable. We can only try to monitor and hope that everything goes well, but we will never be able to decide over life and death – all we can do is learn to cope with death and mourning.

The Mother's Instinct/The Parents are Involved in the Decision

For the doctors it is very difficult to judge how much security the parents need. You should therefore communicate very clearly the extent to which you can endure the period following the due date with a sense of self-responsibility, or would feel safer with surveillance. Unfortunately, the fear of legal consequences is very prevalent among doctors, particular in the field of obstetrics. Without technical monitoring methods, it is very difficult for an obstetrician to prove that a child was faring well at a particular point in time, that on a particular day there was no clear indication that intervention was necessary. With arguments like: "We could not detect any sign from the child" no doctor will be able to stand his ground before the law. Only figures, facts, laboratory results count. As parents, you therefore really have to see both sides and communicate your point of view clearly to your doctor. The fact that children give us a sign, and that expectant mothers have a sure instinct for when their child is in danger, is something very many midwives and women know. But instinct and feel-ings cannot be translated into statistics. As in the case of Mrs. F.-K. ...

... she rang me up on a Wednesday, six days after her due date: "Now they're starting that rigmarole of constant check-ups again, like they did with my first child. I'm supposed to come in for a check-up every two days, and if the baby isn't born by Sunday the doctor wants labour induced. What do you think: I can wait, can't I? After all, my daughter was born nearly two weeks past the due date. But after the birth the midwife said she was clearly not postterm. I'm so sick and tired of running to the doctor's practice all the time. In the case of my daughter the doctor didn't make such a fuss." I couldn't really tell her much in response, but I wanted to know: "What were things like with your menstrual cycle? Or do you know the date of conception?" "You see, that's the point; I just know that my children come a little later, because I have a very long cycle and I ovulate much later, but the doctor is stub-bornly sticking to her calculations. She never once listened to me when I told her it would come later

anyway. So that's why I don't feel like going there every day and letting her put me under pressure. The baby will come when it's good and ready." I had become acquainted with Mrs. F.-K. in the antenatal class and I knew that she was a very self-confident woman and I could believe what she was telling me. I advised her to talk to her doctor again, to explain everything and tell her that she herself had no trouble waiting, that she felt calm and sure of herself and was entirely prepared to take responsibility for whatever happened. She should go ahead and tell her gynaecologist that she certainly would not accuse her of neglect and assure her that she would accept the offer of intensive monitoring at the slightest feeling of unease or uncertainty. Mrs. F.-K. was grateful to me for confirming her point of view, and one week later the baby was born, healthy and ripe, without induction, but also without the slightest signs of being postterm. The doctor had called the woman's behaviour irresponsible because the latter had not allowed herself to be talked out of her conviction and her patience in waiting for the child. She, the doctor, more or less tacitly tolerated the woman's decision. But now she has one patient fewer, because the mother told me: "I'm not going to go through this hassle when I have my third child. I've already started asking around. After all, there are other gynaecologists."

I am always very reassured when it is clear to me that the parents are firmly anchored in their religious faith. These families are very sure of themselves. Their faith and their trust in God are so strong that they do not allow themselves to be misled, and they wait patiently. Again and again, I have heard people like this say: "Our Lord Jesus will know when our child is supposed to be born. He didn't create us to die but to live." In these families, I learn what it means for people to find support in religion. For me as a midwife, it is pleasant to attend to such parents. As in the case of Mrs. R. …

… she was pregnant with her second child and the doctor already asked her several days before the due date if he shouldn't stretch the cervix a bit to make the baby come sooner. The pregnant woman flatly refused his offer. When she had exceeded the due date by ten days, she asked me, in the calm voice that had become so familiar to me: "You also say that the children come when the time is right, don't you? My husband and I have no trouble waiting but the doctor is getting more and more restless and says he can't take the responsibility anymore, which we never expected him to do in the first place. Our Lord will take it for us." She merely wanted me to confirm her in her opinion. Four days later she gave birth to a healthy, strong boy. Two years later, the same thing happened again – Mrs. R. was a week past the due date with her third child. And her third child, the heaviest of all, was also allowed to be born when it was ready to be born. Once again, she refused to be talked out of her patience and religious faith by her "responsible" gynaecologist.

It was an exceptionally positive experience for me to attend to this family the third time around during their early postnatal period at home. I was infected with some of their calmness and conviction. It was a very harmonious phase, borne by faith, and not only by my competence.

Joint Decisions

Naturally, the midwife in attendance will often have to intervene and tell the parents that it is absolutely necessary to have a CTG or OCT carried out. But midwives and obstetricians should make an effort never to decide things "over the parents' head" and demand some measure or another, because after all, the unborn child is the child of the parents, and from the time of the birth onward they constantly have to be capable of making decisions for their child. To my mind it is downright wrong not to leave any power of decision to the mother but then, six days after the discharge from the hospital or when the first illness or the first accident comes about, to tell her: "It's your child. You have to decide what form of treatment you want." I see it as my job as midwife to inform the expectant mothers and fathers and offer them decision-making aids, but I am never authorized to decide for them and their child.

This was something I had to experience in the case of Jeanette …

… almost two weeks past the due date, I was compelled to try to persuade her with a considerable sense of urgency that she should go and see her doctor because I thought the baby's heartbeat was a bit too slow. The cardiotocography confirmed that everything was OK and on the telephone she told me she was relieved, but did not intend to go to the next appointment her doctor had advised her to go to. I merely replied: "We'll see; we'll talk about it when the time comes. If the baby hasn't been born by Monday morning, something will have to happen, because both of you are sure about the date of conception and I don't want to do anything foolhardy. So on Monday, you go for a check-up!" This must have sounded like a threat to Jeanette, because on Sunday night she gave birth to her son. He showed clear signs of being postterm. We both had to admit that the other had been right, that children know themselves when it's high time for them to be born but also that my concern and my warning had been justified.

Inducing Labour

When there are clear indications such as fear, bad premonitions, restlessness, constant ineffective contractions or worrisome examination results, labour has to be induced.

It really can happen that a uterus is incapable of producing contractions, a condition known in medical terminology as uterine insufficiency. But there is no doubt in my mind that in many cases the women are not actually suffering from this hormonal dysfunction. In the majority of cases where induced labour is indicated, there are undoubtedly emotional reasons for the problems, or some confusion about the correct due date. True uterine insufficiency is extremely rare.

Induction of labour is nearly always conducted only in the hospital under the strictest CTG control. For home birth parents, this means that a hospital birth can no longer be avoided. There are a small number of independent birth centres which cooperate with doctors' practices and carry out labour induction in their own facilities.

Here again, I am of the opinion that parents should be involved in the decision, because perhaps the baby knows exactly why it hasn't wanted to leave the womb yet, and perhaps it is worth your while to think everything through again.

Labour-Inducing Methods

Oxytocin Infusion

An infusion of oxytocin is the most common means of inducing labour. This hormone is produced by the woman's pituitary gland, and in cases of insufficient production it can be administered in synthetic form. It is absolutely essential that the baby be monitored closely. You should be aware that the oxytocin infusion takes control of the woman's hormone system from the outside and that she is likely to feel the contractions much more intensely as a result. The need for an analgesic, or pain reliever, is accordingly higher; in many cases the only means of coping is with an Epidural. The reason for this is that, if the body were producing its own oxytocin, the release of serotonin and endorphins would also be increased, i.e. the body's natural analgesic production would be stimulated. The intravenous administration of oxytocin disrupts this system. Very many women report that from the moment the oxytocin infusion began, they could no longer cope with the pain of the contractions.

It is my impression that a woman can sense very well what her body is capable of and what disrupts its natural processes, but the medical-obstetric practices will not be reformed unless and until studies have been conducted on this aspect of childbirth.

Amniotomy/Artificial Rupture of the Membranes(ARM)

Another method is the artificial rupturing of the amniotic sac, the so-called amniotomy. Labour pains generally begin within a few hours after this intervention. It should be well considered, because labour must then be carried through to completion since the child is no longer protected from germs. The danger of infection increases almost hourly. The child is severely restrained in its mobility by this method and may get "wedged" into the pelvic inlet. The sealed amniotic sac gives the baby 'elbow room' since it can turn and bend its head much more easily if surrounded by water. This is a very important factor in the labour process, because the mother's pelvis does not provide much space. In the mid-nineteenth century there was a very important dictate in obstetrics: hands off the amniotic sac! It was strictly forbidden to rupture the membranes. How times and habits have changed! I can only advise all mothers and fellow midwives: leave the course of labour to nature. Avoid rupturing the membranes where at all possible. In the context of home births, this old precept still applies for me as much as ever, and caution with regard to this method has proved to be the best approach in my home birth experience. Children find their way much more easily, and the birthing women are much better able to come to terms with the pains of labour, since the pressure of the baby's head is reduced by the amniotic fluid. The labour pains feel "softer" and the women can cope with them better. The intervals between the contractions often last longer, and the overall labour will take longer, but after all, patience has always been the most important virtue a midwife can have. I try to explain the effect of the contractions where the membranes are intact by pointing out that there is a great difference between applying pressure to a hard object with my bare fist or with a cushioned fist. The retention of an intact amniotic sac is presumably one of the reasons we don't require pain relievers during home births. Naturally, we midwives are well aware that there are obstetrics situations in which the rupturing of the amniotic sac is unavoidable, and you, the birthing mother, will place your trust in us in such moments. The important thing is that impatience alone must never serve as an indication for this measure.

Vaginal Tablets

The administration of *Misoprostol vaginal tablets* is a method of inducing labour which has become very widespread in the past few years. The vaginal suppositories, also available in the form of vaginal gel which is applied to the cervix, contain the contraction-stimulating hormone-like substance prostaglandin, which is produced in various tissues. This is a very effective means of forcing labour. In the context of this method, pregnant women often report, however, that their contractions were extremely strong and painful. Midwives and mothers say that labour is very fast and that everyone involved has difficulty coping with the rapidity of the events. These suppositories are certainly often applied for the simple reason that it sounds relatively harmless when the obstetrician tells the birthing mother: "We'll just insert a suppository near the cervix; maybe that will get the process going, alright?" Now that women have begun to refuse oxytocin infusions since they are aware that it intervenes in the course of labour and increases the contractions, more use is made of this newer method which appears quite harmless. But as I say, its effects should not be underestimated. In my opinion, it even has a decisive disadvantage in comparison with the oxytocin infusion: it is not possible to dose the vaginal suppositories or the gel. Once it has been administered, its effects can no longer be influenced. It is much easier to control an oxytocin infusion or, if the effects are too strong, discontinue it altogether.

The "Ripe" Cervix

The prerequisite for all of the labour induction methods described above is that the due date really has been exceeded and the cervix has ripened and is ready for birth. It is extremely important to check one more time that no mistake has been made in calculating the due date. I frequently go through the maths one more time with the mothers in the last minute and realize that, on the basis of the date of conception, the due date has only been exceeded by a day or two and there is no reason to worry. Do not keep the date of conception a secret if you are certain about it. On the contrary, urge your gynaecologist or midwife to take it into consideration.

Determining the Due Date?

We should really think about it very carefully whether we can allow ourselves to determine a child's date of birth. We probably have no way of judging what it means for the child to have to be born on some particular day. Presumably it will have an influence on the rest of its life. If we believe in astrology, then it is irresponsible simply to decide on the date of a human being's birth ourselves. As is so often the case in life, we should weigh all the pros and cons. It truly sends shivers down my spine when I think back to the years when births were literally programmed. I can only hope that the obstetrics profession will never again revert to such experimental methods. Back then, the motto was: "Tomorrow afternoon at around 4 pm everyone would have time for the birth of this child; let's see if we can arrange it." There is no doubt in my mind that this approach caused a great number of labour-related risks.

But if everything has been checked, monitored and controlled and the mother, father, midwife or doctor is seriously worried, the birth of the baby should be induced without hesitation. As in the case I once experienced with a woman named Simone …

… Simone, her husband and I were all looking forward to the home birth we had planned for. We had gotten to know each other in the context of the birth of her first child and were now waiting for the third. But the waiting was endless. Despite regular premonitory pains, Simone simply did not start having true labour pains. Her cervix was already partway open, the baby's head in the optimal position for birth. But the baby simply did not want to come out. One day after the other passed, and the due date had already been exceeded by eleven days. On Wednesday morning I suddenly had the very certain feeling: today something would have to happen with Simone. We can't go on waiting any longer. When I arrived at her house, I felt my instinct confirmed. It was clear to all of us that the baby was trying to tell us something. We checked the due date for the umpteenth time; it had clearly been eleven days ago. The examination results were unchanged; the fetal heartbeat, which I checked with a small ultrasound device, was strong but too fast in my opinion. A phone conversation with the gynaecologist in attendance confirmed my worries: the hormone levels had fallen significantly. We decided that Simone should go to the hospital and have an OCT (oxitocyn challenge test) carried out, as had already been arranged by phone. Our worries were confirmed. The fetal heartbeat did not bear up under the stress of the OCT. They were weak for a brief period, got stronger again but gave cause for concern. The doctors ruptured the amniotic sac, the contractions soon set in forcefully, and Emil – a healthy baby boy – was born several hours later in the hospital. He had a true umbilical cord knot as well as umbilical cord entanglements. Our decision was right; we had understood the baby's signals even before knowing the results of the lab tests.

Alternative Methods of Inducing Labour

One of the most frequent questions that come up in cases of postterm pregnancy is: "Do you know of any natural methods of getting labour started?" Women often ring up in quite a worried state, because there seems to be no alternative to having labour induced.

Sometimes, however, I have the impression that the women are simply no longer in a position emotionally to endure any more waiting. The pressure of wanting to give birth – or thinking they should – gets stronger and stronger. The women are powerless and often don't know what else they can do: on the one hand they are aware that it can only be a matter of days, and that the child itself knows what the right day is for its birth. On the other hand they are simply fed up with waiting, asking and hoping. This phase often turns into one of the hardest tests of a pregnant woman's patience. She doesn't dare do anything or go anywhere; she keeps the household in tiptop condition because maybe the baby will come that night. The house is always cleaned up immediately; she asks herself over and over whether there is enough food on hand so that her husband won't have to go shopping right after the birth. For days, the neighbour has been calling constantly so as to be available immediately to take care of the older child if necessary. Every morning at the bakers' shop, the woman from the next block is amazed: "You still haven't had that baby! I thought you were already past your due date. And the father's patience is likewise tried. He also feels that he can't stand it anymore when his colleagues greet him at work with typical male humour, saying: "So I guess there won't be a baby after all. Looks like all you did was lay an egg, but not conceive a baby." The situation is stressful, because his workmates aren't always understanding when he breaks out in sweat every time the phone rings and he already sees himself driving through all kinds of red lights because for days the midwife or doctor has been telling his wife: "Once the contractions start, everything is sure to happen very fast; everything is so ripe for birth. Your husband can hopefully get here fast, can't he?" Due to the fact that it could "happen" any minute, fathers have to give up some of their accustomed habits. This is sure to represent a major problem for many a husband. Even before it's born, the baby is intervening in the father's habits. Becoming a father means sacrifices and a bit of inconvenience.

It's not unusual for fathers to say; "What should we do; my holiday is over in ten days, and I can't stay home any longer after that. My colleagues can't postpone their holidays. There's got to be something we can do to get the baby to understand that we are soooo looking forward to its birth. Have you got any advice for us? We don't want to do it with force, just give it a gentle push. That's allowed, isn't it?"

Thus there are a great many circumstances which prompt expectant parents to come by the midwife's practice and ask about natural methods.

Prerequisites

I would like to preface the following words of advice and reports on induction experiences by telling you that these natural methods will only have the desired effect when there is a true readiness for birth, i.e. when the cervix is ripe and the baby is in the correct position for birth. A further prerequisite is that the due date has been re-checked, that the pregnant woman has contacted a midwife and talked to her about the possible methods.

Nipple Stimulation

A very simple and natural form of aid is nipple stimulation. This method has already been in use for several years in obstetrics wards as a form of oxytocin challenge test. Midwives in independent birth centres and naturopathically oriented maternity wards say that for them it represents an effective means of inducing labour.

The woman or couple is requested to rub both nipples energetically for the duration of one minute, then wait two or three minutes and then rub them again. The uterine muscles will thus be stimulated to begin contracting. When a few contractions take place within the next half hour, it is a clear indication that the uterus is ripe for birth. During this time, the fetal heartbeat is monitored with a CTG. If the heartbeat is normal, it can be assumed that the placenta is still providing for the baby optimally. The repetition of this somewhat strenuous procedure over one to two hours is very likely to bring about labour pains, as studies conducted in the U.S. have shown.

Enema, Fasting

An enema accompanied by fasting: an old-fashioned, harmless and effective method. The midwife will carry out the enema, and the expectant mother should drink lots of fluid throughout the course of a day. This frequently leads to the spontaneous commencement of labour pains. An enema with warm water stimulates the intestinal peristalsis and the uterine muscles react with increased contractions.

Natural Prostaglandins

Another effective and entirely natural method is the administration of the natural prostaglandins which are contained in semen. As I have already mentioned in the section on sexual intercourse during pregnancy, these tissue hormones have a contraction-stimulating effect, but only when the pregnant woman's body is ready to give birth. Many parents are surprised when I tell them: "The way to get labour going is the way the baby was conceived." Most women and men say that their book about pregnancy and childbirth advised against having sexual intercourse in the final weeks of pregnancy. I try to set them at ease and explain to them that it will not have any adverse effects for the baby if they sleep together. Maybe it's even nice for the baby if it is sent on its way out into the world with an act of affection. If the contractions are a bit too weak, it almost always suffices to show the baby the way out with this "love method". As was the case with Mrs. S. …

… ten days past her due date, she asked me for advice: "Do you know of anything I can do? I'm supposed to go into the hospital tomorrow or, at the latest, the day after to have labour induced. But we would rather avoid getting an oxytocin infusion if possible." As I always did in this situation, I told her: "The way to get labour going is the way the baby was conceived." "Are you actually saying we can sleep with each other again? My husband keeps suggesting that to me but I was worried it might not be alright. Thank you!" And that was the end of our conversation. The next day there was a message on my answering machine at the midwife's practice: "Thank you for your advice – our little Vanessa was born last night."

An elderly gynaecologist whom I unfortunately met only shortly before he retired used to recommend this natural prostaglandin method to men with a knowing smile: "You know, Mr. Smith, what you should do is take your wife out to a candlelight dinner with a good glass of red wine. You know how women like things, and then, well, the rest will come about of its own accord and you'll see, tomorrow the baby will be here. But don't call me too early; I don't like getting up in the middle of the night!" In other words, it is ideal if the woman can really relax and is very strongly stimulated during intercourse, because then her body will likewise release plenty of prostaglandins. The labour-inducing effect of this substance is widely known. After all, the effect of vaginal suppositories discussed above is also to be attributed to this particular quality of prostaglandins. Naturally there are women who don't want to have intercourse, and there are also cases in which a midwife shies away from recommending it to an expectant mother because the latter makes the impression that she is not accustomed to being addressed openly on the topic of sexuality.

⑤ Herbal Medicine

One effective means seems to me to be a drink containing various spices. It does not bring about any results within a few hours, but usually takes one or two days to work.

What I recommend here is that you prepare *Hebammentee Zimt/Midwives' Tea Cinnamon* for yourself. The ingredients for one litre of tea are: one stick of cinnamon, ten cloves, a small piece of gingerroot and one tablespoon of verbena tea (Verbena officinalis). The spices are simmered over a low heat for ten minutes and the verbena is brewed separately and then poured into a teapot with the spice infusion. This beverage should be sipped throughout the day at a lukewarm temperature. It stimulates the uterine muscles to begin contracting. It helped, for example, in the case of Eunike …

… her first three children had all been born a week before the due date. Now, in her fourth pregnancy, she believed she had already exceeded the due date by six days. During a conversation she was very worried, because she had been having irregular – but very light – contractions every evening for one to two hours. It was clear to her that she would never be able to give birth to her child with such light contractions. She was extremely ill at ease, because even though the first three children had been born a week before the date, according to the midwife who had attended to her they had always been ripe and not had any vernix caseosa. She wanted to give birth to her child now; she was certain that the time had come. "What do you think we should do?" she wanted to know. I advised her to brew herself the above-described tea with cinnamon, cloves, ginger and verbena leaves. I was called to her bedside the following night. A radiant Eunike awaited me: "It really helped; I have regular, strong contractions." She made such a casual and cheerful impression on me that I was almost tempted not to believe her. "That's how women look when the birth isn't going to come about for many, many hours", I thought to myself. But even midwives can be wrong. The family's fourth child was born two hours later. In the place of the above-described spice beverage, many of my fellow midwives also like to recommend the classical Yogi Tea blend with cinnamon, cardamom, ginger, cloves and black pepper.

Aroma Therapy

The abovementioned ingredients of the spice tea – cinnamon, cloves, ginger and verbena – are available in the form of essential oils in the well-known *Ut-Öl/Uterus Tonic 𝒟®* (although the verbena in this blend is the essential oil of the Aloysia tryiphylla). We midwives apply this blend as abdominal massage oil or enhancement for a hot bath. The pregnant woman should massage herself with it several times a day. The contraction-inducing effect can be achieved by moistening your abdomen with hot water, which will accelerate the absorption of the oil, or by making a moist warm abdominal compress after applying the oil. Before the administration of the oil, you can take the hot hayflower steam sitz bath described above. Within about one to two days, this method has already led to success in several cases of postterm pregnancy. Sometimes it suffices for the midwife to carry out a targeted foot reflex zone massage with this oil. My midwife friend Johanna told me about a postterm multipara to whom she had paid a house call for the purpose of carrying out the routine antenatal check-up. Immediately after an abdominal massage and foot treatment with *Ut-Öl/Uterus Tonic 𝒟®*, the woman began having labour pains and Johanna was glad that, as always, she had all of the utensils she needed for a home birth in her car.

Homoeopathic Remedies

It has frequently proven possible to administer homoeopathic remedies to help women begin having contractions spontaneously before having labour induced medically. Once again, I would like to point out that this treatment can only be carried out by a midwife or doctor with experience in homoeopathy. No experiments or self-treatment are to be carried out with these substances.

The homoeopathic medicines I have used most frequently for this purpose to date are: *Caulophyllum, Cimicifuga, Kalium carbonicum, Nux vomica, Pulsatilla, Sepia.*

I had a very interesting experience …

… in connection with one of my first home births. Little Konrad announced himself with a breaking of the water. If labour pains did not begin very soon, it was clear to the mother and me that they would have to be induced in the hospital. In view of her unripe cervix (it was still long and firmly closed), I gave her Caulophyllum, which she was initially to take hourly. Just a few hours later, she already had slight contractions and the cervix had softened a bit, but was still closed. The expectant mother was sad and tears ran down her cheeks because there was no major change in sight. She wanted to avoid going to the hospital at all costs, and was prepared to do everything in her power to be able to have her first child at home.

I then advised her to take Caulophyllum and Pulsatilla alternately at shorter intervals. Thanks to the mother's patience and the effect of the remedies, her cervix opened within the course of several hours, since the contractions had become more regular and stronger. I was quite amazed that we were able to welcome this baby to the world at home, because in my still somewhat inexperienced midwife's eyes the cervix had initially been very unripe, and it seemed completely inconceivable that it could open in such a short time.

… It was a very satisfying experience when a doctor's wife asked me for advice. Her husband had some knowledge of homoeopathy, but couldn't find a suitable remedy. The gynaecologist in attendance was of the opinion that the birth of the twins should now finally be induced since the due date had already been exceeded by five days. The parents wanted to avoid induction if possible, but the woman was waiting longingly for labour pains, which is quite understandable in a case of Gemini pregnancy (pregnancy with twins). When she told me her symptoms it was clear to me that what she needed was Kalium carbonicum. This remedy had the desired effect; the expectant mother soon began having contractions and gave birth to two strong, healthy children. I have often successfully administered this remedy in cases of pregnant women who suffer from back pains and outbreaks of sweat at night, and who make a rather weak impression but still have themselves completely under control.

When Nothing Helps

Of course, it does happen now and then that none of the contraction-inducing methods listed above help, neither nipple stimulation, natural prostaglandins, nor the most carefully selected homoeopathic remedy. This was the case with the second child of a good friend of mine …

… the parents were completely certain that the due date had been correctly calculated. This was a relief, because they had been unsure in the case of their first child, which had taken its time until finally deciding to come out into the world two weeks after the expected date. Now ten days had already passed since the prospective due date. Again she had had constant contractions, but never true labour pains. The condition of the cervix improved daily, became increasingly riper for birth, but the contractions still left a lot to be desired: either they stopped again or were simply too light to make the birth of a child conceivable. Again and again, we tried to find a suitable homoeopathic medication, applied the moxa method, prostaglandins, an enema; but nothing could move this baby to want to be born. The

expectant mother became increasingly worried and impatient, and her mental state was also no longer the best. We decided that it was necessary to have an OCT carried out in the hospital in order to make sure the baby was still faring well. This was fortunately the case and the OCT gave us no cause for worry. The routine administration of a "harmless" spasmolytic (an antispasmodic pain reliever) was accompanied by considerable side effects, and labour had to be induced by an artificial rupturing of the membranes. The baby was clearly not postterm and the mother visibly relieved to have managed the birth. Why this baby could only be born with this massive intervention will always remain a mystery. Whether there are children who really do need a longer period of gestation, or whether this mother suffered from a deep emotional problem which I failed to recognize is something that perhaps nobody but the child knows.

If I had been convinced of the effectiveness of a castor oil cocktail back then, I would have known that it was the only means of avoiding the artificial breaking of the water and all of its consequences.

Castor Oil Cocktail

It is simply incredible how reliably strong labour pains set in after the administration of this cocktail in cases of true postterm pregnancy (!). It is even used very successfully in many hospitals. In numerous cases in which labour was to be induced artificially, the baby was born spontaneously after all thanks to castor oil. I advise the expectant mother to prepare a blend of 20–30 ml of castor oil with a glass of apricot juice and a shot of hard liquor and to drink it. Often whisky or a bit of champagne is used in the place of the liquor. It doesn't matter, as long as it contains alcohol, because otherwise the oil won't dissolve in the juice. And it is important to use apricot juice, because otherwise this method can lead to a threatening loss of potassium, which in turn can bring about a breaking of the water. But if plenty of apricot juice is taken and the dose of castor oil not exceeded, the blend often has no more than a mildly laxative effect. Within three to six hours, strong contractions almost always set in. Especially when the cocktail is taken in the evening, the labour-inducing parasympaticus takes effect. The hospital personnel are not always happy about this point in time, but the parents are. And anyway, deliveries at night are still the nicest. At night nobody just happens into the birth room on account of some formality or other. If the castor oil cocktail fails to work, the mother must assume that the baby simply doesn't want to be born yet. In the case of Marianne, though, it was a suitable means of inducing labour …

… she was pregnant with her third child and, as had been the case with her two sons, already far exceeded the due date. I was beginning to get restless, because no homoeopathic medication led to any mentionable contraction activity. During her last pregnancy, Cimicifuga had been the substance which had led to the birth of the child. Now it was exactly two weeks after the due date. She was prepared to do anything, because she wanted to give birth more than anything, but avoid going to the hospital at all costs. I also suspected that she might be suffering from true uterine insufficiency, because her children were all very big and during her last birth I had had to give her an injection of a labour-inducing

drug – the only one I had ever used in a home birth situation. These considerations led me to send her to the hospital on Monday morning to have labour induced. At the last minute, however, the possibility of using castor oil occurred to me. In view of her ineffective contractions, I advised her to add a drop of the essential oil of verbena to the cocktail. Marianne took this blend in the afternoon, at 9:30 in the evening she thought she might be having light contractions, and at 10:00 she told me they really were labour pains but still very bearable. We agreed that she would ring me up again when the contractions got stronger. On instinct, I drove to her house anyway, and at 11:05 a postterm little girl weighing 4,500 grams was born. We were all completely astonished at the rapidity of the birth, especially the father, who simply couldn't believe that the birth was about to happen because has wife had been in labour quite a long time with the first two boys. Little Veronika was initially quite indignant about life outside the womb – I had hardly ever heard a newborn scream so shrilly. But we were happy about those screams of course – after all, the mother had been spared labour induction with an oxytocin infusion.

In my opinion it was the drop of verbena that had triggered this extremely strong contraction activity. For that reason, I never again recommended verbena as a supplement. Many of my colleagues interpreted this story differently, however, and made a point of using this extra drop. I would like to voice an urgent plea not to regard essential oils as harmless plant extracts! On the contrary: they are extreme concentrations of plant-based active substances, and we are often groping in the dark when we take them. The addition of one to three drops of *verbena 10% in jojoba wax* can be tried in the second castor oil cocktail, but must always be taken under a midwife's supervision, as is the case with the cocktail in general. It is essential that the fetal heartbeat be checked regularly.

If the abovementioned prerequisites are all fulfilled and this traditional method is applied, most children have no choice but to set out for life outside the womb.

unsuspected forces
downward
outward
earth and light
let go
you and me

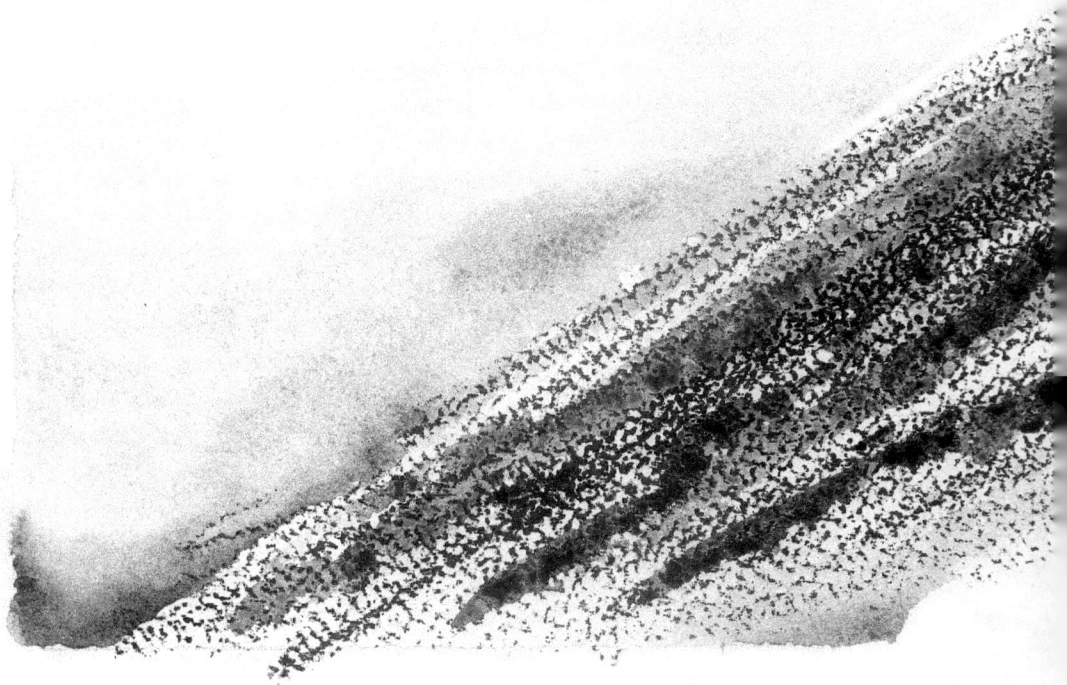

CHILDBIRTH

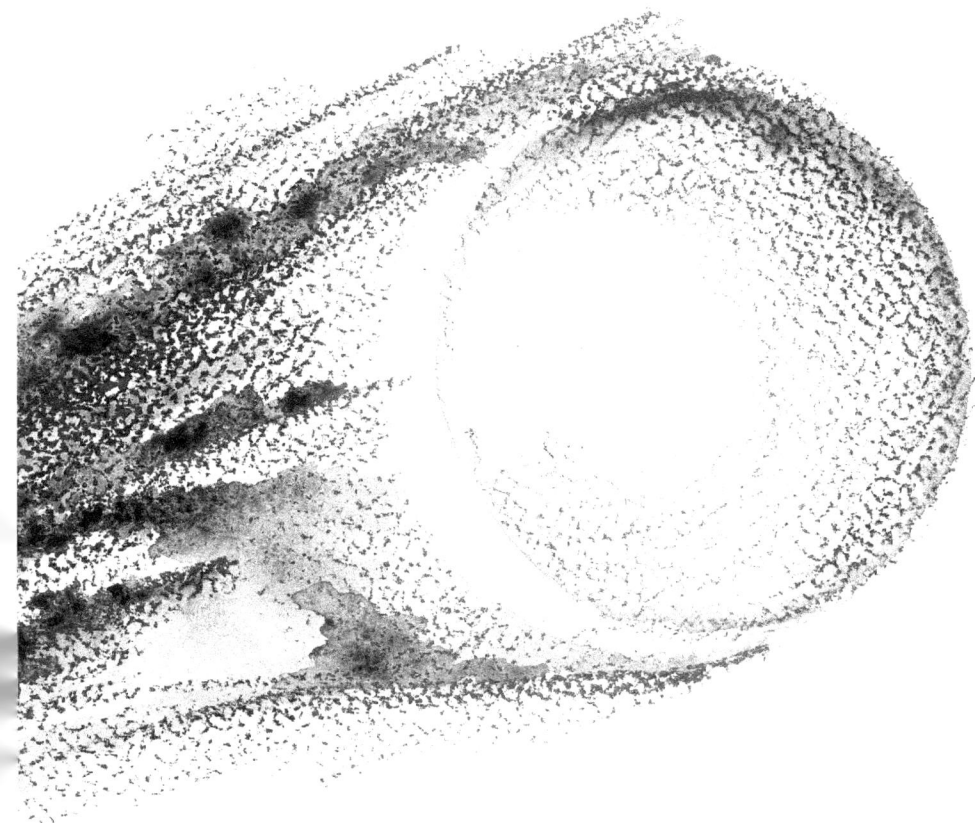

THE BIRTH EVENT

Natural Childbirth

Before I begin to discuss the signs that herald childbirth, I consider it important to define birth – the event of human childbirth. I would like to draw a comparison with nature so that you know what I mean by natural childbirth. Again and again, I notice that this term is used to refer to all kinds of things. And I often have the impression that it is simply "fashionable" to want natural childbirth.

For me it is extremely important – especially at the antenatal classes carried out jointly with the fathers – to introduce the concept of "natural childbirth" as a mental image. A great many men want their children to undergo childbirth naturally, and do not want them born under drug-induced conditions. Unfortunately I often hear men say: "Other women have managed to give birth to children; mine will accomplish it too." Sometimes I have the impression that men are just not capable of really imagining childbirth and the pain associated with it. But then, when the time has come and the woman is lying in the birthing bed, moaning and trying to breathe through her contractions, birthing her baby with screams, the man suddenly can't deal with the fact that this is something entirely natural. Midwives who work in hospitals often tell stories of the kind that I remember all too well from the period when I worked in a hospital myself: that in many situations it is the expectant father, of all people, who worriedly asks his wife whether she wouldn't like to take the analgesia offered by the doctor after all. The men are the ones whom the midwives ask with begging eyes to help their wives so everything is over faster. For this reason, it has always been important to inform the men not only about the 'mechanisms' of birth, but also – and especially – about what goes on for the woman on the emotional and sensorial level during labour.

For me the birth of a human being is a natural event. By "natural event" I mean the rare, extreme and deeply moving experiences of a human being. The birth of a child overwhelms and fascinates the parents; it is an event they will normally have the good fortune to experience only once or a very few times. A natural event remains in the minds of human beings just as a birth event does, and those who have experienced it later recall that they were overwhelmed by the power and force of nature. Whether descriptions of a storm, a violent thunderstorm, a raging sea, a flood or even the emergence of a new island in the middle of the ocean – all of these occurrences are associated with natural forces and powers. And it is precisely as such that I experience the birth of a child, every time anew. The forces that allow contractions to come about and the cervix to open and push the baby out through the vaginal canal are nothing short of incredible. As women we feel this force take possession of us, and all we can do is allow it to sweep us along, giving our bodies full play. Letting herself go, allowing things to flow freely, letting everything go – as soon as a woman has recognized the necessity of doing that, childbirth becomes something she can achieve; it becomes a positive experience. Naturally there are also gentle, poignant natural occurrences such as the emergence of a tiny plant from the soil. The way the tip of the shoot pushes its way through the soil, the way the earth crumbles, opens first a tiny crack, then wider and wider and makes way for the tendril, that is also birth. The earth can't speak, or do we simply not hear it with our ears? Maybe it also hurts to make way for this shoot. During growth, plants are susceptible to disease, because a lot of energy is demanded of them during that phase. There are women who give birth to their children as loudly as a storm beating the land with its waves. But I also know women who give birth to their children with a great amount of silent energy; their entire focus is directed inwardly and their facial features clearly show the positive energy that is working inside them. I advise all expectant fathers to take a good look at their wives' facial features. Women in labour are beautiful; they are soft and strained, but never distorted or tortured. If this is the man's impression, then he should look at his wife carefully. Particularly during the interval between the pains, it is fascinating to see the relaxed, expectant face of the birthing woman. The words of Katja, who was present at the birth of her little sister, confirmed this observation. She encouraged her mother, saying: "You look so beautiful, just as if you had to do strenuous, good work. You'll see; I'm sure you'll manage everything just fine!"

It is extremely important that all of the persons present at the birth are aware of this natural occurrence, because only then can they understand why the woman behaves as she does and only then will they find the right words with which to accompany her. Natural occurrences can also cause us human beings a lot of fear and worry, especially when we are surprised by them. In situations in which we are lying, lost in thought, maybe even asleep, on an air mattress, surfboard or the like, and floating in the sea, a suddenly rising storm with high waves will scare and unsettle us quite a bit more than if we had seen the clouds in the sky when we were swimming out in the first place. To float on a stormy sea far from the shore – that is one way of imagining the experience of labour pains. What I mean is that an expectant mother can cope with her contractions better if she is prepared for them, if she tries to adapt to the force and the swell – i.e. the contractions – of the birth. An expectant father will be able to place more confidence in his partner's ability to come to terms with labour if he knows that she will find her way out there on the stormy sea, because he has already trusted her to be strong and powerful in other situations as well. It is completely understandable that we human beings become afraid in new life situations and call for help. When cool-headed people in our surroundings encourage us again and communicate clearly to us that this life process can and must be lived through, we can mobilize enormous strength and reach that faraway shore on our own steam. As the partner of this woman in a state of distress, the man will sometimes feel like the person waiting on the shore, sometimes as though he were swimming right along with her. The midwife sometimes takes over the role of the encouraging person, sometimes that of the co-swimmer who remembers what it was like to be in a state of distress herself, and together they will reach the safety of the shore. She often brings a boat or a lifejacket to the woman struggling out there in the waves. Sometimes she calls the coastguard and has her rescued as fast as lightning and treated with medication, but on shore other obstetricians are responsible, because it has also cost the midwife quite a bit of energy to cope with those waves.

Try to prepare for a natural birth by calling images such as these to mind, and you will then perhaps understand the natural occurrence of birth a bit sooner. And thus you are likely to accept that we also need 'obstetrical medicine' and must never dismiss it. Regardless of whether you are planning for a hospital or a home birth, leave all the emergency exits open for yourself and get acquainted with the life-savers.

You will probably be wondering at this point: "Yes, but if childbirth is a natural occurrence, why do so many women have to be rescued with medication and an analgesia?" In response, I would like to repeat my understanding that birth is not a routine procedure but a natural occurrence, and in such situations many people react with fear and panic; after all, many people have died in conjunction with childbirth. It is true that women have been giving birth to children since the beginning of mankind, often without help, but women and children have died during childbirth for just as long. In our high-tech medical world, this fact is easily repressed. Just a few generations ago, even in the more highly developed parts of the world, women had to resign themselves to the fact that the mortality rate among children was high, and that many babies died during childbirth. In old fairy tales, stepmothers are a well-known motif, partly because a few centuries ago the death of the real mother during childbirth was a frequent occurrence.

It always causes me to stop and think when I hear about the high consumption of pain relievers and the huge percentage of birthing women who make use of epidural anaesthesia (EDA or PDA) – sometimes even exceeding fifty percent – or that only six percent of hospital deliveries take place without medical intervention (analgesics, labour-inducing or tocolytic medications) or surgical interventions (episiotomy, caesarean section). The rate of problematic cases in obstetrics was and is surely never that high. I consider these medical measures to be indispensable in cases of home births which must be moved to the hospital because of insurmountable problems, but the rate of such births is only one to two percent. Then there is also a large number of parents whose wish to have the birth at home cannot be fulfilled because the pregnancy is recognized from the outset as being high-risk. Another justification for medically/technically oriented obstetrics is the large number of pregnant women who unfortunately never come to a midwife's practice for antenatal care and counselling because for one reason or another their pregnancies are under medical supervision from the beginning and constant risk control is necessary. Even in these cases, however, consultations with a midwife are possible.

Due to the care taken by every midwife in deciding whether or not to carry out a home birth in each individual case, and due to optimal birth preparation, the rate of interrupted home births is quite low, as mentioned above. But pregnant women can proceed on the assumption that even in the hospitals it would be possible to conduct a greater proportion of non-medically supported deliveries and practice natural childbirth methods to a greater extent. This view has been confirmed by the independent birth centres for years. In hospitals where the maternity wards are women-oriented and naturopathic methods are employed – and are directed by midwives – the percentage of high-risk births is substantially lower. So it can be hoped that in the future – even if only because of the necessity of cutting costs – approaches will change and there will be an increasing number of midwife-directed labour wards in the hospitals as well. Midwife-directed births not only have a lower rate of medical intervention but, as a result, there are fewer consequential costs brought about by side effects. World Health Organization studies provide evidence that deliveries attended to by midwives lead to greater well-being for mothers and babies alike, but require the attentive accompaniment and assistance of the midwife and not the overly hasty employment of medication and machines. It is thus in the interest of expectant parents to obtain a sufficient amount of information and choose the place of their child's birth carefully. The number of medical institutions which are prepared to work with midwives from the outside is steadily increasing. Expectant parents can also ask about a hospital's internal statistics, such as the rates of episiotomies, epidural anaesthesias, water births and caesarean sections. Women giving birth in a hospital have a right to attendance by a midwife, and the latter has a good sense of finding the right balance between patiently allowing things to take their course and intervening with technical means. The basic attitude of midwives is one which respects the right of the woman to self-determination and encourages her self-confidence during birth. I am happy about the fact that, with this book, I have already supported many women in undergoing childbirth the way it is best for them.

Only a small proportion of anaesthetics, analgesia, episiotomies and operative interventions are absolutely justified. The fact that one hospital has only a fraction of the episiotomies, caesareans and epidurals counted in another hospital in the neighbouring town speaks for itself. Even the fact that a central municipal or university hospital takes on a larger proportion of high-risk cases does not justify the extremely high rates of technical and medical interventions.

The frequent medical interventions are not always related to the risks associated with childbirth. Rather, to my mind, they are often a reflection of hospital routine, everyday hospital practices, personnel shortages with regard to midwives and obstetricians, etc. A large proportion of them are probably to be attributed to the training situation of midwives and doctors. On the other hand, the trend towards naturally oriented obstetrics has increased strongly in midwife training programmes. Our profession is bethinking its traditional tasks and the midwife's autonomy. We make every effort to allow childbirth to take its natural course and to leave the mother and baby the time they need.

Many decades ago, when hospital obstetrics were just being developed, there were single pregnant women who were not admitted to most hospitals. At university hospitals, they were literally used as obstetrics "guinea pigs". Naturally such practices are no longer possible, and it is my greatest wish that the days in which women are used as living practice subjects for obstetrics will never return. But how is a midwife-in-training now supposed to learn to carry out an episiotomy or a perineal suture, to employ the suction cup/vacuum extractor and the birth forceps; how are all these obstetric interventions to be taught? It is downright cynical, however, to cite this problem as a justification for the great numbers of episiotomies (though the latter has decreased from a horrendous ninety percent to the present forty-five percent, which is still too high) or Epidurals rates of some sixty to seventy percent which is the average in many hospitals. In several maternity units, analgesia is still routinely administered to one woman in two, despite the knowledge of their considerable side effects for the child. The use of medications containing morphine is still par for the course in many delivery rooms, although there are clear indications that it can not only cause respiratory depression in the baby immediately after delivery, but that later addiction to drugs can be traced back to this practice.

I ask myself again and again why so many parents strive for a natural birth, but the birthing mother then supposedly begs for analgesia and anaesthetics. In addition to the reasons mentioned above, I believe the cause is also to be found in our modern society. During the birth of a child, for the first time in their lives, nearly all young women reach the very limits of what they can achieve, and in the transition phase they even have to go beyond those limits. And to make another comparison to the old days, it seems clear to me that, back then, people were challenged much more strongly by life during childhood and youth. They had to grow into adults under difficult living conditions. Everyday life was associated with physical strain and deprivations. Parents had to fear for their children's lives because the latter contracted serious illnesses much more frequently, illnesses that took them to the brink of death. Women who have grown up more recently usually look back on a carefree childhood, have tended to be spoiled, could afford everything they needed and wanted, were able to take the bus to school and, later on, drive to work, and thanks to modern medicine have never been seriously ill. They were also not burdened by the fear of childhood diseases, because multiple vaccinations had made them immune to those diseases. Now, during pregnancy, and often not until labour is in progress, they realize that, for the first time in their lives, their bodies have to perform true, physically strenuous work. Inadequate awareness of pain is undoubtedly to blame for the "failure" of natural childbirth. Many people are simply not willing to endure any pain at all, the pain threshold has become very low. Amazingly, many women say that during pregnancy they attempted to undergo dental intervention without anaesthesia for the first time, and were very surprised to find that targeted breathing exercises helped them in this situation as well. So really it comes as no surprise – and cannot simply be blamed on the hospitals and their personnel – that the use of medication is only gradually decreasing.

In many cases it is thus quite evidently necessary for women to change their inner attitude in order to put the theory of natural birth into practice. It is likewise important for expectant fathers to familiarize themselves with this topic in order to be able to provide their wives with real help. If they just repeat the viewpoint: "Of course our child will be delivered by natural childbirth" and then, a few minutes later, say: "No, sweetheart, don't do that strenuous work; I'll take care of it", or: "Please don't walk; I'd rather drive you", they're not really thinking about what they're saying. An expectant father should not relieve his wife of the normal work and strains of everyday life, because he won't be able to relieve her of the labour of childbirth. Instead, he should place his confidence in her so that she can learn to recognize her own physical limits during pregnancy. The child will signal clearly to the mother when these limits have been reached.

Once again, I would like to communicate to all expectant fathers that their wives are much more capable of bearing physical strain than you think. During labour, at the latest, you are likely to realize that we women aren't such a weak sex after all, but merely very sensitive and often changeable in our feelings – attributes not to be equated with weakness.

I would like to encourage all women to look forward to giving birth and tell them they can by all means be confident in their abilities to achieve this 'work' and to develop unsuspected energies, which they will undoubtedly experience later on in life – i.e. in retrospect – as something very empowering. It is no coincidence that we sometimes hear people say: "It's amazing; she's changed a lot since she had a baby. Suddenly she defends all kinds of causes and fights for things she never even used to be aware of, or even condemned." This is how the birth of a child changes a woman's sense of herself, as in the case of Mrs. B. ...

... after giving birth to her child she was suddenly able to carry out tasks she had previously always refused to do or passed on to others. She could remember many such situations, for example a hiking trip in the mountains, during which she had gotten to a point – before she ever became pregnant – where she simply could not go another step. Now, several years later, at the very same spot on that steep slope, she remembered the situation during labour when she also had the feeling she couldn't go on, but the midwife encouraged her not to give up; after all, the baby couldn't just stay in her tummy. So just as she had done during that birth, she mobilized all of her strength, pushed herself and made it up to the top of the mountain.

Mothers have similar experiences when their children are sick. Susanne recounted ...

... you were right, Inge, it's not so easy to care for a sick child. I was so worried about my little one, because the fever just refused to go down. And then I remembered that moment during labour when the fetal heartbeat suddenly got slower and weaker; I was also extremely afraid for my child in that situation. Now, this one night when my daughter's temperature was so high, I whispered to her: "Come, we're both very strong, you'll get over this fever and I don't have to worry about you because during your birth the two of us also managed it together." So I spent the night by my daughter's bedside, gave

her sponge baths to reduce the fever and finally, towards morning, her temperature went down. Just like during her birth: she was born at sunrise, and this time she got healthy at sunrise.

Actually, I am frequently amazed about the fact that, in this of all times, people are expressing the desire for natural childbirth again – in an era in which technology, research and progress threaten to destroy the world. In this change of direction in the area of obstetrics I see a chance for the rebirth of mankind. A new age, a new mentality, will always begin with birth. In the desire for natural childbirth and – more and more frequently – home births, I see a wish for safety and peace. Maybe children help many families to reconsider the way they think about things and to ask themselves what the future will bring us. Medical obstetrics has been changing for years in many places. An increasing number of hospitals are taking the genuine needs of the birthing women as their orientation. A constantly growing number of midwives, for example, are introducing homoeopathy to the birth room. This is surely one of the greatest successes of the past years in obstetrics – actually a field dominated by medical practices: from the perspective of the pharmacological pictures of homoeopathic remedies, midwives, women and obstetricians learn that childbirth is something to be experienced, it is achievable and natural, and it takes time.

"Gentle Birth", The Atmosphere during Childbirth

I notice again and again that the term "gentle birth" is mentioned in association with natural childbirth, as if the two concepts were interchangeable. The truth is, they have nothing in common. We can, however, allow birth to take its natural course and try to handle the child gently in the process. Leboyer, the founder of "birth without violence", did not invent this term as a means of saying that the course of childbirth is gentle, but that, during birth, everyone involved should encounter the child in a normal and natural way and do everything in their power to make its transition from the womb to the outside world as gentle as possible. What he is referring to here is the atmosphere in the mother's and newborn's surroundings. The important thing is to arrange the room in such away that it radiates a sense of cosiness and safety. The ideal has been reached when it is a room in which the birthing woman feels good. It is an extremely positive development that more and more hospitals are redesigning their maternity wards and creating pleasant atmospheres there. With fabric, soothing colours, plants, music and aroma oils, a dreary, tiled birth room can quickly be improved in the manner advocated by Leboyer.

When labour begins, everyone present should make an effort to adapt to the 'birth mood'. It should be conveyed to the birthing woman that she is truly being guided and accompanied by those in attendance, that they are bearing her along – in the psychological sense – in her labour and birth-giving situation. The woman in labour should be given a sense of safety and hominess, enhanced with pleasant background music if she wants it. The creation of such an atmosphere also means keeping unimportant things and noises out. A birthing woman needs protection and has to be shielded from external influences such as telephones, doorbells and street noise. People who are not supposed to be present at the birth and would detract from the quality of this intimate situation have to be turned away at the door. Even the most trivial disturbance can agitate the woman in labour. The birthing woman should be able to retreat and concentrate entirely on what is going on in her body. Conversations about the latest news or last or next year's holidays are absolutely uncalled for and out of place.

Every person present must be conscious of the fact that here, in this room, a human being will soon be born: a little child which has come to life in the affectionate embrace of two people and will now be born into that relationship. It should be clear to every birth companion that he or she has the honour of witnessing the birth of a human being. This little person should be allowed to be born in a calm, pleasant atmosphere. That means: no neon lights by way of welcome, but rather candlelight; no cold air but pleasant warmth, so as to spare the newborn the shock of the temperature difference to the greatest extent possible. The room should be at a temperature of about 25 °C/77 °F. The normal body temperature is 37 °C/98.6 °F, and everyone involved should call to mind what a temperature drop of 12 °C/22 °F is like. It means a fluctuation from a summery 24 °C/75 °F to a wintry 12 °C/54 °F. So it's no wonder that the babies undergo a shock and are literally frightened into breathing. This effect is vital for the baby, should not be heightened, however, but rather moderated at all costs. We, the parents, midwives and obstetricians, can help the baby by allowing it to sink into a soft, warm, reddish cloth. For forty weeks, the baby's environment has had an even temperature and been softly illuminated by light filtered red by the muscles and placenta, mixed with the blue shimmer of the amnion (amniotic sac) membranes. The baby is therefore accustomed to being warm and softly bedded in a bluish-red, moist atmosphere.

We cannot spare a person this transition from inside to outside when he or she is born. It is undoubtedly of great importance for the newborn to feel distinctly that a change has come about so that its vital functions become active. But the contractions, the narrow birth canal and the change in pressure already contribute to this process. With a water birth, the transition from water to land can be alleviated. The confinement of the birth canal does not end on hard land, the pressure difference is not so great, but rather the baby comes out in water of the accustomed warmth. The baby can then recover for a moment from all that pressing and pushing. As soon as one of its arms or legs is exposed to the air, it is usually lifted gently out of the water by the mother herself, and permitted to take a look at the world from the vantage point of the mother's warm, wet tummy or breast. Due to the difference in pressure under water, the dilation pain is not nearly as strong for the mother. The birth-related injuries are considerably milder than 'on dry land', if only for the reason that nobody reaches for the scissors quite as quickly, since everything feels different under water and the obstetricians are not as practiced in carrying out the cut under water, particularly in view of the fact that the birth is taking place inconveniently far down.

It is a wonderful experience to receive the just-born child in a secure environment and to feel how quickly it recovers from the stress of birth, begins to breathe calmly and slowly opens its eyes. We should all allow the baby time to get its bearings in the world, to slide gently into the world of light, hardness and cold. We should create a soft transition by being silent and attentive, deeply moved by this wonderful moment; all lights should be dimmed, all voices subdued to a minimum. For me, to experience the birth of a human being means to hold man's incarnation in reverence. There are no words to describe these moments during and after the birth of a child. You have to experience it.

I will never forget my first "gentle" experiences of birth, when I became conscious of what it means to be born and wrapped in sterile white towels. My way of accompanying parents during home birth was still strongly influenced by my knowledge of the hospital routine. For me there was no question that the child had to be wrapped in white cotton towels which had been washed in boiling hot water and now pre-warmed to receive the baby. I was just about to swaddle little just-born Anna-Lena in a warm white towel when her father whispered to me: "Inge, look, we prepared this warm, red, fluffy terry cloth towel especially for this purpose; please use this instead." This moment made a lasting impression on me: the little girl immediately stopped screaming, relaxed, opened her eyes and inquisitively met her mother's gaze. I was deeply moved and could hardly believe what I saw. A short time later I exchanged the red towel for a white one. The newborn's answer was prompt: she cried for a moment, squeezed her eyes shut – and was immediately wrapped in red again.

My understanding of a gentle birth thus consists of: calmness, a feeling of safety, warmth and a reddish environment, leaving the child to its parents, cutting the umbilical cord later on when it is no longer pulsating (providing this postponement is medically tenable); giving the mother the means of receiving the baby at her own speed – not laying the baby on her tummy immediately but waiting until she has recovered from the strain of birth, even if it takes a few minutes; allowing eye contact between the parents and the baby and waiting until they want to take it into their arms of their own accord. As a midwife it is indescribably wonderful to hold the child in my arms, to feel how it enters life, to see the liberated, radiant eyes of the mother and the deeply moved and astounded eyes of the father. And then to have the honour of witnessing how, slowly, a finger, a hand, the parents' four arms reach for the baby and wrap themselves around it.

In my opinion, it is this course of events that Leboyer would like to introduce, and thus enable the child to be born gently.

Duration of Labour

In addition to a positive attitude and an atmosphere in which the birthing woman feels comfortable and at ease, another essential prerequisite for natural childbirth is that no demands be made with regard to the duration of the labour. As long as the mother and child are both faring well, there is no reason to hurry. There are cases in which the baby signals to the mother for days: I'm coming soon. The woman has regular contractions which then stop again just as regularly. The cervix ripens and slowly opens. The birthing woman can have a refreshing night's sleep or experience restful daytime hours. Sooner or later, she will begin to have strong contractions and the baby will be born. On the other hand, there are children who don't go back and forth on the matter for days, but are born within a few hours. As expectant parents, you should prepare yourself mentally for anything and everything. Remember, that in any case everything will turn out differently from the way you expect. And since you presumably don't experience the birth of a child every year, the family and the father's employer will be able to endure the temporary uncertainty for once. We self-employed midwives live with this uncertainty as well – sometimes more, sometimes less calmly.

Operative Childbirth

My readers are surely aware that not all births take place naturally, gently and in the normal way. In this book, however, I would like to limit myself to reporting about natural birth experiences. There is other, specialized literature on operative births carried out with the aid of suction cup/vacuum extraction, forceps or caesarean sections. If one of these obstetrics techniques becomes necessary, then there is no way around it, and the obstetricians have their reasons for making the decisions they make. Have faith that the mother and child will only be subjected to what is absolutely necessary, and that everything humanly possible will be done to help both of them. Just as on a lovely summer day a thunderstorm can blow up completely unexpectedly, what was expected to be a normal birth (spontaneous birth) can suddenly turn into an operative one. Everyone involved, particularly parents, have to be able to adjust quickly to new situations.

If it is highly probable or – on account of existing risks – already determined during pregnancy that you will undergo a caesarean or ventouse delivery, then I would like to recommend that you talk about it with your midwife. She will do everything she can to explain the most important aspects. Parents always have to be informed about possible deviations from the norm.

If pregnancy takes its course without complications, however, you should first inform yourself about normal, spontaneous birth before reading up on exceptional circumstances, and simply look forward to giving birth, because 96 percent of all children know they are supposed to be born head down.

Nevertheless, there are trends which I view critically: fifteen years ago the rate of caesarean sections was still 13 percent, and that of manual birth aids 20 percent. In the meantime, however, in Germany we already have a caesarean rate of 20 to 25 percent, and in many places nearly 40 percent or even more (!), whereas in Scandinavia the caesarean rate has remained at a constant 10 percent. These increases in the statistics really give me pause, especially considering that the female pelvis has not changed, and that affluence and good nutrition represent optimal preconditions for a normal course of labour, as do the close surveillance system that constitutes antenatal care. And in fact, it is not the rate of true risks that has risen – for example premature detachment of the placenta – but rather women's readiness to decide in favour of operative delivery. The rise in the number of operative interventions can be attributed to the policies of both the hospital administrations and the medical practitioners as well as to the parents' fear of normal childbirth, in which the woman's emotions cannot be controlled. What they don't tell expectant parents is that the growing rate of caesareans goes hand in hand with a rise in the number of post-operative problems; the risk of death for the mothers increases, and the consequences of this development for human behaviour in relation to childbearing are unforeseeable.

"Elective Caesareans"

Despite the risks of operative childbirth, there is a new, peculiar, and very questionable trend spreading in Europe these days: the desire to give birth to a child by caesarean section. A method employed until now in cases of emergency is thus becoming routine. It nevertheless is and will remain a complicated, major surgical intervention, the risk of which is much greater for both mother and child than spontaneous birth. Not to mention the psychological burden the mother takes upon herself. What is more, there is no telling what the consequences will be of having an entire generation of children whom we rob of the opportunity and the challenge of taking a strenuous but achievable route. Mothers are often not conscious of the fact that the hours after a caesarean are dominated by the pain of the wound and a bedridden state, that they can't have their babies with them, that the phase of getting to know their child and how to breastfeed it is dominated by infusion tubes, intensive care and painkillers. The women do not experience the natural feeling of happiness and well-being brought about by the production of certain hormones, which are reduced to a minimum by the anaesthesia and the various medications taken. The intimacy with the partner and the newborn is constantly interrupted by the measures required for the proper care of a person who has just undergone surgery. Problems with breastfeeding are therefore often par for the course. And an early- discharge birth is therefore virtually inconceivable, at least in Germany. I would like to point out in this context that, for lack of funds, in many other countries in the world women are discharged from hospital as early as three days after a caesarean, a practice which certainly does not contribute to the safety of mother and child. In Germany the issue is being discussed as to whether a caesarean has to be financed by the parents themselves if it is carried out on request. The interests of scientific medicine, the woman herself and the society all tend in the same general direction, and the future will show what the true concern is: the health and safety of mother and child or a trend, or even a change in the developmental history of childbirth.

The gynaecologist Dorothee Struck of Kiel is likewise repeatedly amazed at how strongly the risks of caesarean are played down by medical practitioners. She says: "Naturally, caesarean sections have come to be quite safe, but the rate of thrombosis and embolism during the postnatal period is ten times higher after a caesarean than after vaginal birth. As a surgeon, I have often stumbled across problems in a woman's abdomen which wouldn't have been there if she had not had a (planned) caesarean in the past. For example adhesions [fibrous bands of scar tissue that bind together normally separate bodily tissues] which can lead to obstruction of the bowels, gaps in the abdominal wall which can develop into hernial orifices, adhesions between the bladder and uterus or other organs. Sometimes cells from the uterine membrane can be displaced to cause endometriosis [the abnormal occurrence of functional endometrial tissue outside the uterus] in the abdominal wall. When operations have to be carried out later in life, for example a hysterectomy or the removal of a section of the large intestine due to cancer, there is a significantly larger number of complications if operations have been carried out previously in the same region of the body. Scar tissue does not heal as well, and adhesions heighten the risk of inadvertently injuring adjacent organs such as the bladder. These risks are all worth taking when there are cogent medical reasons why a child cannot be born in the normal way. Otherwise, a caesarean upon request is only seemingly the simpler alternative, comfortable, plannable, except for the patient with the post-operative intestinal obstruction or the embolus."

Dorothee Struck MD concludes with the intentionally provocative question: "If you want to be able to plan your whole life beforehand, why do you want to have a child?"

THE SIGNS OF LABOUR

Among the most frequent "FAQs" posed by expectant parents are:
- How will we be able to tell when labour has begun?
- When do we ring up the midwife and ask her to come?
- When is it time to drive to the hospital?

Naturally, midwives attempt to answer these questions as well as they can, but I point out again and again that the expectant mother should trust her instinct and in an emergency will undoubtedly be able to judge best when she needs help.

Rule Number One for the entire pregnancy in general and for the beginning of labour in particular is:

As soon as a pregnant woman becomes uneasy and worried and asks for help, she should call a midwife, consult with an obstetrician or go to a hospital, depending on the possibilities and the situation – regardless of whether the contractions are taking place at shorter or longer intervals, whether the waters have broken or bleeding has occurred, whether day or night, whether this feeling of unease arises before or after the due date. The behaviour of the expectant mother is the clearest signal as to whether and when she needs help.

For a woman giving birth for the first time, this is the unknown experience to end all unknown experiences. She finds herself facing all kinds of completely new situations and questions: How do we recognize the contractions? How much time do we have after the contractions have begun in earnest? Will we get to the hospital on time? What if we ask for help too early? What should we do if the water breaks? What does it mean if I have bleeding? What if the child surprises us by being born at home? Is it possible to sleep through the birth of a child? When should I call my husband, when does it make sense to have him with me?

Incidentally, these questions are also of significance for women who have given birth in the past. The beginning of labour is always an entirely new situation for all expectant parents. Once again, they are faced with the worry: How will this baby announce itself? Will labour go faster than last time, or will it take longer? Should we stay home longer this time? Can we wait until the grandparents have arrived to take care of the children? What should we do with the children when labour starts in the middle of the night? Should we have someone come to our house to take care of them or should they sleep somewhere else? The questions concerning the care of the older children should be considered by all parents well in advance, regardless of whether childbirth and the early postnatal period are to take place in the hospital or at home. If a child has never slept away from home or from its parents, problems can arise if the first time happens in conjunction with the advent of the new baby sister or brother. It seems to me to be particularly important that the child knows the babysitter well and that it is a person who is capable of offering a child plenty of distraction, so that the birthing woman doesn't have a hard time leaving her child in that person's care. I recommend to all parents that they contact various friends and acquaintances. Otherwise it is sensible to do what a father I knew did several years ago, when his new baby was in a particularly great hurry …

… the minute he got home it was clear to the father that his wife was already having strong labour pains and it no longer made sense to wait for the grandparents. Without hesitation, he put his son into the car along with his labouring wife and drove to the hospital as fast as he could. Upon entering the maternity ward he put his son into the arms of the first doctor he saw and said "Please take care of him; as you can see, my wife needs me at the moment." The dumbfounded doctor nodded, the midwife took the woman, who was already in the final stage of labour, into the birth room. A quarter of an hour later, the 'freshly baked' father fetched his son again. The doctor said: "That was a completely new – and very appealing – form of obstetrics."

Contractions

You recognize contractions by the rhythmic intervals at which the uterine muscles tense up, i.e. contract. Initially, what you feel is your abdomen getting hard. In most cases, the uterus takes on a clearly spherical form during a contraction. At first this hardening will take place irregularly and be accompanied by pain in the area of the sacrum or groin, similar to the pain felt in conjunction with menstruation. It is important to be aware that the pain is not necessarily felt in the abdomen. Just as you can also have menstrual pain in the lower back, initial labour pains can likewise radiate from your back. The contractions can also be felt in the abdomen, which can harden from top to bottom or beginning at the navel and moving outward on both sides. Another equally likely possibility is that you feel the force of the contractions only in the area of the pubic bone, or that the pangs start there and move to the back by way of the groin. It is rare, but some women say that the pains radiate into their thighs. If this is the case, it will be more difficult to breathe your way through the contractions, but you will surely succeed in coping, because we can reach every part of our bodies with our breath (cf. p. 42).

Sooner or later the intervals between these contractions will develop a certain regularity and the pangs will turn into outright pain. With targeted abdominal breathing, however, this muscle cramp can be made quite endurable. Now is the point in time when you are glad you learned something about breathing during contractions. You will realize that it isn't as difficult as you thought to come to terms with the breathing. Many pregnant women are worried they will have forgotten everything by the time the due date rolls around. And of course it does happen that initially they are so excited that it takes them some time to find the right breathing rhythm, but that's not bad. After all, labour pains last several hours and there will be plenty of time to get adjusted. It's like taking a test: at the beginning, many people have the feeling that their minds are completely blank and then suddenly everything goes smoothly. This is exactly what a woman undergoes when the contractions start: first everything is all wrong and then she starts remembering the exercises learned during the antenatal sessions and the breathing starts flowing correctly all of its own accord, and soon she will understand the benefits of targeted abdominal breathing. Because if she breathes slowly and regularly, the labour pains become bearable and can be experienced. This targeted concentration has a hypnotic effect and the pain really does feel less acute.

As soon as the pregnant woman feels the need to breathe her contractions with a loud Aaaaaaaaaaaaaaaa..........., the expectant father and the midwife can be sure that the birth phase has begun.

Experience has taught me that this phase has been reached when the interval between the contractions is about five minutes, counting from the beginning of a contraction. The contractions themselves will last about forty to sixty seconds, the interval between them only three to four minutes.

When should you leave for the hospital? – False Alarms

Pregnant women are often advised to go to the hospital when the contractions come every ten minutes. As a midwife, my only comment on that is: if you feel like leaving for the hospital several times, nobody will stop you. Experience shows that the contractions that come at ten-minute intervals are usually much too weak, and the women are disappointed when the midwife on duty says: "This could still take ages; with these contractions you can't give birth to a child." This experience often triggers a certain amount of anxiety and tension in the expectant parents, with the consequence that, after going home and waiting for several more hours, they ultimately leave for the hospital too late when the contractions finally do get stronger. Please do not be afraid to ask for help, and if anything is unclear to you, it's better to leave for the hospital too soon twice than once at the last moment. It often happens that women – those giving birth for the first time and those who have given birth before – end up driving to the hospital several times. The only unpleasant thing is the fact that in many maternity wards it is not par for the course to be allowed to go back home again. For this reason, it is always worth the parents' while – as mentioned on page 141, to find out about the policies followed at the hospital of their choice. As in so many situations that can arise in connection with childbirth, the reaction of the staff on duty will depend on the parents. If the father makes the impression that he would rather have his wife in the safe care of the hospital, the pregnant woman will be admitted as an in-patient. But if the parents themselves suspect that the contractions are not strong enough to give birth to a child and all they really want is confirmation of that fact, then they should leave the suitcase in the car. When they arrive, they should explain immediately that they have only come to have the woman examined and would definitely like to go home again if possible.

Thus in my opinion it depends mainly on you whether you can go home again when the cervix is unripe or the contractions too weak. You should always take into consideration that the midwife and doctor at the hospital usually don't know you personally. There is no way the staff can know what your expectations are. Some women complain about having been sent home, while others are unhappy when the opposite happens. Don't assume that all women in this unclear situation will voice the same wishes. Communicate clearly what you want, and that will provide every-one else involved with orientation, and as long as it is medically tenable, you will surely be allowed to drive home again.

A Midwife's Opinion

In order to avoid these problems, many pregnant women ring up an independent midwife or drive to the midwife's practice first; they know the practice hours from having had some of their antenatal check-ups there. Interestingly enough, we mid-wives are often sought in the evenings and on the weekends. On weekdays, many women go to their gynaecologists first. And it is also not unusual for us to be asked for advice in the middle of the night. To this very day, I have sympathy for the expect-ant parents in these situations, because I know that for many it is very soothing to be able to talk to the midwife. Usually all they need is confirmation that they are making the right decisions, and often the midwife can give them some helpful words of ad-vice. But the midwife can only make a clear prognosis if she has the opportunity to examine the mother. For this reason, a telephone conversation often doesn't suffice and the pregnant woman either has to come to the practice or the midwife has to pay her a quick house call.

False Alarm

False alarms happen just as often in conjunction with home births as in cases of women who want to give birth in the hospital. The only difference is that, in the case of home births, it is not the parents but the midwife who has to make the trip for nothing. This was the case with Monika …

… she was expecting her fourth child. Initially we were both concerned about whether I was a good choice of midwives to attend to the birth, because during rush hour it took me at least half an hour to get to her house. But since I didn't have any colleagues in the vicinity of Monika's house who conducted home births, I agreed to help her. The parents were confident they would let me know in plenty of time. Then one night, the call came. I was relieved because that meant I'd get there in time. But I was much too early – the cervix was still shut tight and she was apparently having false labour pains. So, my mind at rest, I went back home and back to bed. The next day another call from Monika. The contrac-tions were back, but now she could feel them in the lower back. Off I went again, this time during the noon rush hour. And again I had to console her and explain to her that it would certainly take several days until the baby was born. Fourteen days (!) later, once again a 'contraction call' from Monika. This time she told me that she had had a slightly bloody mucus discharge. We arranged that she would call

me again when she started having contractions. That was the case that same evening, and again off I drive, again for naught. At midnight, finally, the birthing hour had struck, and her voice sounded much different than it had before. Even over the phone, it was clear to me that she was having real labour pains. When I arrived, the first thing she said was: "I never would have thought that I could really forget what labour pains feel like. I think you'll be able to stay this time. And she was right, though for a woman who had already given birth three times before it still took a relatively long time until – around five o'clock in the morning – a healthy little girl was finally born thanks to the joint efforts of her mother, father, the doctor and myself.

I have cited this story as a way of encouraging all expectant mothers to call for help as soon as they feel they need it, no matter how many false alarms they have already set off. And what is more, women having their first baby shouldn't assume that multiparas know everything and are absolutely sure of themselves in their experience. Every woman – regardless of how many children she has had in the past – needs help and is happy when she can ask another woman for help. Women who have already had children before often complain: "I'm so sick and tired of being told: 'I don't need to explain anything to you – you know all about labour pains and giving birth.' Such nonsense, as though I had made childbearing the focus of my life. Just because I already have three children, I supposedly know more than the midwife and the doctor. What are three days compared to my whole life? You forget the labour pains before you know it." Such comments often give me pause for thought and help me to listen to all pregnant women, to their questions, worries and problems with an open ear. I think we midwives probably also have overly high expectations of "experienced" multiparas.

Leaving Time for First-Timers

If the woman is already feeling the contractions at short intervals, i.e. every two to three minutes over a period of two or three hours, then it is undoubtedly time to leave for the hospital or notify the midwife of the birth. If you are having three-minute intervals you can be quite sure that you won't arrive at the hospital too early. These contractions are certain to be very effective already, and the cervix may well have already opened several centimetres. If you have to drive quite a way to get to the hospital of your choice, however, you should get going when the intervals between contractions are five minutes. These pointers are applicable above all to first-time mothers.

Naturally, it is not at all unusual for pregnant women to require a midwife's help when the intervals are still ten minutes. It is possible that they already have the feeling these contractions are strong and effective. In that case, it is the ideal time to betake yourself to the place of birth. As I have already explained, the idea is not to keep a record of the contractions and then call when you have had ten contractions at three-minute intervals, but to get in touch when you feel the need to do so.

Beginning of Labour for Multiparas

In the case of multiparas – women who have given birth before – it is not the intervals between the contractions but their effectiveness that counts. Often an expectant mother has had irregular or weak contractions for hours, but knows from past experience that she never gave birth with such contractions. Then suddenly, with the first strong contractions, the Aaaaahhhh … experience sets in again: she remembers, oh yes, that's exactly how it was, it was only possible to cope with the contractions by exhaling with a loud "Aaaahhhh", and these contractions are just like the ones that accompanied past births. It just doesn't happen without "labour" in the truest sense of the word, and the latter can only be achieved with targeted breathing. Naturally, even multiparas hope that maybe this child will come very fast and without all those painful contractions. In this context, I am reminded of Gabi …

… she was expecting her sixth child and during one of my preliminary visits she told me: "Just imagine, Inge, I dreamt I woke up and the baby was under the blanket. I had given birth without labour pains and without the slightest effort." We both had to laugh, and I remarked: "Wishful thinking, eh?" When the time came for the birth, I was called to the forester's lodge, set scenically in a romantic valley, on a rainy Sunday morning (these are the positive aspects of home births; we midwives have many experiences of nature, not only natural childbirths, but lonely valleys and secluded, idyllic farmsteads where you feel all of the seasons with sun, rain, snow, wind and weather). In the midst of her strong contractions, Gabi was reminded of the births of her first children. The dream really was nothing more than wishful thinking. "I guess I'll never have a baby just like that, under the blankets, without feeling anything and all of its own accord," she groaned. As in the case of her previous births, she did not identify the contractions as true labour pains until the cervix had already opened seven centimetres, but, as always, there was still plenty of time to make all the preparations.

Rupture of the Membranes: The Water Breaks

A very common sign of the beginning of labour is a rupture of the membranes, i.e. an outflow of the amniotic fluid/liquor. Unfortunately, there are no reliable rules for behaviour in this situation either. Sometimes I feel bad about the fact that we midwives often have to answer with words like: maybe, possibly, it could happen that, perhaps, etc. But that's how it is in nature; there are no clear rules which can be followed. And because childbirth is a natural occurrence, and not an illness and not a commonplace event, it cannot be expected to come about in a strictly established sequence like a technically controllable mechanism. Whenever we human beings are confronted with natural occurrences, we have to be prepared for surprises and entirely new situations. This requires a high degree of flexibility, but is also a reflection of life in all its liveliness.

The Unforeseeable Event

The breaking of the waters is a completely unforeseeable event; it occurs without the slightest sign of warning. Many women think they feel something popping in their abdomen, and then the water is already flowing out. The pregnant woman thus never knows when to expect this to happen, and she cannot prepare for it. A rupture of the membranes can take place in a variety of ways:

It is possible that amniotic fluid is already trickling several weeks before the beginning of labour, in which case you must go to the nearest hospital immediately, without the slightest doubt or hesitation – regardless of the time of day or night, and whether you are having contractions or not.

The water can break on or around the due date before any contractions at all have set in, and thus represent the beginning of labour. The uterus usually reacts within a few hours by beginning to contract.

In this situation, parents are very concerned and often ask: "If there aren't any contractions yet liquor keeps flowing out, the baby's environment is completely dry, isn't it?" But I can console all expectant parents by telling them that nature has not made any mistake here. The amniotic fluid is produced by the amniotic membranes as well as by the baby's kidneys. In the final stage of pregnancy, thirty percent of the fluid is renewed every hour, and every two hours the entire amount of fluid is exchanged between the mother and child. So even if there is a loss of amniotic fluid, new fluid is being produced constantly. There is no danger of the uterus drying out on the inside.

Trickling of Amniotic Fluid

You may recognize a breaking of water in the constant outflow of a small amount of fluid from the vagina, initially perhaps a tablespoon full and then just drops or nothing at all anymore. The cause for this can be a fine tear in the upper section of the membranes (a so-called hindwater leak); another possibility is that there was a tiny bit of amniotic fluid beneath the baby's head (rupture of the forewaters), and after it flows out the head presses against the cervix from the inside and essentially "seals" it.

A Gush of Amniotic Fluid

On the other hand, the expectant mother may feel a substantial amount of warm fluid flowing out of her vagina all at once and without warning. She will automatically try to tense up her pelvic muscles to stop the flow, as though trying to stop the passing of water. But she will notice immediately that she doesn't succeed. The amniotic fluid flows and flows without stopping – sometimes until the birth of the child. The latter is only possible, of course, when there is a lot of fluid. Often the gush soon ebbs and turns into drops. In other cases, amniotic fluid flows out only during or at the end of a contraction.

If contractions have already set in, many expectant mothers observe that, after the outflow of such a large amount of fluid, the labour pains occur a few times at longer intervals, but then increase again quite soon with regard to intensity as well as duration. I would therefore like to urge all expectant parents to notify the midwife without hesitation if the water has broken and the contractions have begun.

If you are still at home and plan to give birth in the hospital, it is now – if not before – that you should leave. I often experience women who resist the trip to the hospital, telling their partners: "Calm down, this is how it's been the whole time; maybe it will just stop again, the way it did yesterday. Just because the water has broken doesn't mean the baby wants to be born immediately." The expectant fathers should not allow themselves to be deterred from talking their wives into driving to the hospital or, in the case of a home birth, notifying the midwife.

Remember that the intensity of your wife's breathing is the best barometer for the progress of the birth. But please, in all the excitement, don't do what I once experienced a father doing …

… I was a novice midwife, was on night duty, waiting at the gate for the parents who had rung up and told us that the woman was having contractions and already losing amniotic fluid. I was able to identify the car from the way it was being driven: "Those are sure to be the birthing parents; that was fast." The car stopped, the father got out, went to open the back door of the car, let out a yell, looked over at me and called out as he got back in the car: "Oh my God, I forgot my wife, she's still at home! Please wait, I'll be right back!" How fortunate that the expectant parents only lived a few blocks away, because within ten minutes they were back, everyone laughing or moaning, as the case may be. Their healthy baby was born two hours later.

Better to be safe …

Incidentally, I highly recommend that, on the days before the estimated due date, the pregnant woman keep a small towel, toddler nappies, nappy inserts or a few sanitary pads with her at all times. Because it can happen that the water breaks while you're shopping, in town or visiting a girlfriend. It's embarrassing, but it's completely natural! Take precautions and be prepared for surprises. That's the way it is with children: even before they're born, they constantly confront us with new, unexpected situations. The following happened to a former schoolmate of mine:

… the estimated due date had already come and gone several days before. Her husband wanted to go to the town festival that took place every year at the fairgrounds. She didn't feel like staying home, and accompanied her husband. They had hardly been at the fairgrounds an hour when warm amniotic fluid began running down her thighs. She was completely surprised and happy at the same time, because finally the birth of the child was almost close enough to touch. Since she didn't have anything with her, her husband quickly went and got some napkins from a beer stand and then they hurried

excitedly to the nearest exit. When she related all this to me, she made a point of telling me again what a strange feeling it had been to feel the warm, wet amniotic fluid, the feeling of emptying out and not being able to do anything at all about it. Contractions set in immediately with the breaking of the water and their daughter was born the same day. The second time she was expecting a child, the due date was in the same month, and once again they were at the fairgrounds, this time with a pad in her panties. And as incredible as it might sound, once again, Alexandra's water broke in that very same setting. This time, however, she wasn't so surprised. The expectant parents were highly amused and drove straight to the hospital, because the suitcase had already been stowed in the car. It was quite a happy occasion when the second little girl was also born during the Allgaeu Festival Week.

The Water Breaks in the First or Second Stage of Labour

The membranes can rupture during the first hours of labour, i.e. the first stage, or not until the end, shortly before or during the second stage. In the latter case, the membranes can truly be said to burst. We midwives are frequently taken by surprise and get quite a shower when it happens, since we are usually sitting right at the "scene of the action" and are in the process of massaging the perineum. The woman in labour first has a sensation of pressure which suddenly decreases, as though a balloon had burst. Then she has a pleasant feeling of warmth and wetness and a reassuring sign that the baby's head will soon appear. This breaking of the water shortly before the actual birth of the child is described by women as a kind of climax and feeling of elation. Unfortunately, in labour wards, very few women experience it, since there the amniotic sac is artificially ruptured during the course of labour. In home obstetrics, this sensation occurs frequently, since we intervene in the events of birth as rarely as possible.

By the bursting of the sac and the "shower" for the midwife when a birthing stool is being used, the woman in labour can recognize herself that 'labour' will soon be over. As experienced by Uschi …

… she was still raving about it several hours later: "The bursting of the membranes was like a starting signal for me; it was like immersing myself in the deep waters of childbirth. Everything got warm and wet, the initial pressure disappeared, and then it got very strong. I felt the baby's head filling my vagina; it stretched, it burned, you urged me to be careful, let it come slowly, and then – with a certain amount of pushing – panting – pushing – the head was born. I hope I never forget that elated feeling of wetness, warmth and birth."

Identifying the Amniotic Fluid

The expectant mother can clearly recognize the amniotic fluid and distinguish it from urine. It *smells* different; more specifically, it has a slightly sweet odour. One pregnant woman described it as follows: "It smells just simply like human being." If you are unsure, I recommend dabbing the entrance to the vagina with a bit of toilet paper.

Then it is clear that the fluid is dripping from the uterus and not from the bladder. After all, the suspicion that it might simply be urine is well justified. Towards the end of pregnancy, many expectant mothers have the feeling of being "leaky" – incontinent –, since they lose a few drops of urine every time they sneeze, cough or laugh, due to the strong pressure and the position of the baby's head. After childbirth, this problem is sure to disappear again. But don't forget to carry out intensive pelvic floor exercises in order to keep these symptoms from reoccurring after several years in the form of bladder or vaginal prolapse.

The *colour* of the amniotic fluid is usually whitish-clear to slightly cloudy yellowish. As a way of explaining to parents what amniotic fluid looks like, I recommend filling a glass with water and adding an egg white and stirring. The mixture looks deceptively like "liquor" (amniotic fluid). Sometimes it will have a slightly greenish cast. In this case it is advisable to notify a midwife as soon as possible or drive to the hospital.

At the end of pregnancy, the *amount* of amniotic fluid measures slightly less than one litre (about 33 fluid ounces or somewhat more than a quart) on average. It can vary greatly, however; the norm ranges from as little as 300 ml/approx. 10 fl. oz. to as much as 1500 ml/approx. 55 fl. oz. And even when the water breaks, only part of the fluid flows out.

The Functions of the Amniotic Fluid

The amniotic fluid fulfils a number of functions for the baby. To begin with, thanks to the presence of the fluid, the unborn child learns to suckle and drink and its kidney functions are already activated before birth. In a sense, it also represents a part of the baby's nutrition. In addition to percent water (accounting for 98%), the amniotic fluid contains protein (500 mg) and glucose (22 mg) as well as urea, sodium, chlorine and lactic acid. It is therefore hardly surprising when newborns whose amniotic sac has remained intact until the last contractions are born with a kind of satiation. In the initial hours of life, these babies often get far less hungry and thirsty.

This difference in behaviour is quite obvious in home birth settings: children whose amniotic sac is not artificially ruptured and whose stomachs are not suctioned are usually calmer during the first forty-eight hours, don't require any fluid intake, and lose far less weight. As always, though, exceptions prove the rule. Here again, we have a clear indication that it is sensible to do without such interventions as the early rupturing of the membranes. Even if labour takes longer as a result, not an hour of it is in vain. And anyway, it's really only a few hours of our lives that we devote to childbearing, and by being patient we offer the child an optimal start in life, determined by itself and its mother in harmony with nature.

Another important function of the amniotic fluid consists in acting as a kind of shock absorber during pregnancy, protecting the mother from the baby's movements and the baby from outside influences.

The water provides the baby with space to move and develop and protects the umbilical cord from kinking, which would stop the blood from circulating properly.

The membranes and the amniotic fluid envelop the baby like a silken, water-filled cloak. The baby is thus optimally protected from infection, can move freely and will undoubtedly miss its waterbed when it's outside in the dry world. When it cries, it won't always be on account of hunger, but also because of a longing for something it will never experience again.

Preventive Measures When the Water Breaks

As soon as the amniotic sac is open, a direct path to the child has been created – which can unfortunately be used by pathogens and other germs. For this reason, hygiene and cleanliness are absolutely essential following a rupture of the amniotic sac. For the expectant mother, this means she should keep herself scrupulously clean and not expose the vaginal area to any unclean substances or objects. I therefore recommend the following to women whose water has broken:

⟨⟩ Method of Rinsing with Essential Oils

Every time you go to the toilet, rinse yourself with a one-percent solution of *Dead Sea salt* containing three to five drops of the essential oil *lavender extra*. Lavender has a strongly disinfectant quality. If you should happen to have *Rose-Teebaum-Essenz/Rose-Tea-Tree Essence ᗡ®* on hand, you can also add three to five drops of that blend. Wear clean panties which have been washed in boiling hot water and change your sanitary pad/nappy insert regularly. You can also apply a drop of one of the above-named essential oils to them to achieve excellent protection against infection.

Vaginal Examinations Following a Rupture of the Membranes

Following the outflow of amniotic fluid, I would make sure a vaginal examination is really absolutely necessary before allowing it to be carried out. As a midwife I try to examine the birthing woman as rarely as possible/only as often as absolutely necessary. The reason for this is that, no matter how carefully I wash it beforehand, my hand can transport far more germs to the cervical entrance than would otherwise be the case. The constant outflow of the amniotic fluid impedes the advancing germs through the direction of flow, but every interruption also interrupts this natural process.

Antibiotic Prophylaxis

In many maternity wards, if the amniotic sac has already ruptured several hours before childbirth, the newborn is treated with an antibiotic directly after birth due to the concern that it could have contracted an infection. The time span of this treatment varies strongly from hospital to hospital, ranging from eight to forty-eight hours.

The Breaking of the Waters from a Natural Perspective

I am entirely certain that nature knows exactly why 'she' has had to break the water to make this particular unborn baby and this uterus aware that they must both make an effort to begin the labour process. We might always have difficulty understanding the sense of this method, but perhaps we should simply respect it and be more cautious and prudent with our vaginal examinations and have more faith in the natural course of childbirth. If a break of the water really represented such a threat, it would herald the beginning of labour far less often. Nature shows us again and again that women bear children in order to preserve the species and not to endanger it already right at the beginning of life. I have already pointed this out elsewhere in this book. As parents, you should consult with competent persons regarding the sense – or lack of sense – in conducting prophylactic treatment with an antibiotic.

At my first house call, an "early-discharge" father in the early postnatal phase remarked quite indignantly …

… *"I don't understand it – the doctors said my wife wasn't even allowed to take a bath anymore, not to mention getting out of bed, because they said the danger of infection was so great. But within a few hours she was examined by several people a total of at least ten times. I think it was even more. In any case much too often. That's a total contradiction. As though all those hands and surgical gloves didn't represent a much greater danger of infection. And to top it off, they wanted to protect that baby by giving it an antibiotic, and told us it was grossly negligent of us to go home now in view of the danger of infection." I did not want to judge whether the woman had been examined too often or not, because I had not attended the birth. But I do assume that it could have been avoided at least part of the time. All I said was that it would have been better to clarify this question at the time, to which the father replied: "You know, I was simply too inhibited, and too caught up in the situation. And anyway, it surely wouldn't have done my wife any good if I had started discussing the pros and cons of the hospital staff's professional procedures with them." Of course I couldn't agree with him more, because the birth bed is the absolute worst place for discussions. He did intend to go back and talk to the personnel about these events in retrospect, but I never learned what had become of this plan. The baby, incidentally, was completely normal during the postnatal period and did not develop any infections.*

All parents, obstetricians and midwives should be aware that, in the domestic milieu, the danger of the newborn's contracting an infection is actually lower than in a hospital. In the latter environment, an accumulation of typical hospital pathogens and germs brought in from the outside by the great number of people cannot be avoided.

It will naturally not always be easy for the parents to make the right decision, and for the hospital personnel, the fear and worry about the danger of the baby's contracting an infection is likewise well justified.

The Position of the Birthing Woman

One of the questions most frequently asked in the antenatal classes as well as later, in the acute situation of the waters having broken, is: "Do I have to be transported lying down or am I allowed to get up?" This is a matter of extreme importance for expectant parents and, as is so often the case in connection with pregnancy, childbirth and the postnatal period, there are differing opinions and answers. Particularly on this subject there are two fundamentally different assumptions in the science of obstetrics. Adherents to the one point of view say categorically: "The woman must be transported in a lying position and may not get up again until the birth, since the danger of an umbilical cord prolapse is much too great." The others, however, are convinced that: "Naturally the woman can get up; as a matter of fact she should get up, because the baby's head will seal the cervix through the use of gravity." But which mode of behaviour is the right one? If we take a closer look at this matter, it becomes obvious that of course the woman can get up. Nature made it possible for a woman's water to break in a standing position and without the slightest warning. Nature knows that she may well have a small child to look after and is pregnant with the next child at the same time. That is simply part of the everyday life of a mother. The toddler has to be changed, the six-year-old comes home from the playground crying because it has skinned its knee and at that very moment the water breaks. What should the mother do: lie down immediately as it says in the medical textbook, leave the toddler screaming and the six-year-old waiting outside the front door and hope that a good angel will appear and notify her husband or Grandma? This is a very unrealistic idea: a pregnant woman who lives out in the country, remote from the village or any neighbours, would not even be able to go to the telephone if she followed directions such as: "In the case of a rupture of the amniotic sac, lie down immediately and don't get up again. You must be transported to the hospital in a lying position as quickly as possible." I hope that all expectant parents will recognize for themselves how entirely illogical these statements are. Advice such as this was first voiced in the era when people began talking about the care of women during childbirth as a branch of medicine; and it was voiced by men who have never been pregnant and have never had to experience for themselves how nonsensical and quixotic their recommendations are.

For these reasons, the rule of thumb I follow – regardless of all warnings concerning umbilical cord prolapse – is: a pregnant woman can assume a vertical position even in the case of a rupture of the membranes. In this case she should follow her instinct. As soon as she feels the need to lie down or to stand, her body knows why it is sending that signal, and she is well advised to comply. Naturally, she must know her body well and be able to interpret its needs and signals correctly.

Umbilical Cord Prolapse

In order to prevent an actual umbilical cord prolapse – which, incidentally, occurs extremely rarely – every woman can and will instinctively feel her vagina following an outflow of amniotic fluid to determine what has just happened. If she does, there will be clear signs indicating this condition. If this exceedingly rare complication has occurred (which, amazingly enough, is usually only observed in birth rooms in cases of women giving birth in a lying position), to the extent possible, the expectant mother should immediately kneel on the floor with her pelvis pointing upwards (knee-elbow-position) until help has arrived. Here the risk for the baby really is extremely high. Only few babies can survive this situation, because if the umbilical cord is compressed, the baby cannot be saved. In my opinion, however, there is no general guarantee against this or a similar fate. Everyone knows that we are constantly accompanied by the possibility of taking ill or dying. And we look forward to tomorrow despite this knowledge. The fact that there are emergency situations in the life of a human being is also something everyone knows, but we prefer to concentrate on life rather than on death. It would undoubtedly be very good for our society to learn to talk about suffering, illness and death openly again. In various chapters in this book, I have pointed out again and again that childbearing and birth, dying and death are borderline areas with only thin lines between them and that every expectant mother will accordingly be faced with these truths regularly in one form or another. I would therefore like to request of the expectant fathers: Take your wife's fears and worries seriously, seek advice and come to the consultation with a midwife together so that we can answer your questions and allay your concerns and happy anticipation of the birth and the baby can prevail once again.

Methods of Establishing Contractions

If a so-called prelabour rupture of the membranes occurs and there is no sign of any labour pains, the question naturally soon arises: "What can we do to get the contractions going?"

Naturopathic Treatment

In this case I can recommend the same measures already described in the sections on "Inducing Labour" and "Alternative Methods of Inducing Labour" on pp. ■f. In other words, in addition to trying the effect of natural prostaglandins, you can try to support labour with essential oils, spices and homoeopathic remedies. But be sure to ask your midwife because otherwise you run the risk of applying useless methods and wasting time unnecessarily – time during which the mother and baby are not monitored. Already in antiquity, birthing women consulted "wise women".

Mucous Discharge/Mucous Plug

One frequently occurring sign that labour is beginning is the discharge of mucus, which is observed by many women several days before the contractions begin. As is the case in the menstrual cycle, shortly before childbirth this mucus changes from a milky, sticky substance to clear, transparent, viscid one. A prerequisite for this natural change is a healthy vaginal milieu.

Mucous Plug

Sometimes pregnant women say that suddenly a handful of clear, gluey mucus has been discharged. The latter can look like a real plug, which explains the name so frequently used in literature on childbirth. As I have already discussed repeatedly above, women are not machines and the signs of beginning labour are just as varied as human beings themselves.

Several hours after (or perhaps already before) the appearance of this mucous plug, the expectant mother will feel pangs in the area of the sacrum or lower abdomen, similar to the pains accompanying menstruation. On the other hand, several days can elapse from the time of this discharge to the commencement of labour pains. In the old days, it was understood as a sign for the expectant mother to prepare the linen and the birthing room and notify the women who would be attending to her during birth and the postnatal period, since in the pre-telephone era it often took several days to contact everyone.

Bloody Mucous Discharge

Many pregnant women observe a dark red, bloody mucous discharge. This can occur when the cervix is already slightly open one to two days before labour pains set in or, sometimes, during the first stage of labour. This colouration of the mucus indicates that it is mixed with "old" blood and there is thus no cause for concern. On the contrary, it is a positive sign, since it means that the cervix is gradually opening up further and the membranes are becoming detached from the edge of the cervix. The amount of mucus can be sparse or abundant. This sign can be interpreted as the baby's second "attention-getting mechanism". In antiquity, women had no calendars and there was no-one who could predict – on the basis of hormone tests or vaginal examinations – that she could count on the commencement of labour in one to two days or the next few hours. Back then, people had to rely on signs such as these. These days, many expectant mothers are unfortunately not informed about these initial signs and are either frightened by them or – even more frequently – don't even notice them. They undergo regular vaginal examinations from the due date onward, and perhaps the mucus sticks to the surgical glove of the obstetrician. I would therefore advise a woman always to ask if such signs are visible. And incidentally, they can also occur after sexual intercourse.

Bleeding

Light Bleeding

At some point in conjunction with regular, usually light contractions, a minimal amount of bleeding occurs. You will find a very little bit of fresh, bright red blood in your panties or sanitary pad. This is one more reason to keep a couple of sanitary pads or nappy inserts in your handbag towards the end of pregnancy, because you can never be sure when bleeding or a breaking of the water will occur. Women who tend to bleed very heavily during menstruation can have constant slight bleeding throughout labour. No medical textbook will tell you this; it is just something I know from my years of professional practice. This bright red bleeding is a sign that the cervix is opening. It should never be as strong as menstrual bleeding, however, only a so-called "drawing" is within the norm. It is undoubtedly advisable – and all pregnant women feel the need – to consult a midwife or doctor in the case of bleeding. I would only like to impress upon you once again that bright red blood in the form of a stripe on the sanitary pad is nothing to panic or even worry about.

But as is always the case in life, when a human being sees red, his attention is heightened, all of his senses become alert and focus on what happens next. And that is exactly how it should be. Be alert and watch for other signs that could indicate the beginning of labour, such as:

a bright red trace of blood
pain at regular intervals
regular hardening of the uterus
nausea, constant urge to empty the bowels

It nearly always takes only a few hours until true labour pains set in.

Bright Red Bleeding and Regular Contractions

If you should have regular, moderately strong contractions at approximately five-minute intervals – the kind you have to breathe your way through – and notice that bright red blood is discharged, this is the appropriate moment to call the midwife or drive to the hospital. Experience has shown that slight bleeding occurs when the diameter of the cervix is about five centimetres and again when it is about eight centimetres. Therefore you should take into account that it is advisable to ask for help in the case of fresh red bleeding, even if the contractions are still quite bearable.

Strong Bright Red Bleeding

If you have **strong, bright red bleeding**, i.e. of menstrual strength or stronger, with or without clots of blood, there is only one option:

Go to the hospital immediately –
regardless of when the due date is,
and regardless of whether or not you are having contractions.

Do not allow yourself to be deterred by any inconvenient time of the day or night or any other indispositions. If it takes your partner more than a quarter of an hour until he can come and fetch you, then call a neighbour, a taxi or an ambulance. It is not necessary for the expectant father to drive through red lights but you shouldn't wait until the suspenseful detective movie on TV is over either. It is advisable to ring up the hospital and let them know that you are on your way to the maternity ward with strong bleeding.

Strong bleeding, i.e. stronger than menstrual bleeding, fresh and bright red, in gushes or clots, is nearly always a sign that the placenta is detaching itself prematurely. For this reason, it is urgent that you place yourself in the care of a doctor, because in all probability the child will have to be born by caesarean. Don't let these lines scare you into thinking you have to tell your husband that he should always be on call or demand of Grandma that she be ready to spring into action for weeks on end. The probability of placenta detachment is just as low as the likelihood that you will break your leg when you stand up. So stay calm. Life has many an acute situation to offer, but we only really experience very few such serious and threatening moments. The most important thing for the final weeks and days before labour starts is: remain calm and composed; have confidence and faith in the child. We know there are often heavy thunderstorms in the springtime, but after a long winter we nevertheless look forward to a time of growth and blossoming. That is how it should be after a long pregnancy as well.

Nausea/Vomiting

Many children take leave of the womb with the same gesture that accompanied their arrival: by causing their mothers nausea and vomiting! Women frequently tell me: "This can't be true; I have exactly the same queasy feeling in the pit of my stomach again, today of all days, when I'm also feeling pain in my lower abdomen. Labour won't get under way when I'm so nauseated, will it?" This isn't always the case, but it really does happen quite often that expectant mothers once again have a feeling of nausea in conjunction with labour pains. Usually it passes quickly.

In some cases, vomiting is almost like a starting signal for the commencement of labour. The woman has to vomit once and the menstrual-type aches turn into regular contractions.

Even more frequently, women in labour will have had regular, strong contractions for quite a while already and then have to vomit between the contractions one to several times. This is extremely unpleasant, but there's nothing to be done about it. For us midwives it's a positive sign, because we know that in these moments the cervix widens. So despite the bothersome spitting up, try to be encouraged, because when all canals are open, the baby won't be long in coming, and the birth canal will open as well. I well remember a birth situation that took place several years ago …

… Mrs. M. had strong contractions, the cervix had dilated to a diameter of six centimetres when I examined her less than an hour earlier. Suddenly the birthing woman became extremely nauseated and lost her entire midday meal. At the same time it seemed to me that she felt a certain pressure on the perineum, as I could tell by her behaviour. I gave the father the bucket and said: "You help your wife; I have to go and fetch my things." I consoled the birthing woman by saying: "That's good, just let it all out, your baby will certainly be here soon." "Tell me, what kind of a midwife are you?!" the expectant father snapped at me, "my wife no longer knows what she should do first, right herself and spit up or concentrate on the next contraction. She's about to start crying, she has terrible labour pains and all you've got to say – with a radiant face – is 'That's good!' You help her!" Despite this vehement reaction on the part of the father, I had to smile and tell him soothingly: "I'm really sorry that your wife has to vomit, but you'll see, the baby really will be here quite soon. The second stage of labour will begin any minute; your wife is one of the fast types. Let's talk about it later. Now we should attend to your wife and the baby that's on its way into the world." Actually I was quite glad that he had been so short-tempered, because it reminded me to use the preparatory sessions to draw all expectant parents' attention to such labour-accompanying circumstances.

So when all bodily openings open up, take it as a positive sign, don't hold anything back, and the baby will be able to leave the womb quickly. That's really the way it is: first a couple of tears flow, the mother's nose starts to run, soon many a birthing woman feels the need to let the world know loudly that she is in pain, then perhaps she has to pass water, a bit of blood seeps out of the vagina, the bowels are emptied and shortly thereafter the baby's head appears at the entrance to the vagina. This opening up sometimes occurs little by little in the course of several hours; in other cases the signs don't come until half an hour before the actual birth of the child, but then almost simultaneously.

Diarrhoea

A healthy and frequent sign of the beginning of labour is diarrhoea. The healthy woman's body recognizes that it has to purge and empty itself before the birth of a child. Our body knows that a full intestine only robs the baby of elbow room unnecessarily. For the baby it is additional work and effort to have to push the intestinal contents to the side or cause them to empty by applying pressure. When diarrhoea occurs, it is almost always followed by the setting in of contractions, since the uterine muscles are activated by the intestinal peristalsis. Active bowels and aches in conjunction with the hardening of the uterus at increasingly frequent intervals therefore really are a positive and reliable sign that labour is beginning.

THE STAGES OF LABOUR

Labour is divided into two major stages, of which the first comprises the active phase and the transition phase, followed by the second stage which is the final, strenuous culmination of labour. In the English-language literature on the subject, the delivery of the placenta is frequently referred to as the third stage.

The First Stage of Labour: The Active Phase

The active phase lasts from the time the contractions set in, i.e. when the cervix is only slightly dilated, until that dilation measures about seven to eight centimetres in diameter. For the midwife, the cervix can almost no longer be felt at all when she conducts a vaginal examination, and she will announce that the transition phase is starting. The active phase can vary greatly in length and depends, among other things, on how the birth is being conducted. In natural childbirth it is possible that twenty-four hours or more elapse from the first regular contractions until the cervix has dilated completely. Naturally, this phase can also be over in four hours. Many parents begin counting the hours at the first slight signs of labour, but get another good night's sleep and then say the birth took three days. There are also stories of quite a different nature …

… "Did you hear? Anita had a baby boy; labour only lasted an hour and a half, her husband said. When it really got going in earnest, the baby was born with three contractions. I'm glad it went so fast for Anita's sake." When I hear stories like this I can only smile to myself; usually I know the background, whether over the phone or from paying a house call. That was the case here as well. The father had apparently forgotten to add that his wife had already had regular, moderately strong contractions every evening for several days before the birth, that on the day of the birth she had had contractions constantly at ten-minute intervals, but that those contractions hadn't attained the necessary effectiveness. Thanks to a little piece of advice from me, the contractions finally started occurring at shorter intervals and increasing in strength in the evening. Apparently the friend had overheard when the overjoyed new father mentioned that from the time they left home until the birth it only took one and a half hours. Something I find quite interesting is that for men, the actual "starting signal" of the birth is not until the beginning of the second stage. This is probably to be attributed to the simple fact that men cannot know what women undergo when they breathe through their labour pains for hours on end. From their point of view, nothing is happening. Only when the work of pushing begins, the strain and force of which is very obvious, is there really "action" and only then do the men really comprehend that the birth is taking place. Everything else, the waiting, the efforts to cope with the contractions, the patient hoping and praying, is nothing more than "women's talk".

My reason for telling you this story is to impress upon you that reports about labour and childbirth can be extremely misleading and that, if you are an expectant mother yourself and would like to hear a realistic account of how long the birth lasted, it would be better to speak to the new mother herself. We women are confronted again and again with the fact that men see, feel and remember childbirth in a manner much different from the way we mothers do.

There are undoubtedly also situations in which we women describe a man's experience much differently from how they actually experienced it. My main point is simply that I think it's important for expectant mothers to talk to other mothers about how the latter experienced labour. Men can best gain insight into the events of childbirth not only by talking to other Dads at the pub but by really learning about childbirth and all its stages and phases. It is for this reason that I place a great deal of emphasis on introducing and explaining the function of the "active phase" during the antenatal sessions.

The active phase, as I expressed above, can vary greatly in length. It begins with regular contractions at five-minute intervals and ends with a dilation of the cervix to a diameter of eight centimetres.

The First Stage of Labour: The Transition Phase

The transition contractions are the strongest labour pains. They are required to open the cervix those last two centimetres to a diameter of about ten centimetres. As you can imagine, not all newborns have the same size head. The head of a smaller child might be able to slip through an opening of nine centimetres in diameter, while a big, bouncing baby might need eleven centimetres or more in order to leave the protective and meanwhile extremely confined womb.

The force of the contractions is very strong at this point, and the intervals between them very short. I often observe, however, that this phase also comprises a few very pleasant longer breaks for recuperation.

The Baby Makes Its Way through the Birth Canal

For the baby, this phase means managing the transition from the womb to the mother's pelvis, the transition from being pushed passively to becoming active itself, by sliding down and turning its head. In the confines of the maternal pelvis, which is softly cushioned with muscles, the baby has to carry out a quarter turn of its head and contort its body to make its way from the uterus into the pelvic cavity and finally to the outside. Many children manage this transition from the pelvic inlet into the sacral cavity without the slightest effort; many of them are already looking for this route from the beginning of the first stage of labour, whereas others do not recognize that they have to move downward until the cervix is almost completely dilated. For us human beings, what this means is that being born is associated with "coming down" and "having to twist our bodies" in order to see the light of the world. Many adults are capable of imagining that this process is not easy. But surely it is good that our path into life begins this way, because it gives us the certainty that we will make it through the "downs" that are just as much a part of life as the "ups". For the baby, the transition phase means to feel not only the confinement and the uncertainty but also the force with which the uterus propels and urges it forward. This is exactly what people go through when they are in a difficult phase of their lives: they have to be held and pushed along by the people around them in order to progress past the down phase. Naturally, there are also people who recover from hard times and push onward and upward of their own accord and with little effort. And there are likewise children who make their way through the transition phase quickly. They "dive" into the depths and overcome this phase within a few contractions. This transitional moment is frequently audible in the slowing of the fetal heartbeat and the words of the midwife, who says something like: "Aha, the transition effect. Don't worry, the baby will recover again in a few seconds. Now you've almost made it; labour will be over soon. In a few seconds you'll feel the urge to push."

What I mean to say is that the birth situation depends partially on the baby's behaviour. It can happen that you, the birthing woman, will not be aware of this transition period, especially if it only lasts for a couple of contractions, and will then almost be surprised by the urge to push. It is equally possible, however, that this phase of labour will take quite a while, will drag on for an hour or two, demand another huge batch of patience, and that you will be longing for that bearing-down feeling. Often the midwife will even assist you during the vaginal examination by gentle pushing the cervix over the baby's head during a contraction and telling you to try pushing. You, the mother, will recount later on that you did not experience any urge for the final stage of labour. Whether or not the attending midwife will have to undertake such action cannot be predicted beforehand. Have faith that the midwife will wait for the right point in time before she intervenes. I have to confess that, for me as a midwife, this phase of the birth often requires the highest concentration, because on the one hand I have to restrain myself, and on the other hand I don't want the birthing woman to be subjected to these massive contractions for any longer than necessary. For me the transition phase means finding the right balance between having faith in the woman's self-help mechanisms and intervening at the right moment so as not to subject the mother and child to any risks and manoeuvre them into a situation in which they expend energy unnecessarily.

It is often not easy to help women at this moment, but in my opinion all midwives and obstetricians should be as patient at the end of a phase of labour as they are at the beginning, in order to enable the baby and the mother to "do it themselves". Sometimes I have the impression that – already in the transition phase – the baby reveals its true character, that it can slide through the birth canal quickly and resolutely or make its way slowly but surely, or sometimes leave all the work to its mother.

The Birthing Position

Something I consider particularly important in every phase is that the birthing woman has the opportunity to move about freely. To be free means to recognize and choose for oneself what does one the most good. Naturally, the mother's position helps the baby substantially in making its way through the birth canal. The mother instinctively assumes the position that is best for the baby. Presumably there really is a kind of invisible communication between mother and child. The fact that women have been making use of gravity for centuries – and that lying on one's back slows labour down – has already long been acknowledged. Even if the woman's position sometimes looks strange or complicated for those of us attending the birth, it is amazing how precisely this position can lead to considerable progress in the birth process within just a few minutes. As a means of promoting the progress of labour, a change of position is always preferable, because it is considerably less painful than any manual intervention or manipulation of the cervix.

Of course the woman sometimes has to be encouraged by the midwife to get out of bed, get into the bathtub again or perhaps assume a kneeling position, because women of today no longer have the same experience with childbirth that their great-grandmothers may well still have had. It really is the task of the midwife, the woman's husband and the other people assisting her to encourage her to change to a different position during the intervals between the contractions. Merely asking whether she would like to change positions certainly will not suffice, because the birthing woman no longer wants to make any decisions; all she wants to do is devote herself entirely to what is going on inside her. So it takes the right amount of sensitivity to encourage the woman to assume a different pose without bothering her in her "work". But that's what we midwives are here for. In a home birth setting, where continuous care is provided, this is rarely difficult because the woman, midwife and partner are "broken in" as a team; they've already known each other for several months and practiced together during the antenatal class sessions. The surroundings are conducive to childbirth and it's no problem to change from the crouching to the all-fours position and maybe everything has been taking place on the floor for quite a while anyway, and the floor has accordingly been laid out with mats and pads to make it more comfortable. In the hospital you always have to take into account that the woman literally has to "climb down" from the bed, that the floor is rarely inviting, a look under the bed not always amusing and the bathtub really only allows the lying position – which is dictated by the tub's form. A birthing tub should be like a birthing room: inviting, spacious and warm. And it shouldn't matter whether water splashes onto the floor or not. Freedom of movement means: no matter where she is, whether in the water or the dry air, the woman in labour should feel safe and not have to worry about the bed being too narrow or too short, the bathtub too high or too narrow, the stool wobbly or anything of the kind. To be "free" also means not to be inhibited by any obstacle or any anxiety or to be exposed to the view of uninvolved persons. Here I must quote my esteemed colleague Hanna Fischer, the author of the book *Atlas der Gebärhaltungen* (Atlas of Birthing Positions): "Have you ever made love in this bed, Sir Doctor and Madam Midwife?" With these words she has put the entire truth in a nutshell: the child has come into being in an act of love and its birth should be an act of love as well. And love, as we know, is unconditional! All of these disturbances should therefore be entirely ruled out so that the woman can really let go, literally "turn her insides out" and simply experience intimacy. This might mean that things sometimes get a little uncomfortable for those of us present, but it's not the midwife, doctor or father who is bearing a child, but the woman, who will give birth in the manner most advantageous for the child. You will surely understand, dear reader, that this kind of freedom is actually only to be found in the context of giving birth at home or in a birthing centre, because usually the back of a self-employed midwife is not burdened by several deliveries going on at the same time. On the contrary, she normally has several days in between to recuperate from the bending and crouching she has had to do herself if, for example, the crouching position turned out to be the most preferable for the birthing woman, and the latter has braced herself alternately against the midwife and her partner. I am entirely convinced that this true freedom gives the woman in labour an immeasurable sense of safety. Intimacy doesn't just mean there are no rules and no dictates, but also no monitoring machines, no pre-established routine checks and no norm values which decide when labour is supposed to be over. The desire to have as great a degree of (medical-technical) safety as possible, however, quite often presents the baby with an insurmountable obstacle. Childbirth is not dependent on the ability to monitor the fetal heartbeat, and the birth canal is not just an anatomically correctly formed, immobile female pelvis, but a fascinating interplay of hormones, emotions, time and space between mother and child.

The Woman in the Transition Phase

During the transition phase, not only the personality of the child becomes evident but also, even more distinctly, the woman as she really is. In this phase of birth, the woman's true disposition reveals itself with all clarity. It is no coincidence that, in some languages, there are expressions for childbearing meaning something like: "turning oneself inside out". Women who have mastered all important situations on their own in the past will also go through childbirth very independently. The persons attending will accordingly feel somewhat like outsiders; the partner should be present, but there is nothing – nothing at all – he can actually "do". His wife might say: "Stay here, don't go away, but leave me alone". In this way she clearly communicates that she is able, and wants, to give birth on her own. She will give birth with the same strength, self-confidence and conviction she "brings to bear" in all of the decisions she makes in life without asking others. But women who have never taken action independently in life, have always allowed themselves to be led by others, and need someone to lean on and help them, will be happy – will truly need – to be able to lean on someone and receive help from active, massaging hands. As they have done in previous situations in their lives, these women will communicate their feelings very clearly. In the transition phase at the latest, the birth will be accompanied by words like the following on the part of the woman in labour: "I can't go on, I want to go home, I don't want a baby. I'd rather die than go on with this." Or, equally possible: "This is so terrific, it's crazy. I hardly know myself anymore; I never want it to end. It's completely unbearable and simply incredible all at the same time!" In any case, the birth atmosphere will become very emotional. Several days after the birth, for example, Mr. W. told me on the phone: "It's fascinating; I never knew my wife could be so emotional. Now I know why you can't describe childbirth, but just have to experience it."

For a woman in labour, the transition contractions mean going beyond herself, exceeding the limits of what she can achieve, experiencing a previously unknown side of herself – at least if it is her first child – and opening herself completely and entirely for the baby. There are people who regularly seek their own limits and go beyond them in sports. Once they manage that, they quickly reach the goal they are striving for. But precisely in this situation they need a coach who knows what they can expect and demand of themselves. Applied to childbirth, this means that in the transition phase, perhaps for the first time in your life, you will have to exceed your own limits, and that you will likewise need a coach and fans to cheer you on in order to master the birth. You can't give up midway through, the child wants to be, has to be born.

The persons attending the birth, the expectant father, the midwife, possibly a doctor, have to accompany you through the transition to the final stage of birth very actively, with their hands but especially with words and voices, because ultimately you have to give birth alone. All you need is support and encouragement that you will manage it, because the end, the goal, is the feeling of having to bear down and, ultimately, seeing, hearing and holding your baby.

As a woman and midwife I am aware that, for every woman, the experience of achieving this – being compelled to and being able to achieve it – will have an enormous effect on her life. As long as she lives, it will be a source of great strength for her. But I also know that for many it seems almost impossible to make it through this phase of the birth. The mere awareness that strangers may be witnessing her most intimate feelings can make it impossible for her to overcome her inhibitions and open herself entirely – due to her natural feelings of shame and shyness. The transition phase is like the physical ecstasy otherwise only experienced in conjunction with sexuality, and only with one's beloved partner. Many people don't manage to let go entirely even in that situation. And insight into these emotional depths is simply not granted to strangers. It is actually understandable when a woman has such great inhibitions that they keep labour from progressing in strange rooms and in the presence of strange people, and ultimately the doctors have to intervene. In this situation, recourse must very often be taken to medical aids so as to keep labour from coming to a standstill.

The Atmosphere in the Birthing Room

In the birthing room, the mood will likewise change considerably in the transition phase. A calm, meditative situation will turn into a powerful, energy-charged, emotion-filled birth atmosphere which seems to herald the incredible event which is about to take place. In order for such a mood to develop, it is important that the woman not be disturbed and can be sure that no-one will enter the room unexpectedly. If her surroundings allow intimacy, then intimacy can be experienced to the very depths of her emotions.

The Function of the Contractions: The Turtleneck Principle

In order to help people visualize the contractions in the active and transition phases of labour – when the cervix is opened by the force of the contractions – I like to tell the turtleneck pullover story ...

... to understand this mechanism, the expectant father should imagine that his wife has accidentally washed his favourite pure wool pullover in hot water. Now he tries to pull this stiff, matted pullover over his head. Initially he'll have quite some difficulty even just getting the top of his head into the turtleneck collar, but he'll manage with effort and patience. This would be a way of depicting the false and premonitory pains which serve to shorten the cervix to the point where "the cervix has effaced" as it is expressed scientifically. The father in his turtleneck pullover will notice: "It's rather tight but there's enough space for my head." Then he will very carefully try to pull the sweater farther and farther over his head, and his wife, who is witnessing all this, will say: "Be careful, otherwise the collar will tear. You have to pull evenly on all sides." When he does this, the "cervix" will surely dilate to a diameter of about five to six centimetres. I can imagine that the father will soon lose patience, however, and say to his wife: "Help me, will you? You pull in the front and back and I'll pull on the sides. That'll help more than all your great advice!" This is how it will be during "real labour" as well: at a diameter of about five or six centimetres the woman will lose patience, the force of the contractions will increase and she won't be able to bear it when someone gives her well-meaning pointers. She either wants real help or to be left alone, but she doesn't want any clever advice. Meanwhile, back at the "turtleneck birth", with four hands pulling, more and more of the head will soon become visible. When the turtleneck collar covers the father's head with nothing more than a wide edge, the father will call out: "I knew it! It still fits! One more good push and I'll be through!" No sooner said than done: his head pushes, the four hands pull, and father's head has overcome that tight turtleneck collar. During the birth of the child,

this would be the point at which the cervix is dilated to a diameter of about eight centimetres. It won't be long now, just a few more contractions – the transition phase – and then the second, or expulsion, stage begins.

The Second Stage of Labour

During the second stage of labour, the cervix is completely dilated and the contractions literally push the baby through the birth canal.

The Mother and Child during the Second Stage

When the baby reaches the pelvic floor, it completes its quarter turn and its backward bend of the head. Its head is facing the coccyx and the intestines and it fills the entire cavity of the pelvis minor.

For this reason, the woman in labour experiences a sensation of very great pressure on her rectum, to which she yields with a reflex-like reaction of wanting to push the baby out. This sensation is like having to go to the toilet and empty one's bowels, only much, much stronger. No woman can repress this urge to press. Often, however, particularly first-time mothers are surprised by the fact that the pressure is initially limited to the rectum and, out of a feeling of shame, try to hold back. Again and again, quite startled, they say: "Honey, I think the baby's is coming out the wrong orifice! What should I do?" The midwife will hear these words and remind the woman in labour that it is really only the pressure of the baby's head on the intestines, which have already been emptied by means of an enema or the body's natural purgative process. At this moment the woman will be happy to have evacuated as much as she did, and otherwise she won't care and the midwife will worry about cleaning up. In any case, no-one present will be disturbed, and they will continue encouraging and vehemently urging the birthing woman to yield to the urge to push and press, and to push right along with the contractions. Then the baby's head will propel its way forward to the vaginal orifice, from which it can and will be born. A participant in an antenatal class once described this feeling to the other expectant mothers as follows: "You have to imagine, the opening of your vagina is as big as a lemon and in the birth canal there is a baby as big as a watermelon, and you have to push the watermelon through that opening. And you'll be able to!" When the mother helps push, it animates the baby to stretch its head, brace itself against the pubic bone with the back of its neck and overcome the curve of the birth canal in the direction of the vaginal orifice. The baby has to make the transition from a maximum degree of flexion to a maximum stretching of the head. Since this is a very strenuous and unaccustomed process for the baby, it naturally cannot take place within a single contraction. If it is the woman's first child, this course of events will probably take longer than if it is her second, third, etc. In this phase, the woman's pelvic floor must likewise stretch to a maximum and make room for the baby's head. By this point, at the latest, she will be glad she has been doing plenty of pelvic floor exercises in the past weeks and preparing for birth with hayflower steam and perineal massages in order to have a pliable, soft pelvic floor for childbirth. With every further child, the hope and likelihood that the expulsion stage will proceed more quickly are greater since the muscles have already stretched that far before. The softness is not purely physical, however, but – to an even greater extent – psychological. At the phase of stronger and stronger stretching and greater and greater tension, the woman in labour knows that she also had enough space to let the last baby through. She knows: "I have already given birth to a child and this one will also find its way and overcome the confinement of the birth canal."

The "Birth Slide"

As a means of helping pregnant women in the antenatal class to picture the baby pushing and being pushed through the vagina, I cite the following example. I begin by showing them the shape of the sacral cavity and the birth canal with the aid of a cloth model of the pelvis. In the process, it becomes very clear that the birth canal is like a playground slide. I advise them to watch a first-born child trying out a slide for the very first time. Often the mother wishes she could sit herself down right behind the child and – depending on its disposition – either urge it to go slowly or encourage it to slide down fast. Children often brake when they get to the bottom, and slides are often constructed in such a way that the ride slows down automatically towards the end so that the child doesn't zip right off the end and hurt itself. Children often even want to be caught at the bottom by their mother or father. Second or later children, on the other hand, will simply sit down on the slide and call out: "Watch out, I'm coming, catch me Daddy!" Even if this is not what happens in one hundred percent of all cases, it can be observed quite often. And the mothers in the antenatal groups almost always confirm my observation. To give them a good impression of this "sliding feeling", I have each of them go through the baby's movements with their fist in the cloth model, and "slide through the pelvis" with a quarter turn, a bend and finally a stretch of the head. I received encouraging confirmation of this method of mine when Annette told me the following immediately after the birth of her child …

… her fourth child had been born very easily and quickly, which was unusual for her because she had always had trouble with the last phase of birth. I praised her and we were all very happy that the final phase had gone so well this time around. The new mother beamed at me and said: "Do I really have to have four children in order to understand what happens at the end? Today, thanks to the cloth pelvis and the 'slide' example, I was able to imagine exactly how my baby was passing through the pelvis. It was an excellent example, very easy to understand."

The Last Bit of Work

Like the other phases of labour, the second or expulsion stage can thus also vary in length – from two or three contractions to an hour or even longer. It is surely dependent on how much effort the baby makes itself, or whether it leaves all the work to its mother. As long as mother and child are both faring well, it is possible to wait patiently even in this last tight phase. As already mentioned in the section on the transition phase, it requires a great amount of experience in obstetrics as well as great sensitivity for the midwife to maintain her patience. Her task now is to communicate to the mother that she is capable of giving birth and that she has enough space to allow the baby to pass through. It is necessary – and usually sufficient – to motivate the woman so that she mobilizes her final reserves of perseverance. It is undoubtedly of great importance to allow the child to find its own way, while at the same time not subjecting either the mother or the child to any danger. Everyone – the birthing mother, the expectant father, the midwife and the doctor – must keep recalling that the birth of a human being is a natural process which does not require any intervention but only a lot of human "moral support" as well as the competence to recognize when the natural occurrence is headed for disaster.

The Hormonal Self-Regulation Mechanism

Every woman is capable of giving birth. This sentence, however, sounds as simple as the hormonal system which makes it possible – and which still has never been exhaustively researched – is complicated. This system is what creates the conditions not only for conception but also, later, for childbirth, through the production of female sexual hormones.

Towards the end of pregnancy, the female organism produces the contraction-inducing hormone oxytocin. This substance triggers rhythmic muscle contractions in the uterus and, by the way, is produced by man and woman alike during sexual intercourse. This is why it is referred to as the love hormone; it possesses certain addictive properties and brings about animal-like behaviour. At the same time, it also has an analgesic effect, because in conjunction with oxytocin the body releases pain-relieving substances in the pituitary gland – more specifically: endorphins and encephalins, natural opiates which trigger feelings of satisfaction, well-being and euphoria. In birthing women, they can lead to what is virtually orgasmic behaviour.

As soon as the mother is forced to turn her attention outward or carry on discussions about some medical action or another – i.e. her sub-conscious and 'archaic brain' are no longer active but the intellectual cerebrum is activated or the woman just simply feels stress, i.e. produces adrenalin, the formation of endorphins is inhibited. Relatively little is known about the neurotransmitter serotonin, which is produced in the brain, spinal cord and – according to more recent research – the intestinal mucous membranes. This substance evidently also promotes feelings of happiness and well-being, but is likewise blocked immediately by stress. As it has been for countless millennia, childbirth is achievable by the woman if she is left in peace, experiences no stress and accordingly does not have a high adrenalin level, if she feels well and receives affectionate attention, particularly in the form of back and abdominal massages, which also help to raise her serotonin level. Her favourite music and favourite aroma also influence the sensitive conduction and hormone system by way of the limbic system in the brain. The memory, also located in this region of the brain, remembers the explanations given during the antenatal class, and the woman can relax entirely, in turn creating good conditions for the effects the contraction hormone oxytocin can have in a uterus well supplied with blood and a soft pelvic floor. As already mentioned above, the release of the contraction hormone brings about increased production of endorphins, which makes childbirth achievable despite the pain. And in the intervals between the contractions, the birthing woman's face takes on a relaxed, even dreamy, euphoric expression which never ceases to amaze those around her. The alternation between pain and relaxation corresponds to the natural law of polarity upon which we can rely with great confidence. This elementary law according to which opposites belong together and are mutually determinant – for example pain and well-being, illness and health, day and night, above and below, ups and downs, right and left – are based on the law of plus and minus, the magnetic fields of the planet which keeps the earth in its orbit. The polar rhythm of life thus also facilitates childbirth: contraction – interval; long interval – strong contraction; that is a very healthy and lively rhythm which prepares the mother and father for life with the child, for all the ups and downs which they will experience with this guest on the planet Earth.

We midwives know: as long as the woman wants to give birth with her intellect; i.e. as long as her cerebrum is active – and this is apparent in her behaviour: she talks a lot and reacts to external influences –, the birth process is not acute. It is only when the woman has arrived inside herself, groans, sighs, even sometimes scolds her husband or the midwife, complains loudly about herself or the child, that we know: now things are getting serious! At the same time, we also know that within a few seconds the same woman can be desperate with pain if she has been given labour-inducing infusions with synthetic oxytocin or vaginal ovules containing prostaglandins and her natural hormone system has been disturbed, the release of endorphins blocked and she screams out for an analgesic or anaesthesia. The woman is robbed of her natural reward and satisfaction hormones, she is overcome by pain and the desire just to end the birth as quickly as possible is so overwhelming that even the personnel in attendance and the expectant father forget that every discussion on the subject of "But you said you wanted natural childbirth …" will only drive the adrenalin level up and worsen the pain until finally recourse must be taken to an epidural, or, worse, a caesarean under general anaesthesia.

Verena Schmid, who practices midwifery in Italy, thus asks the interesting question: is this why many women only have one child, because they are no longer permitted to feel the natural pain of childbirth? Is this why so many woman have no desire to have another baby?

Quite in contrast to the little old mother I once met, who confided in me …

…"You know, if the doctor had had his way about it I would only have had one child because they predicted that another birth would be fatal for me. But you midwives are women too, and you know that longing is stronger than reason. So I went and had three more children and I'm still alive today. But you know, the trouble the first one and then again the third one caused me was made good by the second and the fourth, which were both easy births, and today I go through life with all of these memories and wouldn't want to miss a single one of those experiences."

So it really is true, I thought to myself when I heard that story: childbirth really does release unsuspected energies and make women strong for life. Whether it is the mother or the baby who is more strongly shaped by childbirth is a question for thinking minds.

THE BIRTH OF THE CHILD

A Midwife's Guidance

The midwife in attendance will talk to you, the birthing woman, in easily comprehensible terms. She will talk to you with a calm, soothing voice and, if necessary, with clear, unequivocal words. She will make an effort to give you instructions as to what you should do during this phase of birth in order to create the best possible situation for the child and yourself. Naturally, the midwife will also let things take their course and leave you alone if you are doing the right things instinctively and what you are doing is good for your child. Trust the midwife to guide you in pushing the baby out. During the expulsion stage, the midwife will begin massaging your perineum to make it soft and pliable. That will make it easier for the baby to overcome this obstacle. Many colleagues consider it a positive challenge if the parents make a point of requesting that she do what she can to make sure the perineum is not injured. But please don't give the midwife any directions; she will be able to tell whether the perineum needs to be cut or not. Show her that you have faith in her abilities. In this phase of maximum dilation, what is important is to follow the midwife's instructions precisely, exert pressure when it is necessary and remain as relaxed as possible when the perineum needs time to stretch. The birth of the baby's head will follow, an event that will be accompanied by sharp, burning pain – a pain which can nevertheless be described as positive and expedient.

Pregnant women can prepare themselves mentally for what it means to feel this pain – and fathers can learn to understand it better – by doing the following: you know that the sensations of the mouth are very similar to those of the pelvic floor. With two fingers of each hand, take firm hold of the corners of your mouth all the way to the mucous membranes on the inside of the cheek and open your mouth like a wide-mouthed frog. At the same time, pull your cheeks outward with all your might and try to attain a maximum dilation of the oral orifice. This is exactly what the passage of the baby's head will feel like for the birthing woman, except that the perineum will have been well prepared. Next, you can rub *Dammmassageöl/Perineum Massage Oil 𝒟*® into the corners of your mouth and then repeat the procedure. How does it feel now? Above all: good when you let go again!

During this moment of birth, almost all women have a great need to let off steam by uttering a liberating yell or to try to endure the tension with the panting or blowing techniques they have learned.

Over and over again, I am amazed at how well women cope with this brief but intense feeling of stretching. It is no doubt extremely important to have faith in the woman that she can cope, and repeatedly assure her that there really is enough space in her pelvis and that she really can stretch and open herself.

If you don't believe that the baby's head really is visible as the midwife claims, that it really is protruding into the vaginal orifice, then feel for yourself. For many birthing women, it is an overwhelming feeling to touch and stroke the baby's head. Following this gesture of welcoming, you as the mother will be all the more able to summon your last reserves of energy and push the baby out with the greatest effort. Very often, the midwife even has to remind the woman to be careful and allow the baby to pass through her perineum slowly. I still see the situation before my mind's eye, when Andrea …

… was already at the point of giving up after just a few contractions – it was the beginning of the expulsion stage – and groaning: "I can't go on; I'll never manage this. Help me!" Moments like these are always horrible for me, because at this point we can't go to the hospital anymore; we're left to our own devices. Now there is no machine; no doctor with a suction cup can relieve the mother of the work and pull the baby out. In these situations – as in the case of Andrea – I try to remain entirely calm and confident, at least on the outside, look the mother in the eye and tell her quite unequivocally: "You know that you have to give birth to this child. You can do it; there is absolutely no doubt in my mind. Come on, touch it with your fingers, it's already almost out, and if you show it the way and push hard, you'll be done very soon. Now please push!" And the experience of touching the baby's head worked wonders. With radiant eyes and the words: "It's really true, it's really the head, how wonderful! Yes, Inge, I'll try, I'll manage it." With enormous energy and effort, Martin was born a few contractions later. I was very relieved that I had managed to motivate the birthing woman at the right point in time.

It cost me a lot of effort and powers of persuasion to get Kirsten to slow down …

… she kept reaching down with her hand to see if she could feel the baby yet and suddenly I could hardly hold her back. She called out: "It's coming, it's coming, I feel it, I want it now!" With soothing words I was able to subdue her in her ecstasy and tell her not to push quite so hard and let her first child pass through the perineum slowly so that it would remain intact.

Naturally, there are also women who cannot conceive of touching themselves in this moment. That is just as normal and perfectly alright. And there are midwives and doctors who shy away from encouraging the woman to do it. In these situations the midwife will say that she can clearly see the baby's hair. She will describe that she sees just a few dark strands or thick locks of black hair. One colleague of mine kept trying to convince a birthing woman that the baby was already quite visible and it would surely take no more than a few contractions and out it would come. But the mother didn't believe her and groaned, exhausted, "Sure it is, you already told me hours ago that it would only be a few more contractions and four hours have passed since then. I don't believe anything anymore." Without a moment's hesitation, the midwife took a pair of scissors, cut off a lock of the baby's hair and gave it to the mother. This clear, tangible sign restored the trust between the mother and the midwife and the baby really was born after only two more contractions. No matter how, it always helps immensely to give the birthing woman a positive report on the position of the head. Whether by having her touch, giving her a lock of hair or holding up a mirror for her to look in – what is important is that the mother can recognize for herself that the baby is already visible. I would advise all of my colleagues to offer these various possibilities and, naturally, leave it up to the woman in labour herself how she would like to convince herself of the progress of the birth.

With the final contraction, the baby's face passes over the perineum and its head then slowly turns to the side. Very often, the baby already lets out a little cry or sometimes even a loud yell at this point. If the perineum has been cut, the baby usually slides out immediately. Without an episiotomy it takes a bit longer. The mother, the baby, the midwife, everyone has to wait for the next contraction. This time the shoulders are born, causing the mother another feeling of stretching, and then she feels her baby sliding out:

"A child has been born! The most wonderful feeling on earth!"

How the Partner Can Help

BEING THERE is everything – and going with the flow

In the partner antenatal classes I ask the expectant fathers how they expect to benefit from the course. They nearly always say: "I'd like to learn what I can do during labour. I expect you as the midwife to tell me what to do." As I have mentioned frequently in the preceding chapters, the most important thing you as an expectant father can "do" is: just be there! You should remember that you can't *do* anything, but that the entire act of giving birth has to – and can – be mastered by your partner.

I find it perfectly alright if a father does not want to be present during labour, for whatever reasons. As a midwife I simply accept it. But in the past few years it has become par for the course for men to be in the birthing room. And the midwives have gotten so accustomed to their presence that, if a father wants to go out of the room, they ask, quite astonished: "What? You want to leave?" Don't let yourself be talked into staying against your will. You must decide for yourself whether you would like to welcome your child when your partner does, or feel overwhelmed by the situation, or are of the opinion that childbirth is woman's territory and men have no business being around.

If you do not want to be present, you should by all means see to it that your wife has a good woman friend with her during labour, preferably one who has already given birth herself. A woman needs encouragement and sympathy throughout labour. She should never have the feeling of being alone.

Another Helper

At home births, in addition to the woman's partner she often has arranged for a good friend – a woman or sometimes a man – to be present to provide additional support. When the birth takes place at an independent birth centre it is often a second midwife or a midwife trainee in her third year, getting practical experience as part of the requirements for completing the course. The expectant father is very relieved and grateful and accepts this help gladly. Often these additional helpers stay somewhat in the background and only participate more actively when they notice that the main helpers are beginning to run out of energy. The father can take a break any time and "refuel" by eating, drinking, getting some fresh air or just relaxing. The birthing woman will immediately benefit from this renewed energy. For the midwife it is a great help if sensitive helpers are present. A hospital midwife is often equally happy about it, because she often has to attend to several births at once. After all, the midwife is also responsible for all kinds of secondary details such as making telephone calls, notifying the doctor, or examining other in-patient pregnant women. An expectant father or friend of the birthing woman is very rarely sent home again by the midwife.

If you have decided to accompany the mother during labour, don't allow yourself to be turned away; just stay. Be guided entirely by the needs of the birthing woman.

The First Stage of Labour from the Helper's Perspective

During the first stage of labour it is sensible to busy yourself with some little job you have to do, book you have to read, or the like, and assure your wife: "If you need me then call me; I'll be with you immediately." Don't keep asking how long the intervals between the contractions are because that will put the birthing woman under pressure to perform. What you need now is a good balance between being attentive and being relaxed. Be aware that it might be necessary for the birthing woman to interrupt you in what you are doing at any moment. You should be able to abandon everything at the drop of a hat if your wife suddenly needs help. As soon as she begins making conscious use of her breathing techniques it would be best to stay in the room. From this point on, many women appreciate a massage during their contractions. They are glad when you run her a warm bath and breathe through the contractions with her. For you as the expectant father, being present during the first stage of labour means: doing the breathing exercises together, making sure there's enough fresh air, offering the woman something to drink, putting her favourite music on, walking back and forth with her in the hallway step by step, kneeling on the floor with her when it's necessary. See to it that your wife can assume whatever position she wants to. Normally, the body of the mother knows exactly what position will be the most advantageous. An intermittent examination or monitoring of the fetal heartbeat should not keep the woman from continuing to move the way she wants to. This doesn't mean she's not allowed to lie down. There is no one correct position for birth, just like there is no one correct course of events during birth. Every woman has her own way of behaving in the manner best for her in conjunction with the birth of this particular child. Unfortunately, in many obstetrics wards the birthing women's freedom of movement is still quite limited, but you have already visited the hospital and know what to expect. If you want to try to get your way in this regard, be diplomatic. Remember, no professional likes to be told what's best by a layman.

The Helping Hand/Breathing

Sooner or later, the most important thing will be to have your massaging hand at the centre of the labour pain and to help by breathing out. During this phase, speak to the woman with the deep voice so familiar to her, slowly chanting the words: yeeeeeeeeees – ooooooouuuuuut – aaaaaaaaaaaaaaahhh – soooooooooooooft – wiiiiiiiiiii-iide. Signal to the birthing woman again and again that she can open and widen herself. During the intervals, remind her comfortingly that every contraction fulfils its purpose and brings the baby closer to you little by little. Try not to talk constantly, however, but allow yourself to be guided by your wife's behaviour. Adapt yourself entirely to her needs.

The Transition Phase – Feeling, Breathing, Being There

Beginning with the transition contractions, if not before, the birthing woman will appreciate your breathing with her and, if necessary, helping her maintain her breathing rhythm by demonstrating it to her. Particularly when she has pains in her lower back – as is often the case during the transition phase – it will do her good to "show her the baby's way out" with one hand, using slow downward strokes and applying gentle, slightly increasing pressure. This downward massaging movement should be synchronized with her exhalations. Be sure never to massage in an upward direction. Again and again, the helping hands should show the birthing woman the direction in which the contractions are supposed to take effect – downward and widening. The greater the diameter of the cervix, the more advantageous it will be for your hands to conduct a gentle massage in a downward and outward direction. In many cases, the woman loves it if her partner's hands slide over her buttocks every time she breathes out. If the massage is strenuous for your hands, it means you're doing it right.

See to it that your partner has warm buttocks and warm feet. Warmth will help her to relax. If she doesn't want to be touched, at least try to hold her feet and brace her heels. Often this gesture is more pleasant for the woman in labour and does her more good than any other physical contact.

As a person attending a birth, do not be afraid to take the birthing woman into your arms. It is a wonderful thing to experience when a woman is literally held during labour.

It is equally possible, however, that she really only wants you to be there and that there is absolutely nothing you can do to help her in any way. Throughout my years of conducting home births, I have never once experienced this. Maybe it has something to do with the way the persons attending deal with the birthing woman. On the other hand, it is almost always the case that towards the end of the birth the woman turns her attention increasingly to the midwife. You as her partner should not be frustrated, and not withdraw, but encourage her in her instincts. Usually, fathers come to terms with this change quite well and recognize that the woman is now seeking competent help. It is in the nature of the event that, during this phase of birth, a woman needs another, a wise woman to help her.

Don't feel like an outsider, but remain integrated in the overall birth situation. During the final, strong transition contractions it will help your wife if you speak the words of letting go and letting out more distinctly than ever, virtually urge her: "Come, oooooooooooopen yourself, wiiiiiiiiiiiiiiiiden yourself, the baby wants to get ooooooooouuuuuuuuut." Or, during exhalation, join her in calling out: "Coooooooooooome!" It is very important to praise her and confirm to her that she is doing her work well. Encourage your wife by saying: "You can do it, yeeeeeees. You're strong. You're going to manage it. Think of our child." If she says during the interval that she just can't go on, remind her of all the great, strenuous work you have already jointly achieved. It will help her and give her strength. And if you frequently dab her face, forehead, throat and neck with a refreshing washcloth, it will also provide her relief.

The Pushing Phase – The Birth of Your Child

During the expulsion phase, the act of giving your partner the "backing" she needs not only has symbolic significance, but becomes a physical necessity. Sit, stand or crouch behind her and let her lean on you. In many hospitals the fathers are allowed to do this, and if that has not been the case until now where you are, you'll just have to be the first! During a home birth it is completely natural for the partner to have close physical contact with his wife during this final phase. It will soon be clear to you whether the midwife's words alone suffice, or whether it would be good and appropriate for you to give your wife additional verbal support. You could say, for example, "Come on, push! Let the baby out. You have enough space. You can do it." I can still hear my husband saying into my ear – apparently I was pushing in the wrong direction! – "With your belly, come on, push with your belly, downward!" I was immediately able to apply my strength in the right place. If the birthing woman tries to clench her teeth, then it is your job to remind her clearly: "Don't keep everything back, let the child out, come on, open your mouth, then the baby can come out!" With these words you will remind your wife of the pelvic floor exercises in which she was made aware of the direct connection between tension in the mouth and in the pelvic floor. In other words, she knows about the negative consequences of clenching her teeth and, conversely, the positive effects of opening her mouth. She only has to be reminded and encouraged and she will sense the strength and commitment you are putting into trying to help her. If the midwife doesn't tell you about the baby's progress of her own accord, just be curious and ask. In this final phase the woman needs as much positive support as she can get. As her partner, try to be the midwife's and doctor's interpreter; speak the language your wife will understand. Sooner or later you will realize that you are really part of what is happening, that you are a witness to the birth of your child. You will be overwhelmed, moved, close to tears, drenched in sweat and relieved after this strenuous experience:

»*Your baby is here! She gave birth to it. The most wonderful feeling on earth!"*

One marvelling new father remarked: "Birth – it's as though heaven and earth touched. And I was allowed to watch it happen."

Natural Remedies during Labour

During the antenatal classes and the consultations with a midwife, people very often ask about natural means of supporting the course of childbirth. There are a number of homoeopathic remedies and essential oils which can be administered to help the birthing woman with labour. Other holistically oriented methods are naturally also valuable, such as Bach Flowers, foot reflex zone massage, acupuncture and Reiki.

If a home birth is planned, the midwife explains to the woman during the very first talk that she will not be confronted with pain-relieving medication or with labour-inducing substances since their possible side effects are not only undesirable but moreover can only be controlled clinically. For most parents who decide in favour of giving birth outside the hospital, one of the main reasons for planning midwife-led labour is the fact that chemical-medical substances will not be used. They want to avoid the medications used in the hospital. A birth room in which pain relievers are ready and waiting is almost as tempting as a well-stocked pantry when you're fasting.

⊙ Homoeopathy

Expectant parents who would like the birth to take place in a hospital try to obtain as much information as possible in order to support labour with naturopathic methods themselves. A surprising number of mothers and fathers request information about homoeopathic remedies because they have been having themselves treated homoeopathically in hospital situations for a long time already or have gathered know-how themselves and set up a homoeopathic home medicine chest. In response to such requests I have always been happy to give the parents a list of the remedies that might be indicated. Since I know most of the parents and how much they know about homoeopathy, it is not difficult to give them the right advice. In cases in which the parents don't have the slightest knowledge of homoeopathy, it is impossible, however, to convey such knowledge to them within a short time. After all, the removal of an appendix also can't be learned during a consultation with a surgeon. I would like to point out once again that the teachings of classical homoeopathy by Samuel Hahnemann are comprehensive and that true classical homoeopathic doctors working on this basis are of the opinion that this method of healing is something it takes a lifetime to learn. I have been gathering knowledge of and experience in this field since 1981 and I can only confirm that point of view. I would therefore hereby like to urge all expectant parents who read this book: look for a midwife or doctor trained in homoeopathy so that you will receive the right support – through personal contact – and the remedies suitable for the individual pregnant woman. If you have the opportunity to plan birth in an independent birth centre or hospital in which you will be attended to by obstetricians trained in homoeopathy, take advantage of it. This is no longer very difficult, at least in Germany, where homoeopathy has become popular in obstetrics. And I would like to urge all of my colleagues not to try to learn about homoeopathy from books but to obtain their knowledge in well-conducted seminars. And once again, I would like to tell all of my readers very clearly: knowledge of homoeopathy cannot be obtained from books; the pharmacological pictures have to be heard and experienced. Not every homoeopathic remedy is appropriate for every person. The respective temperament, the conspicuous modes of behaviour of the respective pharmacological picture must be conveyed by a specialist in the field in such a way that the people who are to be treated with this remedy can be recognized. Particularly in the case of the major homoeopathic remedies listed below, the person should be reflected in his or her entirety. Remember: homoeopathy does not see only the uterus, but the woman in her entirety, in her disposition, in her contractions, in the course of her labour.

If you possess no basic knowledge whatsoever, then just turn the page, because you will only be confused by the descriptions of the remedies' "guiding symptoms". Homoeopathy is based on the correspondence between the remedy and the symptom, just as only a certain key will fit a certain lock. It is always the remedy that best matches the clinical picture which must be taken. I am consciously providing brief, precise symptom descriptions so that you will not be distracted by superfluous words and observations.

All parents with previous knowledge of homoeopathy receive the following information, with which particularly the partner of the pregnant woman should acquaint himself, because he is the one who will have to find the most suitable remedy for the symptoms observed during labour:

Aconitum –
sudden, acute fear of death, excruciating contractions, all mucous membranes dry. With regard to the newborn: anxiety about the child; major birth shock.

Arnica –

in cases of non-locatable labour pains, the entire body feels exhausted and the bed feels too hard; after birth to heal injuries (placenta wound, injuries to the vagina or perineum), can be administered after every birth!

Belladonna –

strong contractions: suddenly there – suddenly gone, very forceful; the birthing woman refuses to be touched, her complexion is beet-red, usually her whole body sweats, she makes an irritable and angry impression.

Caulophyllum –

no contractions but waters have broken, ineffective contractions: too short and too fast, nevertheless exhausting to the point of agony.

Cantharis –

the placenta fails to detach (frequent administrations of the remedy).

Chamomilla –

the pregnant woman is impatient, finds the contractions unbearable and wants an anaesthesia or epidural, she refuses all help and makes an aggressive and almost hysterical impression, often already at the beginning of labour.

Cimicifuga –

she talks a lot, fears the worst and sees everything very negatively: "The baby won't come out." The contractions are ineffective, like a cramp from hip to hip.

Coffea –

unbearable pain, faintness during the intervals; a remedy particularly effective shortly before the final contractions when the perineum is stretching.

Gelsemium –

restlessness, fear of what is coming ("What are they doing with me?" – "modern hospital atmosphere"), shaky weakness accompanied by nervous excitement, wants to be held.

Kalium carbonicum –

strong contractions, pain in the back, needs firm pressure and massage, craves warmth, strong self-control – can't let go.

Nux vomica –

overwrought and distressed, annoyed by the labour pains, cannot endure much pain, has never gone without pain-relievers, extreme nausea, feels pressure on bladder and bowels, can't bear draughts, craves warmth and demands anaesthesia.

Pulsatilla –
weepy, has inadequate contractions, postterm situation – "she can't let go", craves fresh air, wants to go for a walk, everything is changeable: her contractions, her mood, her position.

Sepia –
seems worn out, has had to take care of various other urgent matters before coming to the hospital, loves to take a warm bath for hours – wishes she could give birth in the bathtub, painful, agonizing, downward-pushing contractions accompanied by sharp pains in the vagina.

With these remedies as accompanying measures, it is possible to support a birthing woman in such a way that she feels she can go through with and accomplish the birth. I would like to emphasize that it is not possible – and would essentially also not be sensible – to make the contraction pains disappear with homoeopathic remedies. Natural methods support natural childbirth, and the latter is not without pain. At this point I could tell you a great number of stories about all of the globuli listed above. But I would rather quote a colleague who works at a hospital on a free-lance basis: "Since we have been working with homoeopathic remedies in the birth room, I hardly use any Dolantin (a morphine-like analgesic) anymore. Our doctors are amazed at how quickly the women deliver their children; the anaesthesiologists know we only need them for epidurals in hopeless situations. The statistics of the past years show what we midwives have been claiming for a long time: uterine atony (secondary haemorrhaging) has dropped to a minimum. I'd like to hear someone say that's not proof of the effectiveness of homoeopathy!"

There is no doubt in my mind that the homoeopathic remedies are what make low-risk childbirth at home – or in general outside the hospital – possible, allow mothers to experience the natural course of labour and grant children a carefree – and medication-free – start in life.

🌀 Aroma Therapy/Fragrances Used during Labour

The most suitable aromas are *verbena, jasmine, Roman chamomile, lavender extra, clary sage, cloves, rose, ylang-ylang* and *cinnamon*. To the joy of birthing women, midwives and doctors alike, these scents already envelop many obstetrics wards in a pleasant birth atmosphere. The fragrances often give the bleak and impersonal rooms a touch of nature and security. A sense of peace, warmth, trust and a subtly sensual, often slightly erotic atmosphere develops. Everyone present associates femininity, strength and perseverance with these aromas. All persons accompanying and attending to the birthing woman become aware that this woman can and will give birth. Due to the fact that the essential oils listed here are among the types that are more costly and difficult to dose, I created the sensual *Entbindungsduft/Childbirth Aroma 𝒟®*. This blend creates a pleasant aroma during the antenatal sessions, it helps the men tune into the topic of femininity and, during labour, helps the women remember the exercises learned in the antenatal class without a lot of explanations which would only distract her unnecessarily. Moreover, this essential oil blend has a relaxing and hormone-regulating effect. If the midwife deems it necessary, she can add clary sage, cinnamon, cloves or ginger oil to it during labour.

⑨ Massage Oil for Use during Labour

Since I myself am so convinced of the effectiveness of the fragrant essential oils, I wanted to make the benefits of these oils available to all expectant parents. In addition to the *Dammmassageöl/Perineum Massage Oil 𝒟®* I therefore decided to concoct an oil for massage during contractions. That is what led to the product *Geburtsöl/ Childbirth Oil 𝒟®*, which has enjoyed great popularity ever since I started working with aromas and has meanwhile come to be used widely. The power of the aromas can be experienced with an entire range of sensory perceptions. With massage oil the woman feels the effect by way of the olfactory organ – the nose – and the tactile organ – the skin – which also experiences the attention of the massaging hands. Millions of cutaneous receptors make direct contact to the brain stem and trigger the release of hormones. Countless midwives are convinced of the benefits of this massage oil, which can be ordered at the Bahnhof Apotheke in Kempten, and always have a bottle of it with them at the birth bed. During a seminar, a colleague of mine gave me an enthusiastic report on her first overwhelming aroma experience…

… "Recently I had a couple in my care who really took me to the limits of my abilities. No matter what the partner did, it didn't help the woman. It was really no wonder – he was so clumsy. Unfortunately I couldn't tend to the birthing woman very much because I had another one to take care of at the same time. It seemed to me that in view of the helpless partner and the nearly hysterical woman, the only thing that could help now was an epidural. In my own helplessness and hurry, I put a bottle of oil into the man's hand and told him to massage his wife's back with it. It had been standing on the windowsill for weeks, where it had been forgotten by another couple. When the other woman had finished giving birth, I returned to the couple. Before I even entered the room I noticed the peaceful mood, and when I went in I was absolutely amazed: the pregnant woman was relaxed and concentrating on breathing through her contraction, and the man was sitting on the bed and massaging her back. At the end of the contraction she looked up at me, beaming, and thanked me for this wonderful oil. Since her husband had begun rubbing the oil into her back the contractions had become much more bearable and she no longer wanted to be without his hands – it was simply a boon to be massaged by him. The man was still quite astonished about the fact that his wife now needed his hands so urgently; an hour ago the opposite had been the case. And the baby was actually born less than two hours later without an epidural. During the postnatal period the mother kept telling me that she certainly never would have experienced normal childbirth without that oil. And now", said my colleague expectantly, "I would like to learn a lot more about the effects of essential oils."

The *Geburtsöl/Childbirth Oil 𝒟®* used for coping with the contractions and so convincingly described here contains the essential oils of jasmine, clary sage, rose and the blossoms of the ylang-ylang tree. They have been blended with jojoba wax and other high-quality plant oils. If you would like to find out more about the way the various oils work, I recommend my book *Original D® Aroma Blends: Essential Oils for Living, Giving Birth, Dying.*

I am sure that with the administration of *Geburtsöl/Childbirth Oil D®* for massages during the contractions, a sense of safety, security and trust in the natural course of birth can be conveyed to all of the persons present. The woman in labour can allow things to take their course, her partner has faith that she will accomplish it, the obstetricians allow the woman to act as she deems necessary and regain their respect and reverence for the process of childbirth.

I was happy about a phone conversation I had with one mother …

… in which she told me that she was quite amazed about the effect of the massage oil on the team of doctors, because the aroma not only spreads onto the skin of the woman but also throughout the room. She described how a doctor burst into the room and was about to ask grumpily how far the cervix was now … And broke off in mid sentence, suddenly radiated a sense of contentment and friendliness at the same time and said "What's going on here? It smells mighty fine here on midwives' territory today! And that baby will surely want to be born today too!", thus signalling his readiness to wait patiently. With a cheerful look on his face he then left the birth room again. Now it was the midwife's turn to be amazed, and she remarked: "What's happened to him? I have never seen that man so cheerful, and he actually left the room without determining the degree of dilation. That has never happened once in all the years I've been working here." The consequence was that the midwife made a note of where she could purchase the Geburtsöl/Childbirth Oil D® in the hope of experiencing a working atmosphere such as that one more often.

My most intense experience with *Geburtsöl/Childbirth Oil D®* took place during the home birth of little Cora …

… her mother is a very strong and resolute person who made it clear to me that she didn't want any massages or rubbish of that kind, she just wanted to be able to have her baby at home in peace and quiet, without other people meddling. When I arrived, the birthing woman was sitting upright, cross-legged and meditating. She was making a great effort to breathe through the contractions as perfectly as possible and not lose her composure. When I timidly asked her whether I should massage her at the centre of the pain, she energetically declined, saying that it wasn't necessary. As it became increasingly clear to me how much she was struggling with the contractions, I simply rubbed a bit of the oil gently into her lower abdomen without asking her. It took just one contraction and then she whispered to me softly but enthusiastically: "Oh that feels wonderful, please keep the oil and your hand there." A few contractions later it wasn't me who was actively massaging her anymore, but the birthing woman herself, on all fours and moving her belly back and forth in my hand. Now she was able to let go and it was obvious from listening to her that the baby would soon be born. She opened all of her emotional doors and we experienced a wonderful birth.

✑ Using Aroma Therapy during Labour

Naturally, all of the essential oils I am about to mention below can also be used in the aroma lamp. During home births, it is the birthing woman's favourite fragrance that fills the room. In the hospital, it is better to use the aromas in the form of bath salts or massage oils so as not to burden the midwives and other personnel to an excessive degree. And you should also take into consideration that perhaps the pregnant woman in the next bed is calm and collected, in which case Roman chamomile, for example, would be inappropriate for her.

- *Geburtsöl/Childbirth Oil 𝒟®* has a supportive, pleasant effect during labour if you administer it in the form of bath salts. Emulsified in plenty of Dead Sea Salt and one to two tablespoons of honey or cream (in the hospital you can use evaporated milk), it develops a strongly relaxing, pain-relieving effect. Through the use of Dead Sea Salt – you can use up to one kilogram – the bath will also have disinfectant and circulation-stabilizing qualities. The birthing woman will feel as though she is being held and protected by the water.

- *Lavender oil extra* is an ideal bath supplement in cases of massive contractions or a tense atmosphere. It helps to create clarity and calm. The fragrance of lavender extra will help even the most excited father or nervous midwife.

- Used in the form of a massage oil or bath supplement, *Roman chamomile* is likewise helpful, especially for birthing women who are unusually sensitive to pain and already suffering from strong, cramp-like, unbearable contractions at the beginning of labour. Three to five drops of *Roman chamomile 10% in jojoba wax* mixed with a tablespoon of massage oil will suffice.

- If the contractions decrease in strength and frequency or in cases where they stop altogether, mainly due to exhaustion, it has proven helpful to administer *Ut-Öl/ Uterus Tonic 𝒟®*, which contains verbena, cloves, ginger and cinnamon. I would like to advise all midwives to keep this massage oil on hand in case the woman's energy ebbs during the transition or expulsion phase, making the contractions weaker. Massage the fundus uteri energetically with this oil. The woman in labour will be capable of enduring the birth and the strength of the contractions will suffice to give birth to the child. I would like to request, however, that this oil only be used by midwives and only if indicated – and not because the midwife will soon be going off duty, but only when the birthing woman really needs it. I am quite certain that it is thanks to *Ut-Öl/Uterus Tonic 𝒟®* that I have never had to make use of labour-augmenting drugs at a home birth.

- The midwife will often use the essential oil of *verbena* in the form of smelling salts in order to rouse the woman from her emotional reverie and thus focus her concentration on letting go of the baby entirely. She will become very attentive and accessible and cooperate optimally again. One drop of *verbena 10% in jojoba wax* administered to the forehead, the fold of the neck or the décolleté will suffice.

- A time-tested essential oil for obstetrics situations is *neroli 10% in jojoba wax*, likewise in the form of smelling salts or natural perfume, as in the case of verbena. Its application is also helpful when the father needs first aid. For many fathers, the birth of the child takes such a load off their minds that they become faint. At home births, the tension caused by the responsibility and the active assistance are both much greater, and moreover we almost always succeed in warming up the birth room quite considerably, which likewise leads to unsteady circulation.

- *Neroli 10% in jojoba wax* can also be helpful for the new mother, because women often overestimate their strength the first time they get up again after giving birth. Despite our warnings, they don't wait, but hop out of bed before the midwife can turn around. But they no sooner take a few steps than they find themselves on the floor. Then the good old smelling salts suffice to get the mother safely back into bed. A word of well-meant advice: midwives know what they're talking about when they ask you not to get up from the birth bed without doing exercises to stabilize your circulation first.

- Added to *Geburtsöl/Childbirth Oil 𝒟®*, the essential oil of *rosemary* is an ideal support during labour – used for a foot massage or, mixed with salt, in the bathtub – in cases of birthing women whose blood pressure is too low. It is always amazing to see women who have been suffering from insufficient contraction activity and fatigue in connection with low pressure suddenly start having strong contractions and master the birth with vim and vigour.

- Rubbing *Rose Hydrolat* onto the forehead, back of the neck or upper body provides very pleasant refreshment during labour or after the birth. Expectant fathers can perhaps pleasantly surprise their wives with the refreshing hydrolat of rose or orange blossoms.

The Third Stage of Labour: The Afterbirth

Childbirth is not entirely over when the baby is born. The first moments of joy and relief at having made it through the birth are followed by a final, generally very brief effort on the part of the mother: the birth of the placenta. Unfortunately, in many hospitals, women get an injection of a contraction-inducing hormone immediately after the birth of the baby to ensure that the afterbirth will separate from the wall of the uterus as quickly as possible. Even without medication, however, the placenta can be born within five to fifteen minutes. On the other hand, there are also situations in which it can take an hour or even longer until this final stage of birth is concluded. This can be patiently awaited as long as the mother is feeling well and doesn't develop any circulation problems or bleeding – after all, after forty weeks of waiting it should be possible to wait another hour. What is more, even now, the natural hormone balance should not be disturbed if possible. It has been shown that women who do not receive the obligatory dose of oxytocin experience that the milk flows sooner and their babies are calmer. In high-risk situations, of course, oxytocin can and must be used. But it is quite difficult to understand why childbearing has only been declared a high-risk process since the "technologization" of medicine. It would be far preferable to view every birth as an individual event and act accordingly.

Many obstetricians think they have to help the afterbirth on its way by applying relatively strong pressure to the uterus – painful for the woman – and tugging gently on the umbilical cord as a means of pressing the placenta out. Maybe you as the woman's partner can request a bit of patience and sensitivity. Your wife will appreciate it. I consider it important that women let go of and deliver the afterbirth voluntarily. I believe that nature intentionally arranged it so that, after the extreme stretching of the vagina during the birth of the child, now one soft, light, final stretch takes place so that the mother will remember the soft afterbirth as the last stretching sensation.

The birth of the placenta is accompanied by further contractions, which, however, are seldom as strong and intense as labour pains. Once again, the woman experiences cramp-like pains and – after a length of time which varies from one woman to the next – pressure on the pelvic floor. The new mother will then deliver the placenta as a "soft warm something" with a minimal stretching sensation. The midwife will call your attention to this process, help you through it and make sure that the fetal membranes have passed through the vagina in their entirety. Already for this reason alone, it appears to me to be important that the woman is given the time she needs to wait for the placenta.

Together, we will then check the afterbirth to make sure it is complete. It is usually about the size of a cake platter, is about two to three centimetres thick and – on the side on which it adhered to the wall of the uterus – the colour of dark red meat. On the side that had been facing the baby, it is covered with fetal membranes which give it a pearly sheen. The attached umbilical cord gives the placenta an interesting tree-like appearance, the umbilical cord itself representing the trunk, the major blood vessels the large boughs, which divide into smaller and smaller branches and finally form a crown in the placental villi. And just as there are many different types of trees, every placenta also looks different. In many regions it is still customary to this very day to bury the placenta and plant a tree on top of it. Since it is human tissue, midwives have always had to see to it that the afterbirth was disposed of properly. And in the days before waste incineration, the best method was probably to bury it in a deep hole in which a tree was subsequently planted. Until very recently, deep-frozen placentas from the hospitals were used to manufacture medicinal skin creams. But that has also changed, and now all placentas, including those from home births, are to be destroyed by the hospitals. I simply can't understand this ruling! Childbirth has always been – and presumably always will be – an event which takes place in the bosom of the family. And what is more, it isn't possible that there is anything pathological about the placenta. The placenta is regarded by some as something valuable – they would use it to manufacture medicine if they were allowed – and by others as something suspect, material to be destroyed under surveillance.

When we inspect what has been the baby's "pantry", the placenta, we are almost always amazed by the silky surface of the side facing the child and serving it as a cushion to rest on. The colours of the fetal membranes and the placenta are very striking and the parents gain an understanding of why children love soft, silkily translucent shades of red and blue during its first weeks of life.

Throughout my service as a home birth midwife I have never once experienced a mother or father being disgusted by the sight of the afterbirth or horrified by its bloody appearance. They are actually only fascinated by the way nature works. We midwives should also learn to talk about it with respect so as not to scare the parents off with this bloody aspect of obstetrics. In any case, I am grateful to one father who said to me reproachfully once in the early days of my hospital service: "Why are you treating the afterbirth so disrespectfully; you don't have to remove it immediately, we want to see the organ that has been nourishing our baby." This doesn't mean that you as parents will be forced to look at the placenta, or to feel it, but if you would like to do either, you can surely talk to the midwife about it. Because, among other things, this situation is an excellent opportunity to voice your ideas about what should be done with the placenta.

Incidentally, the afterbirth, the final stage of labour, is a bloody affair. Many men are of the opinion that they don't want to witness a birth because of all the blood that supposedly flows during it. Afterwards they are often relieved that it wasn't all that bloody after all. But that's because, after the birth, the men are usually preoccupied exclusively with the newborn and don't even notice that their wives bleed following the birth of the placenta. A loss of up to 500 ml/17 oz. of blood is normal.

Natural Means of Support

Here again, there are natural means of support in the event that this final stage of labour takes too long.

The Baby's Sucking Reflex/Stimulation of the Nipples

One of the simplest aids provided by nature is the newborn baby's sucking reflex. As soon as the baby starts making sucking and searching movements, it is time to put it to the breast. Many a child finds the mother's nipple on its own as soon as she takes it into her arms. The sucking serves to stimulate the uterus, which begins to contract. If you discover you have given birth to a child who really doesn't have the need to suckle – there are babies who don't – then you, the mother, or you, the father, will have to think of some other way of stimulating the new mother's nipples. This is undoubtedly the most effective natural method of triggering "afterpains".

Change of Position

If the sucking or stimulation doesn't help and the waiting time is getting longer and longer, the young mother can be encouraged to move around. Just as gravity and movement have a positive effect on the birth of the child, they will also help her to deliver the afterbirth. I learned this naturally effective method from women and not from obstetricians. Naturally, I know that many midwives and obstetricians would not permit this, since it would be extremely unusual behaviour in a hospital birth room. But perhaps it will at least be possible upon request to assume a crouching position on the birth bed. The woman should then carry out intensive pelvic exercises, which are likewise also sure to lead to the birth of the placenta. Naturally, this method cannot be employed if the woman is bleeding strongly.

⑤ Homoeopathy

Homoeopathically, usually one of the following medications is employed: *Arnica, Cantharis, Sepia, Pulsatilla*.

When the woman begins to bleed, I have had good experience with homoeopathic remedies, and only in a handful of cases have I ever had to take a woman to the hospital. I am only listing the following medications, though, so that young colleagues who want to inform themselves about home childbirth hear something besides a lot of warnings and fears.

This situation is one that is feared by midwives in general, but it loses a bit of its terror if we are well-versed in the pharmacological pictures of the following substances to counteract bleeding: *Arnica, Belladonna, China, Ferrum, Hamamelis, Ipecacuanha, Millefolium, Phosphorusus, Sabina* and *Secale*. Once again, however, I would like to draw the reader's attention emphatically to the fact that it does not suffice to read books and have your own selection of obstetrical remedies, but that their administration has to be learned thoroughly, starting at the beginning. Moreover, I would also like to point out again that in the context of home births, there are no means of preventing this acute threat to the mother's life. I can remember every single woman I have ever had to have rushed to the hospital because of profuse bleeding, and it took me a long time to digest each one of those experiences. What I have learned from them, however, is that even this risk can be dealt with if everything has been carefully planned, clear decisions can be made, and the cooperation with the ambulance service and the hospital runs smoothly. No time is really lost through the transport, because the hospital also needs time to get set up for dealing with the situation. After all, the anaesthetics team doesn't wait in front of every birthing room door, but is on duty in surgery or on call and has to be informed if there is an emergency.

I would like to tell you about one of the most memorable experiences I ever had with bleeding …

… when I arrived at the woman's house to attend to the birth, the woman told me she had just carried out an enema with chamomile. The baby was born a short time later. She began to bleed rather strongly due to the separation of the placenta from the uterus, and the bleeding did not come to a standstill following the afterbirth. I quickly looked up what remedies were appropriate in cases of bleeding and I recalled the chamomile enema. Under the pharmacological picture of China it said: bleeding following abuse of chamomile. A dose of China globuli brought the bleeding to a standstill within a few minutes. The woman recovered very well from her substantial loss of blood.

◎ Aroma Therapy

Naturally, a delay in or difficulties with the detachment of the placenta can also be counteracted with essential oils. The midwife can add a few drops of *verbena* to the *Ut-Öl/Uterus Tonic 𝔇®* described above, and use this blend to massage the fundus uteri, a method which will often trigger very effective afterpains. This method should only be employed, however, if the woman has no bleeding whatsoever and tends to feel cold easily.

In the past years I have heard from many colleagues that cool lavender compresses are also effective. A blend of mint, sage, lemon and cypress – the composition of my *Salbei-Zypressen-Öl/Sage-Cypress Oil 𝔇®* – is even better. The oil is rubbed onto the woman's abdomen and then a cold compress is applied on top of it. This measure almost always suffices to trigger afterpains and is preferable to *Ut-Öl/Uterus Tonic 𝔇®*, since *Salbei-Zypressen-Öl/Sage-Cypress Oil 𝔇®* has an astringent and haemostatic effect.

Once the placenta has been delivered, the postnatal phase begins.

STILLBIRTH

WHEN LIFE BEGINS WITH DEATH

As has already been mentioned several times in this book, there is no guarantee that the pregnancy "project" will have a completely happy outcome. Since time immemorial, women have given birth to dead children. Globally speaking, only every second pregnancy brings forth a living infant. Unfortunately, women don't learn that until they undergo the experience themselves in the form of a miscarriage, a premature birth, a dead child carried to term, a postterm child that dies in the womb, a severely deformed, nonviable child, or a child that dies immediately after birth. The mourning is the same, no matter what the point in time. When the baby is a victim of sudden infant death syndrome in the first year of life, it is an equally indescribable tragedy.

It only makes matters worse for a woman to be told by medical professionals or people she knows: "You're young; you can still have lots of children." As if one child could replace another!

For expectant parents it is difficult to deal with this subject. Usually they don't read these lines until it has happened. But perhaps you are one of the exceptions and are taking this into account even though you fortunately have every reason to believe your child will be born alive and healthy. If all of us dealt with the subject of mourning more openly, we'd know how to cope with these challenges of life when we were faced with them.

The first thing you should know is that when you learn of the child's death you have all the time in the world. For this child, time will always stand still! And your life also seems to stand still, or at least to be ticking much slower. Don't let anyone put you under time pressure. The first order of business for you is to let all of your emotions take their course – cry, scream, despair, lapse into silence, rant, sob, howl, break down. And then what you need is peace and quiet. Find a retreat. Find someone to take of your older kids – a friend, a babysitter, a neighbour; someone will have time. Naturally, it is alright for the children to experience their parents' desperation, but they should have someone they can turn to, and who will take care of them accordingly. For you, eating, sleeping and in general daily rhythms will be unimportant.

Don't expect any sympathy from others; other people are usually just helpless. As an expectant father, you will presumably also be at a loss, all the more so the earlier the pregnancy has come to an unfortunate end. The man often doesn't develop a bond with the child until the moment of birth. All the more difficult will it be for the man – in the case of a miscarriage or a premature birth – to find his own emotionality and understand that of his wife. The difference in the way the two persons react emotionally sometimes even places a serious burden on their relationship.

Following an initial phase of peace and retreat, necessary just to begin to grasp the ungraspable, the next thing is the question as to how things will continue:

In the case of a fetus which has died in the first few weeks of pregnancy, sooner or later the body will miscarry without any hectic action being taken. The woman will develop abdominal pains and more or less rhythmical contractions and bleeding, with which she will abort the baby. There is likewise no reason to rush the decision as to whether curettage should be carried out, as is done on a routine basis in many hospitals/doctor's practices. It is possible to determine whether this is necessary with the help of modern ultrasound methods. I have attended to many women who did not want to subject themselves to this surgical intervention. In connection with the subject of curettage, it may help to think about the fact that, all over the world, women abort every day, but in many countries no surgical measures are possible and these women are still able to have children afterwards anyway. Moreover, by carrying out the exercises described in the section on the early phase of the postnatal period, the woman can get her reproductive organs back in shape. Thus even in times of mourning, you need to use your common sense, because action is sometimes taken all too quickly which you would question critically in a normal life situation. You do not by any means have to go to the hospital immediately, but need only have an appointment with the gynaecologist. If you should develop strong bleeding, however, you know that every hospital is open twenty-four hours a day and will always admit you.

If the fetus dies in the womb later on in pregnancy, there is likewise no need to rush. Your body will understand the situation and initiate the birth process within about ten days after the death of the child. The pain experienced is clearly identifiable as labour pains, and it will be a painful birth. In the sensation of pain in this context, the role played by the psyche is anything but insignificant, because – understandably – the woman undergoing such an experience lacks all understanding for this occurrence, which is not accompanied by happiness but by unspeakable sorrow. And the pain of mourning alone is already felt physically to such a degree that the labour pains are the last straw. Here again, give free rein to all of your feelings. Even if you theoretically could receive any amount of analgesics, you should be aware that the physical pain you are feeling is like an emotional pressure valve that will help you to come to terms with the situation emotionally. You can – but certainly don't have to – accept the offer of analgesics and/or an epidural. The sooner the pain reaches the physical level, the faster your soul can heal. With your partner and your midwife, think about what the ideal place would be: your home, an independent birth centre or a hospital. The midwife will know what is common practice at the nearby hospitals and be able to advise you. It is important to know that, even though it is a sorrowful birth, it demands just as protective an atmosphere as that of a living child, and, naturally, a water birth is equally possible. See to it that you can have the kind of environment you need and in which there is space and time for all of your pain. Take time for your decisions and don't let yourself be rushed. In such a situation I once experienced a doctor saying: "Yes, but the woman should come today; she has to be kept under surveillance!" I answered: "But the child can't do anything worse than die, and that has already happened!" He saw my point: "Actually, you're right. Okay, tell the parents they can come whenever they feel the need." As you can see, there will never be a routine for dealing with stillbirths, because fortunately they are very rare. On the other hand, that means that the parents are called upon to consider carefully and come to a decision on their own in a situation in which what they really need urgently is support.

Taking Leave

After the birth of the child, you should again take all the time in the world. Take leave of your child in the manner you yourself think is the best, allow yourself to be guided by your feelings. This is no place for rational thinking. If you want to, it will be a good memory to hold your baby in your arms, put it in its nicest suit of clothes, or simply swaddle it in fluffy nappies. Lay your child in a crib, or perhaps in an affectionately carpentered and decorated coffin, if you have had time to have one made before the contractions started. The act of building a coffin might serve as a valve for the father's tears and pain. A man who had experienced this tragic situation once told me what an important task it had been for him, his labour pains, so to speak. If you already have older children, they might like to give the baby a doll or cuddly toy to take with it on its long journey. It is also important to take the time you have before labour begins and choose a name for the child. Remember that, no matter how briefly your child lived, it did live, and will always be an integral part of your biography. And when the dead have names it's easier to talk about them later on.

It is also good for the midwife to take pictures of your child so that later you can look at them if and whenever you want to. But you will realize that your memory stores pictures wonderfully.

Arrange to have your baby buried if at all possible. In this matter, your self-employed midwife will once again stand by you and provide important support. If your midwife does not yet have much experience with miscarriages and stillbirths, there are sure to be organizations such as the German REGENBOGEN »Glücklose Schwangerschaft« e.V. (for address, see appendix, p. ■) where she can obtain helpful information.

SIDS: Sudden Infant Death Syndrome

If your baby dies of sudden infant death syndrome – known in the vernacular as cot death or crib death – on top of all your pain and sorrow you will have to deal with the law. The police will demand medical certification that the baby has died a natural death. You yourself will perhaps hate these examinations – which incidentally never become routine for the policemen and the doctors, even if they seem merely to be indifferently doing their jobs – or you may experience them as though in a trance. Or perhaps you will have remembered your midwife again, who stood by you through childbirth with all of the fears that accompany it. Now she will be prepared to help you again and support you with her empathy and take you protectively into her arms just as she did during labour; she will simply be there for you. Here as well, give free rein to all of your emotions! It is completely natural to wonder how it could have happened. But remember that the question of blame will not bring your baby back to life. Try to liberate yourself from those thoughts and encounter everyone in the family with love and understanding. There have always been babies that died after a few months of life. They simply choose to leave again, as difficult as it is for us to under-stand. Death is always accompanied by question marks and speechlessness, even if it seems completely unnatural to have to bury your child and not the other way around. Nevertheless, you will have to let go of it. Try to understand it the way a child does: "It wanted to go back to the angels; it's nicer up there!"

You will be confronted with reality all too quickly and have to decide whether the baby can be laid out at home for a few days or be taken to the local mortuary. Maybe your baby hasn't even been baptized yet, or you had planned to let it decide for itself later on what confession it wanted to belong to. Again, there are organizations which help parents in this situation, such as the »Bundesverband Verwaiste Eltern e.V.« (for address, see appendix, p. ■) in Germany.

Let me repeat: in this phase of life, the most important thing is to take your time! Take leave of your child. Hold it in your arms as long as you think it is necessary. Lay it down again when your instinct tells you: now is the moment, now I will put it back in its favourite place. And once you have dressed it in the clothes you most prefer, you can decide when to put it in its coffin. Maybe as you read this you'll think: I could never bring myself to do that! But it will be different from the way you imagine it – life will show you what you are capable of in connection with your child.

The Days and Weeks after the Death of the Child

A midwife is someone you can turn to for help if you go through a miscarriage or premature birth. She can advise you on procedures for weaning and involution (the return of the uterus to its normal size). You can also read about these topics in the sections below on the early postnatal period and breastfeeding. Look for a self-help group in which you can talk about your feelings and experiences with people who have suffered similar fates. Such groups will also provide you with help and support on questions of mourning, e.g. how to deal with and involve your other children, the grandparents and your partner. Every individual has to find his or her own way of coming to terms with the situation. But the mothers are the ones who suffer the most unspeakable pain. Allow your family a different way of mourning.

For the woman, the question as to whether she can get pregnant again, and the extent to which it is physically safe for her to do so, will come up sooner or later. From experience I would like to advise you not to consider this question on a purely rational level. Give your body time and listen to what it is telling you. But also be aware that your body might not mourn as long as your soul. Many women get pregnant again right away. Take into account that the due date calculated for the dead child will be a difficult phase of intense mourning which can even be accompanied by physical pain. I have witnessed the latter above all in cases where the first phase of mourning was not given enough scope, but successfully repressed. The first birthday of the baby carried to term will likewise be a day of sorrow. My concern here is to point out to you that you will not conceive the child you have buried a second time. Give every further pregnancy, every further child the chance to find its own place in your life, alongside the dead child but not in its place!

Ritual instead of Burial

If a child weighing less than 500 g/1 lb. is miscarried, it is not buried by the city but by the hospital, although all parents have the right to a burial. To date, only very few towns have made it administratively possible to bury these children at the cemetery. This means that you have no gravesite for the child, or perhaps you do not want a gravesite at this point in time. Then I would advise you to find a site somewhere in the open country where you can return your baby to nature and the universe within the framework of a ritual. Choose a place where you will be able to visit your child. Whether you choose the leaves of a tree or the petals of flowers to give to the wind or water, or bury a beautiful stone you have found, or a precious stone, or whatever reminds you of the existence of this child of yours on earth, what is important is that you always – at any time in your life – have the opportunity to awaken your awareness of this existence and also consciously let go of it again so that you do not carry the burden of it only in your soul.

Bach Flowers
Rescue drops, a Bach Flower remedy, provide excellent help. I have never gone to visit a mourning woman or family without taking these emergency drops along. Begin by taking one drop undiluted, by letting it trickle out of the bottle onto your tongue. In the days that follow, dilute three drops in a glass of water and take small sips of it throughout the day. The Bach Flowers are wonderful consolation to the soul.

Herbal Medicine
The herbal tea blend *Herzenströster/Heart Comforter*, drunk in small sips, helps the entire family learn to cope with this incomprehensible fate. It contains the nerve-

fortifying, calming herbs damiana leaf, St.-John's wort, lemon balm leaves, passion flower leaves, peppermint leaves, rose petals and liquorice root.

✆ Aroma Therapy

I can no longer imagine coping with such situations without the help of essential oils, because the aroma affectionately envelopes the woman and helps everyone involved to accept the circumstances. Aroma, the language of nature, needs no words – in this situation words are often awkward anyway – and helps you to embrace the irreversible. Particularly the scents of *lemon balm* and *rose* are optimal for this purpose. Years ago, I created the essential oil blend *Trennungsschmerz/Parting Pain* $\mathcal{D}^*$. This can be used in the aroma lamp or, whenever you feel the need, you can draw yourself an aroma bath with it by mixing the oil with honey or dairy cream. The precious blend *Sprachlos/Speechless* $\mathcal{D}^*$ also helps many parents. The essential oils of rose, lemon balm and iris are mixed with jojoba wax and, administered as a natural perfume, provide you with protection and shelter.

✆ Homoeopathy

Here the first-aid remedy *Aconitum* is at the top of the list. Later *Ignatia* and *Natrium muriaticum* can be considered. In this context, it is usually necessary to administer the higher potencies, and it is strongly advisable to discuss the doses with the midwife or homoeopath.

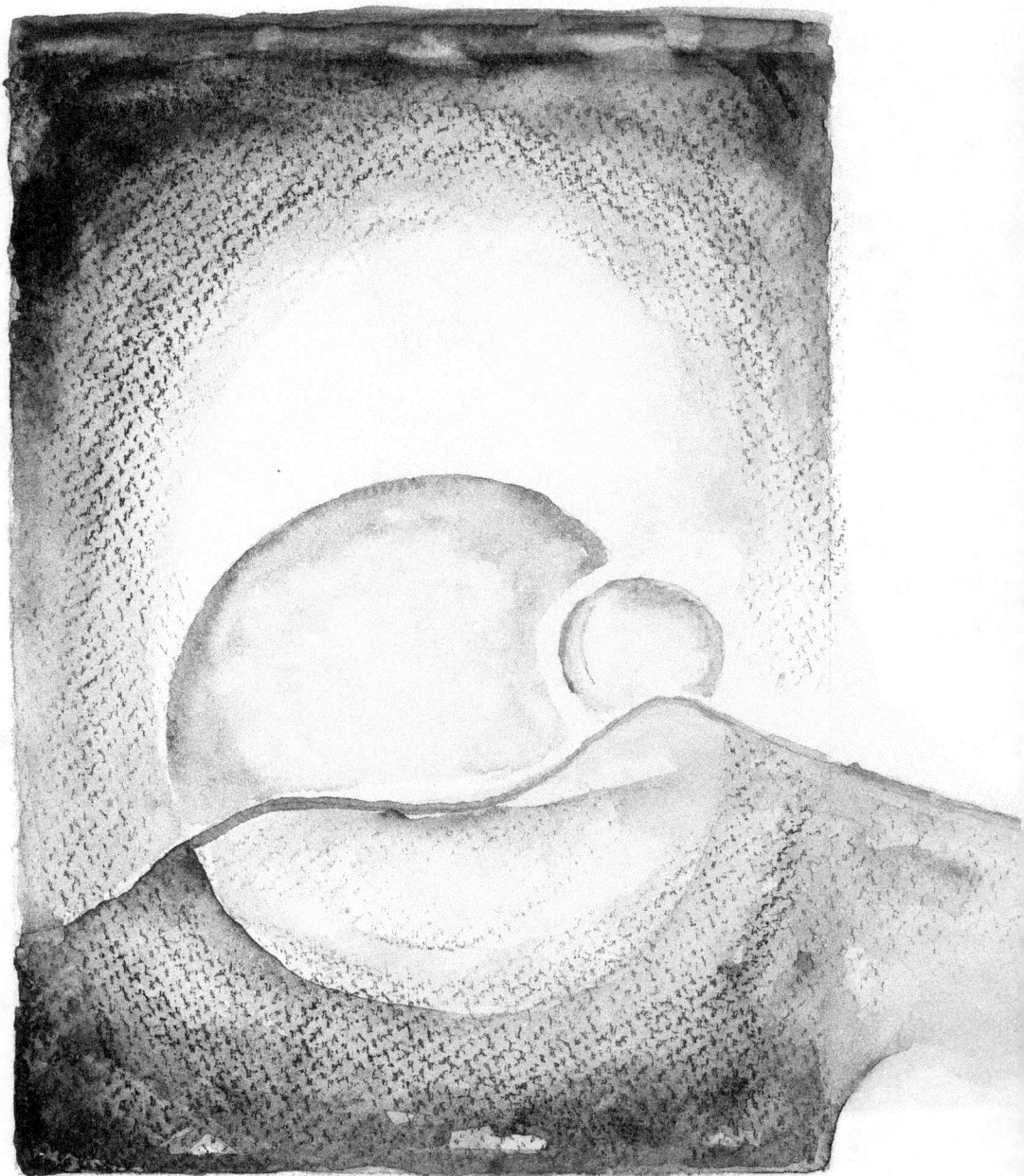

CHILDBED:
THE POSTNATAL PERIOD

empty – alone
the cave again – protection
a little while
we
you and me

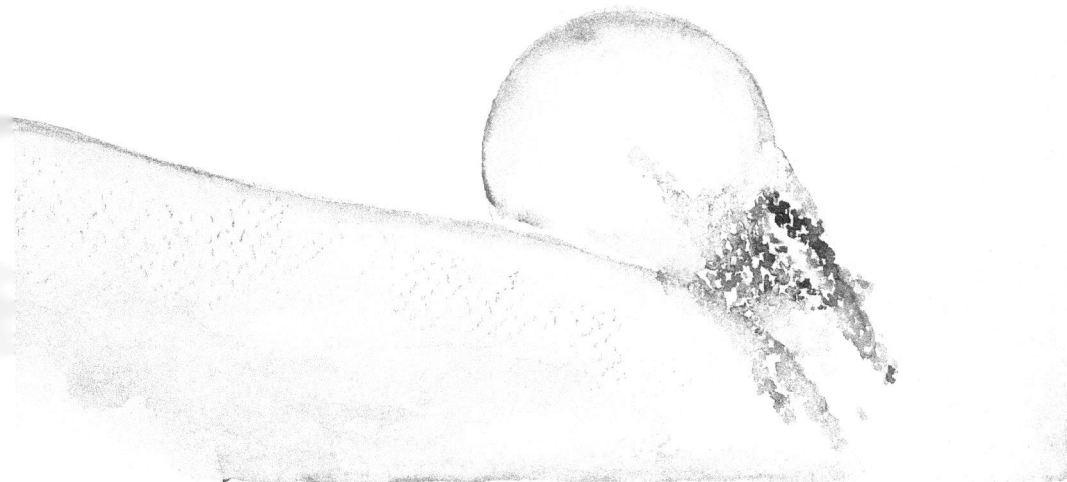

The postnatal period begins immediately after birth and lasts a total of eight weeks. It is a completely natural condition in the life of a woman and has nothing at all to do with illness. It merely represents a special situation. In my opinion it is one of the nicest phases in the life of a mother. She has time to recover from the pregnancy, rest from the strain of the birth and absorb that event emotionally. In addition to recuperation, the postnatal period should give the woman the opportunity to gather new reserves of energy for the coming strenuous months with an infant.

Postnatal Care by a Midwife

Here in Germany, every woman in the postnatal period is entitled to a midwife's assistance. During the first ten days, the midwife is obligated to look in on you once a day, find out how you are faring, check the involution process of the uterus, assist you with the breastfeeding and care of the child and attend to the baby's navel. You can receive this aftercare for as long as eight weeks following birth without any kind of application, red tape or doctor's prescription. You are moreover entitled to consultations throughout the entire breastfeeding period. If the house calls provided for by this system do not suffice, your doctor will be happy to prescribe you additional ones.

If you have given birth in the hospital, all you have to do is ring up your midwife, with whom you are advised to register during the pregnancy, unless you go to her regularly for antenatal check-ups anyway. If you have already had the opportunity to get to know your midwife during pregnancy, it will be like a meeting of old acquaintances, and she won't have to ask you many of the usual questions. The midwife knows you and your personal life situation, knows how the pregnancy progressed, and will now continue attending to you according to your individual needs. Do not allow anyone to talk you out of a midwife's care if that's what you want, because there is no other professional group which is as well trained to attend to a woman in the postnatal period.

The Meaning of the Postnatal Period

The postnatal phase is divided into the **early postnatal period** and the **late postnatal period**. The former lasts until the tenth day, the time it takes for the birth wounds to heal and lactation to commence. It is a time of great intimacy between mother and child. The two of them live in a kind of symbiosis and are inseparable. The late postnatal period ends about eight weeks after the birth and serves the process of adapting to life with the child and the readjustment of the mother's hormone system.

As a means of illustrating this adjustment process, I like to compare the postnatal period with the initial phase in a relationship between a man and a woman, the difference being that now a child is there – which, like an invader, can disturb the balance of this relationship. The first few days are like the period of being in love, with all its euphoria and the feeling of infinite fortune in having found one another. There is no difference between day and night; it's as though time was standing still. After these initial days, however, things gradually get back to normal; fatigue and stress set in. The period of being in love is replaced by the engagement, and days in which the bond is put to the test. Now it is necessary to divide up one's time and slowly readapt to the demands of everyday life. The first arguments and conflicts take place, but they are very brief, because you are still being sheltered by the great fortune of love. The "marriage" phase begins in the second to third week after birth. Now routine can return, and you begin to take notice of what is going on in the rest of the world again. Old habits and desires come up again, though now filtered, so to speak, by the indissolubility of the bond you have entered into with the child. Entirely new kinds of conflicts are experienced in the relationship between the parents, and great sensitivity is required on the part of the father to understand the various moods. The first weeks of life with this newborn child are a touchstone of every life partnership. The children challenge their parents and force them to reorient themselves in their existence and co-existence. In the process, however, the love for the child will flare up regularly and constantly, helping the parents to turn the crisis back into harmony very quickly. Again and again, as during the birth situation itself, demands are made on the parents' staying power and patience, but ultimately the postnatal period will be one of the crowning moments of the relationship. I would like to advise you to view the postnatal period as the first adventure with your child. Because after all, it is a rapidly growing relationship you have entered into, and that is adventure enough. If you have taken advantage of the pregnancy period to fortify your partner relationship, the effort now pays off.

Embark upon the adventure of the postnatal phase with a lot of curiosity, faith and trust; later you will look back on it fondly and often.

I feel a great need to communicate to all mothers the wonderful as well as the realistic sides of the postnatal period, along with as much information as possible, so that this phase in the life of a woman will once again take on a normal status and not be regarded as an illness or ignored altogether.

Parents during the Postnatal Period

When you page through the following sections, you will not find very many personal accounts. There are reasons for this: during pregnancy, many women ask me: "Do other pregnant women have the same experience?" Until the birth of the child, expectant mothers take the experiences of others as their orientation. During labour, however, they realize that what is happening is extremely personal and concerns nobody but themselves, and that it's really true: there is only *this* experience with *this* child! The hours of labour constitute one of the most intimate memories in this partner relationship. And that's how things continue in the postnatal period. Mothers don't want to hear how other women in the postnatal period fare, but seek advice and help for their own specific situation. For that reason, I will rarely have recourse below to personal accounts of other new women's experiences. It is not until the early postnatal period draws to a close that parents gradually become more open to what happens in other families and what is going on in the outside world. Alternatively, it can also take until the late postnatal period before they truly start participating in public life again. I would nevertheless like to share an experience with you to demonstrate how a newborn actually succeeds in making the parents build a hermetically sealed nest around its cradle …

… in the spring of 1990, Hurricane Wiebke raged over the Allgaeu, and it was an adventure just to be out and about. Many a street was blocked, and you were never sure whether you would make it to the other end of a road through a forest. I was happy to have arrived at the parking lot of the woman in childbed to whom I was going to pay a house call, but now I had to put the thirty metres from the car to the entrance door behind me in the squalls and pouring rain. My worries were justified, because I had hardly taken ten steps when a gust caught me and threw me into the dirt of the newly constructed lot. Accordingly, I had dirt all over my knees, my hair, my clothing, my satchel, and everything was sopping wet! I rang the bell and then I had to wait quite a while before the completely astonished father opened the door with a question I had great difficulty understanding: "Where have you been? What happened? Oh, it's raining outside. Excuse me for keeping you waiting but we're glad you're here, we're just in the process of changing the nappies, come right on up." I had to point out to the father that I would really prefer to change my clothing – I was soaked to the skin – and my dirty shoes, and asked if he could at least give me a towel for my hair and something to change into, and then I would be more than happy to come and take a look at the newborn baby. He apologized again and now he helped me out of my awkward situation. When we talked a few minutes later, the parents were completely astonished at the news that a state of emergency had been declared in many places in the vicinity, and I nearly didn't make it to their house. The parents stood together at the window and saw the havoc which had been wreaked around their house and said maybe it was about time they started reading the newspaper again. "I never would have thought something like that could happen to me", remarked the father, shaking his head at his own behaviour as he showed me to the door.

Time, Attention and Affection for the Mother

It is of great importance to me to create an awareness among all women, men, midwives and doctors of the circumstance that the postnatal period is hardly acknowledged in our society as a phase in its own right. In my opinion it has all but lost its place in family life in the past decades. After nine months of pregnancy and the birth, it takes a woman several weeks to adjust to her new life situation – but in many places that fact seems to have fallen into oblivion. A remark I once heard a doctor make still echoes in my ears: a few days after a birth he came to pay a house call and found the mother lying in bed: "Remember, he who rests, rusts [translation of a German saying]. You really must get up!" The mother of four decided not to take this comment seriously and strictly observed her early postnatal phase until the tenth day. In the past years I have had the growing impression that only the physical aspect is perceived. But the fact that a woman also has to come to terms with her motherhood of this particular child on an emotional level seems to me to have been forgotten by many people, including highly trained professionals. A woman in the postnatal period needs more than a bed and something to eat. Nor does it suffice to take her temperature and blood pressure once a day. A trained midwife doesn't need a thermometer or blood pressure meter to tell whether the woman is suffering from a fever or cardiovascular problems. The latter, like varicose veins, can be countered very effectively with physical exercises carried out in bed; it doesn't have to be the notorious stair-climbing. Already during the above-mentioned woman's previous postnatal phase two years earlier, the same gynaecologist had considered stair-climbing a better therapy than being coddled by her husband, or at least he had made a remark to that effect.

With regard to the care of a woman in the postnatal period, it seems to me to be of fundamental importance that everyone involved be conscious of the major hormonal fluctuations to which the woman is subjected during that period. Everyone should be aware that, during labour, she has had to turn her insides out in order to bear the child. Afterwards, every woman feels empty and vulnerable. No sooner did she finally grow accustomed to the baby's movement inside her belly than it is empty, numb and flabby. A feeling of injury and loneliness sets in. That is surely the reason it is now so important to leave the newborn infant as close to her as possible. I remember very well myself that I loved having my children lie next to me with their little legs and arms towards my tummy so that I could feel their little jabs and pokes again. To get through the initial days of emptiness and exhaustion – combined with the feeling of euphoria at having accomplished the birth – what every woman needs first and foremost is love, time devoted exclusively to her, affection and attention, preferably from her partner. For me as a midwife, these elements are just as important as professional postnatal consultation, which should not be restricted to the functions of the body but also take the emotional situation into account. The fact that holistic care is of great benefit to the entire family applies to the postnatal period as well.

THE EARLY POSTNATAL PERIOD

The Postnatal Period at Home and in the Hospital

Since the goal I have set myself is to write this book about natural and normal post-natal phases, I will endeavour to describe my experience with attending to women who spend this phase at home. I highly value the knowledge I obtained during my period of employment in a hospital, where I learned a great deal about caring for newborn infants and women in the postnatal period. But since I myself was fortunate enough to experience the postnatal period at home and attended to other women at home for many years, I know what a normal postnatal process really is. In a hospital, the physical processes are the same, of course, but there they are interpreted as being pathological. Naturally, in this chapter I will also attempt to provide pointers for a stay in the hospital. But as I already mentioned in the chapter on "Childbirth", practices vary from hospital to hospital, although in recent years efforts have been made to make the postnatal period in the hospital more family-oriented. The women have breastfeeding rooms, rooms for receiving visitors, even family rooms at their disposal; breakfast is served in buffet form so that the women don't have to adhere to specific hours. The question remains, however, as to the sense of making the women go from one room to the other as opposed to staying in bed and being spoiled there a bit. Another positive change is the introduction of so-called integrated care. Now no longer is there one nurse responsible for the woman's abdomen and the care it requires after giving birth, and another - the nursery nurse – for her breasts and breastfeeding and the baby. Rather, the women and the babies are now cared for by a single team. Nevertheless, I am of the opinion that a well-organized postnatal phase at home is the most personal.

It is therefore advisable to inform yourself about the practices in your hospital. Until now, it has been customary in Germany to discharge the mother on the third to the fifth day after birth. This period of rest will presumably be shortened even more in the near future, as was already the case in 1982, when in-patient postnatal care was reduced from ten days to six. In most European countries, incidentally, women are discharged much sooner – after only twenty-four hours. As you will remember, the early postnatal period has by no means been completed by then. Discharge from the hospital does not mean that knowledge already several millennia old suddenly no longer applies and women have now developed a new anatomical reaction: it still takes ten days for lactation to correspond approximately to the baby's individual nourishment needs. The infant's navel still frequently needs special care. The uterus can still be felt above the pubic bone after ten days, and the wounds are not yet completely healed. So even if you are discharged from the hospital, don't immediately try to lead life as normal, but give yourself your entire postnatal time. Take advantage of the advice and care of a midwife in your home. We are trained to recognize when the postnatal period has been completed from the functional point of view, and rather than determining that point in time according to the calendar and financial considerations.

Recovery from Labour/A Week in Bed

In the early postnatal period, both the baby and the mother should recuperate from the strains of childbirth. The mother should have a chance to rest after the cumbrous weeks of pregnancy and the strenuous hours of labour. During that week she should lie down as much as possible so that the birth wounds can heal, the pelvic floor can become firm and lactation can get underway. In the coming months you will often remember these days. In the years that follow, you will presumably never have time just to stay in bed unless you are actually sick. Do you know a mother who experiences how her housework is being done while she lies in bed? Who hears the washing machine spinning without having to do anything about the laundry? A mother who can smell tantalizing scents coming from the kitchen without being active herself? All these things you can enjoy in the early postnatal period, with your infant in your arms. Don't let yourself be robbed of this special time in the life of a woman. For the rest of your life, you will look back on your postnatal time with pleasure. In the old days, this was for many women the only holiday they ever had; perhaps that was why the family and the neighbours placed especial emphasis on not disturbing the woman during the postnatal period. According to a poem in the Allgaeu vernacular: "All Joahr kam's Weib ins Wuchebett, sonst hättse koi Erholung ghött ...!" – Every year the woman went into childbed, otherwise she would have had no rest at all...!

Protection and Rest

The mother was protected from the outside world and given the best food available. The "wise women" came and brought nourishment and wise words of advice on the care of the infant. In Allgaeu this is still a widespread custom, but has unfortunately undergone a very fundamental change: now, when the neighbour women come to bring the baby presents, the young mother provides them with an ample meal, though fortunately not until a few weeks or even months after the birth. Another version of the custom has developed in many places: while his wife is recuperating at the hospital, the neighbours provide the young father, with good homemade soup. Now the father gets the attention once lavished on the mother.

Maybe we can manage to restore this custom in its original form and provide the woman in the early postnatal period with food so that she can use her strength and energy for the process of lactation and not for standing at the stove to cook for the neighbours.

To give a woman in the postnatal period this protection is something we must learn anew. Already by the streams of visitors that go in and out of a hospital maternity ward, you can tell that the overall setup has little to do with rest and recuperation. Sometimes I have the feeling the infant is being presented on a silver platter; every visitor wants to hold it and everyone subjects it to his or her sniffles. As the mother, try to protect your child and nip offers of such visits right in the bud. "Rooming-in" has nothing to do with a "silver platter", but is intended as a means of keeping mother and child together. Interestingly enough, there are rarely such visitor problems when women spend their postnatal phase at home, because there people distinctly sense the new atmosphere; they speak in a whisper, and take off their shoes so as not to risk making any noise. Everyone greets the new arrival with a sense of awe. Friends and acquaintances are moreover disinclined to pay a visit in the parents' bedroom. The intimacy of that room is respected, in this particular situation and in general.

During the first few days, most women stay in bed quite of their own accord; their birth wounds virtually force them to do so. One woman expressed it as follows: "My entire body aches, as though I had a massive case of sore muscles. And not only that, but when I stand up I have the feeling my brains are running out between my legs. My circulation just isn't up to it. Before all this happened I had the feeling I could take on anything, but I guess that's not the case." With this statement she hit the nail on the head. It doesn't take long for a woman to realize that childbirth is not only an act of the abdomen but also puts a strain on the circulation and the emotions. Naturally, there are mothers who feel bouncy after a fast, easy birth. Such a woman can take a shower and sit down at the table for a meal with her partner and the midwife. But women like this really are a huge exception, and usually they go back to bed quite voluntarily before half an hour has passed. The truth is, that even if the newly delivered mum hasn't suffered any injury to her perineum or simply has not regained perception of her pelvic floor, she is bleeding quite profusely, a circumstance which puts a burden on her circulatory system and forces her into bed.

The Postnatal Period Step by Step

I have consciously decided to treat bleeding, the lochia, afterpains and the involution of the uterus as an integrated whole, because it is not possible to report to you about the bleeding and describe the involution separately. The human being him/herself is an integrated whole, and cannot be divided up into individual organs and bodily functions. In my opinion, the postnatal period is an extremely good example of how the body represents a single, individual whole, a huge system of wheels and cogs in which the various mechanisms are interconnected and interdependent.

Actually, in this section I would essentially have to discuss breastfeeding and the care of the child as well, because initially the mother and child likewise form a single unit – the separation only takes place gradually. To help you "find your way around" better, however, I have taken the liberty of treating those topics separately. The same applies to the area of wound treatment. To give you an idea of the normal course of events during the postnatal period, I will divide the following section up into the individual days. Naturally, that course of events can vary from one woman to the next. Every woman has her own way of bleeding, her own fast or slow involution of the uterus and her own way of coming to terms with strains on her cardiovascular system. Every "childbed" is completely individual; I can only report on an approximate norm, from which you are more likely to deviate than not – just as every midwife naturally also has her own methods of accompanying the postnatal period. One colleague might still define a certain situation as normal which another would consider cause for concern.

By presenting the events in this manner and this order, I do not mean to convey that the bleeding, afterpains and involution of the uterus are the most important aspects of the postnatal period. On the contrary, the care and observation of the child will take so much time and attention that the processes going on in your body will recede into the background. There are countless books telling you all about how to handle a newborn, and I will also devote an entire section to this extremely important topic, but I don't want to forget the mother in the process, as is so often the case. You will only be able to concentrate properly on the child if you are able to assess and cope with your own bodily processes. And that is also an important means of guarding against problems with lactation and providing your baby nourishment.

Already in the first few days, something fundamental will become apparent, something you will observe constantly in the years to come: if the mother feels good, the children fare well.

The Bleeding Uterine Wound

I would like to begin by describing how the postnatal bleeding comes about: the afterbirth leaves a huge wound behind on the uterine wall, about as large as the palm of your hand. Within the next three weeks, the size of the wound will decrease to about three centimetres in diameter. The remaining uterine muscles have abrasions caused by the detachment of the fetal membranes. Imagine you had a large scab on the mucous membrane of one of your nostrils, and that scab was suddenly torn off – that will give you an idea of what the detachment of the placenta and the fetal membranes is like. Since mucous membranes are well supplied with blood, the wound naturally begins to bleed profusely. Incidentally, in the course of the postnatal period, the overall blood loss amounts to between 200 and 500 ml/7 and 17 fl. oz.

The First Hours

Bleeding

In the uterus, the dimensions are several notches larger (than in the nostril), and the bleeding will be accordingly strong during the first few hours after birth. Most women experience a gush of blood every time they move. It is a strange feeling to bleed after so many weeks of pregnancy and it takes a bit of getting used to. Your words of astonishment have their own function; they remind the midwife to check the extent of the bleeding. Prepare yourself mentally for having to go into the postnatal period thickly "diapered"; probably you will need to use two to three cotton wool pads at a time as well as a small disposable bed pad (incopad). You'll be very glad you bought yourself a big package of thick cotton wool pads or have been supplied with them by the maternity ward. And you'll also enjoy your roomy cotton panties, which keep your "nappy package" from falling apart and provide warmth. You will have to renew the arrangement every three to four hours; this is about how long it will take until the pads are soaked with blood. Don't be surprised if the midwife takes the first time you change the pads as an opportunity to apply pressure to the uterus in an attempt to press out the blood which has accumulated there. It is unpleasant, but will spare you a substantial number of afterpains.

Afterpains

The so-called afterpains are absolutely necessary; they can be described as sharp, cramp-like abdominal pains. They are very similar to the final dilation contractions during labour, except that they last longer. For first-time mothers, the afterpains will probably not be very painful. They are especially important for the uterus, because the strong contractions serve to reduce the uterus in size. In the process, the size of the wound left behind by the placenta also decreases considerably and the bleeding lessens. In other words: the more afterpains, the smaller the uterus and the less bleeding. Women who have given birth before will begin to feel the afterpains shortly after the delivery of the afterbirth. These spasmodic pains are necessary in your case, because after every birth the uterine muscle requires more strength and effort in order to return to its proper size. Be mentally prepared for these pains. You will be able to endure them best if you breathe through them using the same technique you used during labour.

The Involution of the Uterus

The involution of the uterus begins immediately with the detachment of the placenta and the first afterpains. Both processes are supported by putting the child to the breast as soon as possible. During the first few hours after birth, you will be able to feel your uterus distinctly as a spherical shape in the vicinity of the navel. You will be amazed at how your uterus has changed from providing soft shelter to your baby and bumping against the bottom of your ribcage to being empty, small and hard. Mother

Nature really did think of everything. You may find your uterus more towards one side of your abdomen rather than in the middle. It's no wonder; now it has your entire abdomen to itself and feels as strangely anchorless as you do. The uterus really does fall from one side to the other, which is why the midwife will request that you stay in bed. When you lie on your back, the uterus will stay in the middle, and the blood which has accumulated in the uterine cavity can flow more freely. Then the midwife won't have to apply pressure to force that flow of blood.

Getting out of Bed the First Time

It is equally helpful to get up soon and venture your first walk to the toilet to pass water, because then the blood will also flow out on its own and you will be spared the pain of having it pressed out. But please never get up alone and never without doing circulation-stimulating leg and arm exercises first. Be aware of the fact that, due to the loss of blood, you will have circulatory problems and a very hard time keeping your balance, also because your sense of balance has adapted to the weight of the baby.

Before the mother gets up for the first time, *rosemary, neroli* or *Rose Hydrolat* can be patted onto her face, back and legs; they are all suitable means of stimulating the circulation. For a sponge bath, a few drops of essential oil can be added to a washbowl or basin of water, e.g. *lavender fine, neroli 10% in jojoba wax, rose 10% in jojoba wax, rosemary* or *lemon*. The *Original Ɗ® Aroma Blend Hallo-Wach-Öl/Hello-Wake-Up Oil Ɗ®* has also proven most effective.

In my opinion, it is absolutely essential to eat and drink something before you get up. Now, at the latest, you will be glad you brought a little stock of goodies with you to the hospital, if you can't get anything in the ward. In the home birth setting, incidentally, it is often a cosy, festive meal we partake of together before the mother gets up the first time …

… Gisela reported how she had found it difficult to believe her midwife's warnings. The latter finally resorted to the following words: "Imagine you had had a leg or an arm amputated. The body now has to cope with a similar loss." That convinced her.

It is an extremely strange feeling to stand there with a flabby, empty tummy with no baby inside it. You will have the urge to hold your abdomen because it feels as if it is falling into an abyss. You feel as if there is nothing holding you because, due to their overextension during pregnancy, your stomach muscles are completely incapable of contracting. This feeling comes about regardless of whether you have just had your first child or already given birth several times. But it's nothing to worry about; within a week you will have adjusted.

Intimate Hygiene

Try to see to it that you can rinse yourself with a cool to lukewarm solution already the first time you go to the toilet. To this end, use an empty mineral water bottle, a beaked pitcher or pot, which you fill with lukewarm water, adding a teaspoon of the

Original D® Aroma Blend Sitzbad/Sitz Bath D®. As soon as you are seated on the toilet, pour the contents of the vessel slowly onto your pubic hair, from where it will flow over the vulva to the perineum. You can do this yourself, and the midwife or your partner will surely be happy to assist you. By administering this rinse as you pass water, you can avoid or alleviate the burning sensation – the urethra has also been irritated by the process of childbirth. The burning sensation you feel when passing water is often caused by tiny abrasions.

Don't be afraid of that first trip to the toilet, and be prepared to carry out the rinsing procedure with this disinfectant, cooling solution which moreover promotes the healing process, and you will see that it's not half as bad as you expected. It is also helpful to bend forwards slightly with your upper body and spread the labia a bit. That way you can keep the urine from running over the vagina where it could also cause a burning sensation. The rinse also serves to remove small bits of coagulated blood from the pubic hair, and makes you feel pleasantly fresh. If your circulation is stable, you can naturally also refresh your face and upper body. But most women prefer to go and lie down again and have the midwife or their partner give them a sponge bath there.

Day One

Bleeding

On the first day, you should avoid getting up without someone to lean on. Particularly new mothers who have lost a large amount of blood in conjunction with the detachment of the placenta have a tendency to faint. Don't be surprised if, when you assume an upright position or are sitting on the toilet, large clumps of coagulated blood plop out of your vagina. Very many young mothers are badly frightened when this happens, because they have not been informed about it beforehand. There is absolutely no cause for worry, these clumps are completely normal: while you are resting on your back, the uterine cavity – which extends all the way up to your navel – fills with blood, which coagulates there and is only discharged when you sit or stand in an upright position.

Afterpains – Primiparas and Multiparas

In the case of a primipara – a woman who has just given birth the first time – the afterpains will be perceivable as a slight ache, while multiparas – women who have given birth two or more times – will find them bothersome, in some cases even extremely painful. Women who spend the early postnatal period in the hospital are therefore offered cramp-relieving medications, so-called spasmolytica. In home accompaniment I have had to recommend these antispasmodic remedies no more than a handful of times. These were cases in which the mother had had her fourth or fifth child. Amazingly, however, all other mothers get along quite well without medication. This is undoubtedly due to the measures we take to support the natural bodily processes as well as to the mothers' attitude, because these are mothers who follow our advice and obey the needs expressed by their bodies.

Many mothers confess to me – or I have called their attention to the fact – that they don't put their newborns to their breast often, because after breastfeeding the afterpains are simply too painful. This is nature's way of ensuring that, from the first day on, babies are consoled and comforted with means other than the breast. Having to wait patiently is a fate all second-, third-born children etc. share. I don't mean that the babies should be left screaming in their bassinettes. On the contrary: all mothers who spend the postnatal period at home – and in the meantime in many hospitals – have their newborns very close to them. In the mother's warm armpit, the baby feels sheltered and protected. Lips searching for something to suckle are offered one of the mother's fingers, with which the infant pleasurably satisfies its sucking instinct. Calm, soothing words lull the baby back to sleep, and the mother is spared the severe afterpains this time around. But no matter how painful these abdominal cramps are, remember: without afterpains there is no involution of the uterus.

For a multipara, one of the most important means of keeping the afterpains at a bearable level is to maintain a constant body temperature. Since I began advising women in the postnatal period to keep their abdomens warm, it has been my experience that they cope with the afterpains quite well. The postnatal period can no longer be imagined without a hot-water bottle or a warm cherry-stone or herbal sack on the woman's abdomen. When you get up, you should see to it that you are warmly bundled up. Wear big, comfortable, warm panties, no matter how terribly unsexy they are, and use an angora kidney warmer or wrap a wool scarf around your hips when you go to the toilet. Everyone knows that warmth is a good remedy for abdominal cramps. And a scarf will also provide pleasant support for your heavy, empty belly.

The Involution of the Uterus

On the first day, it will still be possible to feel the uterus around the level of the navel. The sphere-shaped organ will sometimes be soft, and then harden up again when you put your baby to your breast. Breastfeeding represents the best way of supporting the involution of the uterus – i.e. its return to its normal size. Another helpful measure is to lie face down as often as possible on the first day. That position will apply pressure to the uterus, the blood can flow out better and the pressure is taken off your perineum, something you'll appreciate if the latter has been injured. You are probably looking forward to being able to lie on your front again at last. Take advantage of the brief phase constituted by the first few days of the postnatal period – once the breasts have filled with milk, the opportunity to lie in a face-down position will once again be over. Take the pressure off your spine and sacrum, put a small bolster under your tummy. The regular evacuation of the bladder is an extremely important prerequisite for the involution process. Make an effort to go to the bathroom regularly, at least before every time you breastfeed. Initially you will not be able to feel whether your bladder is full or empty. Don't worry though, the feeling will come back; it is merely that, after birth, the bladder enjoys the newly recovered space in the abdominal cavity. It fills up and becomes quite large, confining the space for the uterus. The uterus, for its part, attempts to contract by means of afterpains and to find its proper place in the pelvis minor, but the bladder prevents it from doing so. By passing water regularly, you can also spare yourself unnecessary afterpains.

Circulation

After a normal birth and afterbirth phase, a woman can generally take a shower on the first day. Please be careful and observe the following rules: don't try it until you have had a plentiful breakfast. Make sure your partner is within calling distance, so that he can be there quickly to help you if you need it. Adjust the water temperature at a rather cool level and adjust the shower head (if possible) to produce a single stream of water which you direct at your limbs in an upward direction as a means of stimulating the circulation. Please wait a few days to wash your hair; otherwise it is sure to become too strenuous. During the day you will remember to carry out the regular intimate hygiene, the rinse described above, since you will have already long recognized how refreshing it is. If you spend the postnatal period at home and your bathroom is equipped with a bidet, you should use it. Normally your circulation will only give you problems when you stand for a long time, but that is something you shouldn't do anyway. Your place, for the time being, is in bed. If only to benefit the pelvic floor, you should remain in a lying position, because those muscles are simply not yet capable of bearing too great a burden.

Day Two

Bleeding

By the second day, the bleeding should have decreased to the extent that now two pads suffice. The clots of blood are becoming smaller, the largest of them now being about the size of a walnut. But the blood will still be very thin and bright red. Quite often, fibrous shreds of mucous membrane will be discharged as well as, sometimes, small remnants of the fetal membrane, which look like strings of blood.

Afterpains

In the case of primiparas, the afterpains will have become very slight. Women who have given birth in the past will continue to have afterpains, although only after breastfeeding will these pains reach the highest level of intensity. In the intervals between breastfeeding they will already be quite tolerable. The application of a hot-water bottle or a warm cherry-stone or herbal sack to the abdomen before putting your child to your breast is still very helpful and pleasant.

Involution

Thanks to the afterpains, the involution process will progress nicely. Perhaps you will be able to feel your uterus as much as two or three finger-widths below your navel now. If you cannot locate it, don't worry; your midwife will be able to check it when she comes for her daily house call.

Circulation

Your circulation system will certainly have stabilized and you will have no problem taking a shower on your own. Only standing at the changing table for a long time might still cause you problems. Try to avoid standing still, and take a few steps around the room now and then. As on the previous day, however, your favourite place will be in bed. You will surely not forget the regular rinsing procedure when you pass water; for the time being this is the best method of carrying out intimate hygiene.

Day Three

The Lochia

Beginning on the third day, the bleeding will become darker and rather watery. Now the true flow of lochia – the normal uterine discharge of blood, tissue and mucus from the vagina after childbirth – begins. This discharge is actually a form of ichor which does contain germs, but no pathogens, and you can safely keep your child in bed with you even if many people, including experts, claim the opposite. If this were not safe, mother and child could not live in a symbiosis during the first few days. It is also not necessary for the woman to use a separate toilet because, thanks to our modern hygiene facilities, there is no cause for concern. For years I have found that women never place as much emphasis on hygiene as during the postnatal period. This is undoubtedly due in part to the slightly stale, cheesy smell of the lochia. Regular hand-washing, a disinfectant rinse and frequent changing of your pads will provide you with sufficient protection against infection. After all, in the past women didn't die as a result of the germs in their own lochia, but from bacteria transmitted by doctors. Protect yourself from every danger of contagion from the outside, because your immune system is still very weak and will not be able to defend you against foreign germs this soon.

Afterpains

Now the afterpains will finally become less frequent even for multiparas and you will feel them only after breastfeeding, and then only slightly.

Involution

The uterus will demonstrate its individuality. Even trained professionals are often amazed at the extent to which many uteri have returned to their normal size already by the third day. In many cases the uterus can already be felt midway between the navel and the pubic bone – a sign of very rapid involution. On average, the uterus is three to four finger-widths below the navel on Day Three. The most important thing is that the reduction in size progresses tangibly and the uterus moves down noticeably from day to day. This process is different from woman to woman, but should progress continuously.

Circulation

Your circulation is undoubtedly back to normal and you'll no longer suffer from dizziness if you stand for longer stretches at a time; for the pelvic floor, however, it is still not advisable (see the section on "The Pelvic Floor", p. 293 f.). Now you will really like rinsing yourself with a pleasant scent, because the lochia meanwhile have their typical strong odour and it will be especially important to you to smell fresh and clean. You will notice that, due to the readjustment of the hormone system, you will regularly be bathed in sweat; you'll begin perspiring at the slightest provocation. By the third day at the latest you'll want to wash your hair, and there is no reason why you shouldn't. In many maternity wards – or by older women you might have contact to – you'll be warned that shampooing during the postnatal period is dangerous. This information dates back to an era predating heated bathrooms and blow dryers. The one thing you should be careful about is not to turn the water on too hot, since your circulation is still not entirely stable. And you should blow-dry your hair immediately but, again, not with too much heat. Please avoid having wet hair in the postnatal period, because cold and wetness will throw your body off balance and make you susceptible to infection. Since you yourself have not entirely found your centre again, you should avoid everything that could have a destabilizing effect.

Regular Bowel Movements

Most women in the postnatal period have to empty their bowels by the third day after childbirth at the latest. Whether you have a bowel movement earlier, or not until Day Three, will depend on whether you were given an enema before the birth. Another decisive factor is whether you are at home or in the hospital. Women who are at home during the postnatal period rarely require a laxative, and the majority of those that do have had an episiotomy. These women are initially afraid that the suture might be very painful when they empty their bowels. At home, the digestive system normalizes of its own accord, presumably because the young mothers eat the food they are accustomed to and can use their own toilet whenever they want to. Both in the hospital and at home, I advise women in the postnatal period to begin with easily digestible foods and above all to drink enough, because their bodies require quite a lot of fluid to get lactation going and compensate for the profuse perspiration. In conjunction with these various bodily processes, the content of the intestines becomes much too firm and the woman is constipated before she knows it. During the first few days, fear of going to the toilet undoubtedly also leads the woman to repress her natural urge, so that the rectum fills up increasingly and its content becomes harder and harder. Because of the fact that, like the bladder, the intestines likewise have plenty of space now, you don't become aware of this "full" condition until it's too late. Once this point has been reached, it makes no sense to seek relief by taking laxatives "from above", because, after all, the rectum is full. Your best option is to have a microclyster prescribed, which you insert into the anus. This will provide you with gentle assistance in emptying your bowels. If this method does not suffice, have an enema carried out; that always works. In my opinion, it makes no sense whatsoever to give a woman in the postnatal period a laxative every day, because during the first few days, constipation is a natural form of protection for the woman. She cannot and will not feel or achieve anything "down there" for the time being. As soon as the intestines have recovered from the pregnancy and birth, they will function quite normally again. If not, the reason is almost always fear of the first bowel movement, but not constipation in the strict sense. Then it is the midwife's responsibility to make it clear to the woman that all of her organs, including the anal sphincter, function properly, and that she should not be afraid to press gently; all she must do is see to it that the bowel content is soft. Every midwife, nurse and mother should be aware that every laxative taken orally finds its way into the breast milk and causes the newborn child flatulence and stomach aches, as is likewise the case with the mother herself.

The moral of the story is: see to it that you eat the foods you are accustomed to from the beginning of the postnatal period. Incidentally, a daily abdominal massage in a clockwise direction will support the intestinal activity well.

Days Four and Five

Lochia

On the fourth and fifth days of the postnatal period, the lochia will continue to be slightly bloody and similar to the bleeding towards the end of menstruation. Some women report that the bleeding stops at night for the most part but flows heavily again in the morning. Just as there are no norms in life, there is also none for the lochia. The most important thing is that you have a visible flow of lochia, because then you can rest assured that you are not afflicted with retention of the lochia.

The Discharge of the Remaining Fetal Membranes

During this phase, there can be an event which is very frightening for the woman in the postnatal period and a great relief for the midwife: the discharge of the remaining fetal membranes. This was the case one evening for Vera …

… her sister rang me up, very distraught, and told me that the young mother was sitting on the toilet and a piece of the cervix or uterus had come out of her vagina. For a second or two, I was likewise shocked, but then I was able to allay her worries over the phone: "Those are sure to be remnants of the fetal membranes, no cause for concern; I'll come by right away." As I was driving over I thought about whether I could possibly have overlooked anything unusual about the uterine involution process or the lochia, but I couldn't remember anything out of the ordinary. A few minutes later, I was relieved to find that the discharge contained of quite a number of tattered remains of the fetal membranes, which were visible in the vagina. Bits of clotted blood had gotten caught in these tatters, which had accordingly taken on such a strange colour and consistency. With the help of a clamp and a pair of tweezers, I carefully removed the remaining, extremely fragile fetal membranes from the vaginal cavity. We were both moreover relieved when I determined that the uterus was in the correct position. Such events are very rare this far into the early postnatal period, but they do occur. Usually, as mentioned above, the fetal membranes are discharged right at the beginning in conjunction with somewhat heavier bleeding, and often go completely unnoticed. I was happy that everything ran smoothly for Vera for the remainder of the postnatal period.

Don't always just assume the worst, but, like the two sisters, try to reach your midwife immediately; she will provide you with advice and support. Thanks to phone calls like the one from Vera's sister, there is never a dull moment in the life of an independent midwife!

Afterpains

During the postnatal visits, the multiparas now sit up in their beds and radiantly report that the afterpains have finally subsided. They may still have very light pains the first time they stand for a longer period. These pains are merely the body's way of reminding them that the postnatal period is not completely over yet.

Involution

The involution of the uterus tends to stagnate in this phase, since the body now requires a lot of energy and strength for lactation. But it's not a problem as long as the lochia are flowing and the manual examination of the uterus does not cause the woman any pain. By this time the uterus is nearly always to be found between the navel and the symphysis (pubic bone) when felt from the outside. If that is not the case, I ask the woman to empty her bladder, because a full bladder is often the cause of out-of-the-ordinary findings. And I would urgently advise all women who are at the hospital in the postnatal period to pass water before the doctor makes his daily rounds. A full bladder can influence the medical findings to such an extent that the involution process is deemed inadequate and the doctor prescribes medication – Methergine®, an ergot alkaloid – which passes directly into the breast milk and often even reduces lactation. And in addition to strong afterpains in the mother, it also causes abdominal cramps in the infant.

Postnatal Exercises

To help your body back to normal, in addition to making sure you are warm and emptying your bladder regularly, you can also start doing postnatal exercises. The aim of these exercises is not only to restore the pelvic floor to its original state of firmness, but also to stimulate the involution of the uterus. Both in the hospital and at home, the midwife will instruct you in carrying out the respective exercises; initially you can go easy on yourself with them. Amazingly enough, around the fourth or fifth day, every woman in the postnatal period signals a desire to do gymnastics. Naturally, you can begin with light abdominal breathing exercises even sooner. For the pelvic floor muscles, however, it seems to be more effective to wait a few days. According to the latest findings, it is better to wait even longer, and to develop a good feeling for the pelvic floor before the actual exercises begin. I am moreover of the opinion that a woman should rest thoroughly before demands are placed on her figure again. Don't go to a postnatal gym class because you've been instructed to do so, but go when you feel up to it yourself. The important thing is to carry out the exercises regularly for a reasonably long period of time, even if you don't start with them until eight weeks after birth.

Personal Hygiene/Rinsing/Sitz Baths

The personal hygiene measures carried out until now will I hope be enhanced by a sitz bath. The rule as to when you can take your first sitz bath after childbirth varies greatly from one maternity ward to the next. At home, women can usually take one as early as the second day. You can read up on this topic in the section on "Perineal Care" (p. 297). Most mothers very much like to continue with the regular rinsing procedure for quite a while. If your bathroom is equipped with a bidet, you will be as glad to use it after every time you pass water as you were to employ the rinsing procedure during the first few days.

In the context of personal hygiene, you should be careful not to change your own natural scent with too many artificial fragrances. Synthetic aromas not only confuse the child too much, but it is also not known whether the child's body will ever eliminate the aroma molecules. Remember that the newborn child has an extremely sensitive sense of smell and that the human being's memory is closely associated with this sense. Our perception of odours is never again as strong as it is during the first few weeks of life, and the baby automatically stores these scents in its memory centre. It would be a shame if the child could only remember some run-of-the-mill perfume rather than its mother's own unmistakable scent.

Day Six

Discharge from the Hospital

For all mothers who have spent the postnatal period in the hospital, today – at the latest – is an exciting day: you are due to be discharged. Try not to let the day become too hectic. Resist the temptation to stop by the supermarket or visit some friends on the way home from the hospital. No matter how wound up and perky you feel, things will change very quickly once you are home. Remember: the early postnatal phase has not yet been concluded.

Lochia

Women who have been at home for the postnatal period will experience this day no differently from the previous ones. They are glad that the flow of lochia is slowing down, the afterpains are over, and they enjoy caring for themselves and allowing themselves to be spoiled.

Involution

The uterus will gradually make its way downward towards the pubic bone. Now it can usually be felt three to four finger breadths above the symphysis (pubic bone).

Days Seven to Ten

Young mothers no longer stay in bed all day, but get up for an hour or two now and then. The nightgown is exchanged for leggings and a T-shirt or a jogging suit. During this stage, most women prefer to retreat to their bedrooms to nurse their babies. Surprisingly, women who have given birth at home stay in bed the longest. They enjoy the atmosphere as long as possible, because the room still smells a bit like childbirth.

Lochia

In the period between the sixth and tenth day of the postnatal period the lochia turn into a thin, brown discharge. Now, if not before, you will become acquainted with the typical smell of the lochia. After breastfeeding, they may turn red again temporarily. You are no longer using thick cotton wool pads, just normal sanitary towels. Make sure they are unscented, because the scented ones can cause itching and rashes in the area of the vagina. These afflictions usually disappear as soon as you change to a different brand of sanitary towel. When you shop for them, try to get the type without an adhesive strip, because the latter tends to peel off and cause unnecessary pain when the sticky part touches the perineal suture. Incidentally, if you can obtain them, I can highly recommend reusable sanitary towels made of pure, unbleached natural fibres such as cotton or silk (offered by the German firm Kulmine; for address see appendix, p. 460). This type of towel is washed in the washing machine after use, but you'll be doing laundry constantly during the postnatal period anyway. Incidentally, I also recommend sanitary towels made of natural textiles to women not in the postnatal period but suffering from chronic vaginal infections. The natural fibres and holistically oriented medical advice often already suffice to bring about improvement in this situation. I would like to recommend that you stock up on sanitary towels already during pregnancy, since men don't like to have to go looking for the right feminine hygiene product.

Involution

By the tenth day, the involution of the uterus will have progressed to the point where the latter can just barely still be felt behind the pubic bone. From this point on, the midwife will remind you to do your involution exercises regularly. Particularly multiparas request postnatal care by a midwife until the tenth day, because her house call often represents the only opportunity for carrying out the exercises regularly. Other women prefer to be taught the exercises once and then carry them out on their own. Naturally it also depends on how much time the midwife can take for a house call, since it is not unusual for her to have to attend to several women on a single day.

Helpful Measures during the Postnatal Period

As mentioned above, the postnatal period is an exceptional situation in the life of a woman. And we all know that special situations can easily be associated with certain risks. To prevent the early postnatal period from taking a pathological course, I advise every woman undergoing it to make use of naturopathic means of supporting the healing process and the hormone system. You can facilitate the wound healing process and the readjustment of the hormones very effectively with certain tea blends, homoeopathic remedies and essential oils. These natural aids were already known to mothers and "wise women" in antiquity.

It is always advisable, however, to ask a midwife for advice on what roots, leaves or blossoms are best for you, and in what form – as globuli, tea or massage oil.

Herbal Medicine

During the first few days, I recommend that you drink *lady's mantle tea* with raspberry leaves. Lady's mantle grows especially for us women, to provide us with support in all hormonal adjustment phases. The raspberry leaves, for their part, stimulate the bowels and have a detoxifying effect. Even if the qualities of these two herbs have not yet been scientifically proven, the centuries of women's experience with them are a strong argument in their favour. You should, however, limit your consumption of the tea to the first few days after childbirth, because then the focus will be shifting to the firming up of the tissue.

⟨⑤⟩ Homoeopathic Treatment

The intake of the homoeopathic remedy *Arnica* is undoubtedly the most successful method of ensuring normal wound healing and thus of supporting the normal flow of lochia. We midwives observe that women who take Arnica stop bleeding sooner and that the uterus is restored to its normal size more quickly. After the second child, women who take Arnica in a C6 potency are themselves amazed by how much less blood they lose this time around.

⟨⑤⟩ Aroma Therapy

Essential oils are an especially pleasant as well as effective method of supporting the normal course of the postnatal process. Women who own an aroma lamp love to use it during this phase with a few drops of one of their favourite oils. All blossom and wood oils can be used. A woman in a situation like this one needs the support provided by the essences to find her inner balance and stability again. There is a whole range of well-suited oils, especially: *fennel, rose geranium, jasmine, lavender, linaloe wood, clary sage, rose, rosewood, yarrow, juniper, ylang-ylang, cedar, cypress.* As always when you use essential oils, on the one hand your nose will tell you what the right oil is, and on the other hand many of the oils are too intense or too expensive to be used on their own. I accordingly developed an oil blend especially for the postnatal period and have been using it with great success since the late 1980s: the *Original 𝒟® Aroma Blend Wochenbettbauchmassageöl/Childbed Abdominal Massage Oil 𝒟®* containing grapefruit, rose geranium, yarrow, juniper berry and cypress. These oils are an effective means of promoting the involution of the uterus without triggering massive afterpains in multiparas. The *Wochenbettbauchmassageöl/Childbed Abdominal Massage Oil 𝒟®* is also designed to stimulate the purification process and support the firming up of the abdominal skin and muscles. Its chief task, however, is to aid in the healing of the uterine wall. Particularly for this reason, I was interested in making it available to women in the postnatal period and midwives as a ready-made blend. Many of my colleagues, also those who work in hospitals, greatly appreciate my *Original 𝒟® Aroma Blend* when they use it to massage the abdomens of the women in the postnatal period. As one midwife told me: "This blend has become so important to me and helps so outstandingly that I don't lend it out to people anymore."

I am certain that many of the complications described below can be prevented with the regular application of this massage oil. You can begin with the abdominal massage on the first day. The person giving the massage – the partner or midwife – should be gentle at first, because the uterus is still very sensitive to the touch in places. The massage can be carried out a bit more energetically every day. If you – the mother or her partner - have not been instructed by a midwife, try it on your own, guided by your intuition. What is important is to massage the abdomen in the clockwise direction and radially. Then you can knead the abdomen crosswise from the sides and, finally, diagonally, beginning at the ribcage, with alternating hands describing figure-8s and gradually progressing downward. In conclusion, massage the hipbones with circular movements, alternating from one side to the other. You'll see; it will be fun for everyone involved!

Strong Afterpains

The treatments mentioned above will not suffice for the strong afterpains experienced by multiparas. But in order to avoid taking an analgesic – which will make its way into the breast milk – I recommend the following treatments in addition to the above-described methods of heat therapy:

Herbal Medicine

The so-called *Wöchnerinnentee/Childbed Tea* has a spasmolytic effect, since it contains ground ivy, goose grass, lemon balm and damiana leaves.

Homoeopathic Treatment

In addition to *Arnica,* the substances very often helpful in this context are *Caulophyllum, Chamomilla, Cuprum metallicum, Kalium carbonicum* and *Secale.* These remedies should by no means be administered on the basis of self-diagnosis, but be prescribed by a midwife or doctor with training in homoeopathy …

… Marianne had given birth to her third child and had severe afterpains, a circumstance she was quite upset about. "I just want to have my peace and quiet. Don't you have any globuli for me?" A few hours after a dose of Chamomilla, the afterpains had subsided to a tolerable point.

Aroma Therapy

In these circumstances I have had a lot of good experience with the tocolytic (contraction-inhibiting) *Toko-Öl/Toko Oil $\mathcal{D}$®* , with which many women have already become acquainted during pregnancy. This oil, consisting of lavender, linaloe wood and marjoram, can be used to make a damp, warm compress or administer an abdominal massage, preferably before breastfeeding …

… Karin had just had her third baby and was already beginning to suffer from strong afterpains after the birth. When I paid her a house call that evening, she told me she preferred offering her baby tea to breastfeeding it because the afterpains were simply unbearable. That was fine with me. I did not, however, want to comply so quickly with her request for a painkiller. I suggested that she focus on breathing through the pains, massage her abdomen with Toko Oil $\mathcal{D}$® and keep it warm with a hot-water bottle. If all of this failed to bring relief, she still had the option of taking a spasmolytic. The next morning Karin proudly showed me the unopened package of suppositories and reported that the breathing and the hot-water bottle had fulfilled their purpose and, what is more, she had nursed her daughter about every four hours. As a side effect of this afterpain therapy, the initial engorgement of the breasts with milk was much more manageable than it had been in the case of her first two children.

Problems during the Early Postnatal Period

As is the case with all natural life processes, disorders can develop in connection with the flow of lochia and the involution of the uterus. Here it is important to recognize the signs as early as possible in order to increase the chances of naturopathically oriented treatment leading to success. If you wait too long, a true irregularity and illness will develop – i.e. a problem which can presumably only be treated by scientific-medical means, possibly even in the hospital, in order to prevent serious consequences. You as the mother should take all disorders arising during the postnatal period very seriously.

I will base the following discussion on the assumption that you are being attended to by a midwife during the postnatal period and that she is taking all of the necessary measures. She will be able to tell whether your condition is normal or abnormal and will react accordingly. Where necessary, she will enlist the help of a doctor.

Basic Emotional State/Midwives' Knowledge

In my opinion, no matter what irregularity arises during the postnatal period, the chief focus must be directed towards the woman's basic emotional state and the overall family situation. It is absolutely essential to take a holistic approach in the care of a woman in the postnatal period. Attention is not to be paid to the uterus, the breasts or the blood pressure as isolated factors, but to the woman in her entirety, since it is she who has given birth, it is her hormonal balance which has been thrown off course by the pregnancy and labour, and her life energy upon which extreme demands have thus been made. Again and again, it becomes clear to me that if the woman does not get enough rest or has some physical or emotional burden to bear, her body has no choice but to react with a functional disorder. In this phase of life, women apparently have no other mechanisms for calling attention to a disturbance in the self-healing process. Accordingly, I find it important for the midwife to "read between the lines" and be sensitive to the overall family situation, which naturally requires a certain amount of perceptiveness. In these moments, independent midwives are always very glad that they have gotten to know the woman during pregnancy and a certain amount of trust has already developed. Particularly when the physical disorder is rooted in problems of a personal or intimate nature – for example having to do with the partnership between the parents of the newborn child – the mother will much sooner confide in a midwife she already knows. By the time the postnatal period rolls around, if not sooner, it proves extremely valuable for us midwives not only to think holistically but also to practice our professions in this manner, i.e. to accompany a woman through pregnancy, attend to her during childbirth and again during the postnatal period.

Excessive Bleeding

Your midwife or a doctor may have pronounced the diagnosis "excessive lochia". If all necessary medical examinations have been carried out and everything else is found to be progressing normally, excessive bleeding during the postnatal period is, in my experience, a matter of individual constitution. Many women with this condition say that they also menstruate quite heavily. Then the midwife will not be surprised if the same is true during the postnatal period. This bleeding is acceptable provided the woman's general condition and her uterus are examined regularly. Again, the prerequisite is that the mother herself is not worried. The midwife must always take the momentary condition into account in order to know how long she can wait or whether it is necessary to intervene therapeutically. Often the woman will consider the bleeding normal – because that's how it was after the birth of her last child or, as mentioned above, because she always bleeds heavily – and only the midwife is alarmed. In these cases the midwife has to weigh the various factors: the extent to which the woman can decide for herself whether therapeutic action is necessary, and when the limits of inactivity have been reached. The experience the midwife has gathered in the course of the years will play a major role. Let me take the liberty of urging you – my fellow midwife – to be careful; it is better to examine the woman once too often. And you – the woman undergoing the postnatal process – are called upon to accept it if the midwife wants to consult a doctor against your wishes. We midwives are very familiar with these borderline situations, and they are always a challenge for us.

Often the excessive application of warmth is the cause of overly heavy lochia. Accordingly, if you tend to bleed heavily in general you should not take any hot sitz baths or use a hot-water bottle, warm cherry-pit or herbal compress or pad. Be careful with your intake of analgesics, because the latter have an influence on the blood coagulation system and therefore make the bleeding all the heavier.

During my entire period as an out-of-hospital midwife, I cannot remember a single case of heavy bleeding which did not quickly return to normal with the aid of a tea blend, a few globuli or an aroma-therapy oil. In fact, this complication is extremely rare and has, in my experience, always had a very obvious cause. I have never once had to have a woman in the postnatal period hospitalized for this reason. This circumstance is undoubtedly to be attributed to the preventive and individually tailored measures we midwives take when attending to women who are at home during the postnatal period.

⑤ Herbal Medicine

In a case of excessive bleeding, the following tea blend is helpful: *lady's mantle, yarrow* and *peppermint*. Peppermint is an excellent astringent. Remember, though, that it will work as an antidote to any homoeopathic substances you may be taking.

⊙ Homoeopathic Treatment

Here we administer the same remedies as in the case of a disorder in connection with the detachment of the placenta accompanied by heavy bleeding, i.e.: *Arnica, Belladonna, China, Ferrum metallicum, Hamamelis, Millefolium, Phosphorusus, Sabina, Secale* and *Sepia* (cf. p. 250 f).

⊙ Aroma Therapy

Of course, essential oils can likewise be very helpful. The best choice here is *Wochenbettbauchmassageöl/Childbed Abdominal Massage Oil 𝒟®* used in conjunction with a cooling compress or even an ice-cube application. A cold *lavender, peppermint* or *lemon oil* compress prescribed by me over the phone as an emergency measure has often provided relief until my arrival "on the scene". Use whatever oil you have in the house; one of the abovementioned is usually on hand in every household. If you should happen to have *Kräuterkorb/Basket of Herbs 𝒟®* as an essential oil blend in the form of a pump spray, that would also be an excellent choice. The woman can spray her abdomen with it, perhaps make herself a cold compress in addition, and the bleeding will quickly come to a standstill. In view of the fact that this is a measure employed only temporarily to counteract an acute condition, the milk-reducing effect of peppermint oil is unimportant here.

Insufficient Lochia

In cases of insufficient flow of lochia, which usually goes hand in hand with inadequate involution of the uterus, the mothers themselves are never worried but, on the contrary, glad that they don't have to cope with the bleeding. We midwives, on the other hand, or the doctor making his rounds in the hospital, will regard this condition with a furrowed brow. The insufficient flow of lochia with their typical slightly nauseating smell can all too quickly develop into true retention of the lochia, which means that no lochia are discharged at all anymore.

So don't be surprised if the midwife asks you about the amount of flow on a daily basis. You may even find us sniffing at your sanitary towel, because even just the smell of the lochia tells us a lot about whether everything is proceeding normally or not. The examination of the amount and consistency of the lochia is not simply curiosity-inspired disregard for your intimate sphere, but one of our most important duties during a postnatal visit. Initially you will be unaccustomed to talking about your bleeding, but you will surely overcome this inhibition soon.

Midwives' Knowledge

The best method of dealing with the insufficient flow of lochia is to put the baby to the breast frequently. If the flow increases after breastfeeding, then there is nothing to worry about. Incidentally, during my years as a self-employed midwife, I have observed that the amount of lochia almost always decreases when the milk "comes in", and increases again when the breast milk flows. Naturally, the same applies to the involution of the uterus – after all, the woman's body is a uniform whole and cannot be broken down into isolated parts – breasts, abdomen and lochia – for the purposes of examination and observation. On the contrary, it is extremely important always to regard a woman in the postnatal period in her holistic entirety. A word of advice for the midwife: please don't be shaken when a woman goes through the typical postnatal "down". Her breasts swell up but no milk flows, the involution of the uterus leaves much to be desired and to top it off, she remarks that her bleeding has decreased and smells strange. How can the river flow if the entire the postnatal period atmosphere is dammed up? Begin by helping the woman to cope with her depressed mood and give her the opportunity to let her tears flow. Assure her that the problems with her breasts and milk flow will certainly be less severe by tomorrow. The best thing you can do is to help the young mother put her baby to her breast and see to it that the baby drinks its fill so that one breast is completely emptied out. Already these steps alone will help the woman, and within a few hours everything will be flowing properly again. I cannot conceive of paying a postnatal house call without taking the emotional background into account. Understanding, encouragement and consolation help a woman in the postnatal period every bit as much as any medicine.

In the case of subinvolution (delayed involution of the uterus) and slightly foetid (offensive-smelling) lochia, it is helpful to teach the woman certain involution exercises from the postnatal exercise programme. Of course it is important that the mother do these exercises several times a day.

A hot sitz bath or a hot-water bottle likewise often gets the lochia flowing again.

Herbal Medicine

If the postnatal bleeding is insufficient, one way of helping yourself is to drink *Rückbildungstee/Involution Tea*, consisting of one part shepherd's purse as well as two parts each of lady's mantle and lemon balm. I have achieved excellent results with this blend. Please note that you should not drink more than two cups a day in small sips, because otherwise it can cause severe abdominal pains …

… as was the case with one of my first early-discharge mothers on the third day after birth. Her uterus was still about two finger breadths below the navel and she was hardly bleeding at all. I had left her the Rückbildungstee/Involution Tea and advised her to drink it. Later that afternoon she rang me up and wanted to know what she should do; she had such strong abdominal pains. These words set off all my inner alarms and I promised I'd be there as soon as possible. On the drive to her house, my beginner's fear already had me imagining the transfer to the hospital, complete with all the consequences of an antibiotic, an anaesthetic and curettage. In my excitement, I had totally forgotten to ask her about all the other symptoms of a postnatal infection. A short time later I arrived, breathless, at the family's house, where I found the woman lying in bed curled up around a hot-water bottle. My first act was to feel her forehead; with my other hand I felt for her uterus. To my astonishment, her forehead was no warmer than normal, nor damp; there were no discernible signs of fever and her uterus was not to be

found around her navel. To my great surprise, I could feel the uterus halfway between the navel and the pubic bone, and it was not sensitive to the touch around the edges. The woman told me that she had been bleeding strongly again for about an hour, but had already had these cramp-like pains for two hours. I was relieved and happy at the same time. When I asked her how much Rückbildungstee/Involution Tea she had already consumed, she answered: "This is my third pot; I thought it would be good to drink a lot of it." Now it was clear to me what had happened: Mrs. G. had simply drunk too much tea and the shepherd's purse had brought about strong afterpains. We both laughed with relief and told each other about the horror scenarios that had gone through our minds. Since that day I have always urged the women I attend to to drink no more than two cups a day, lukewarm and in small sips.

⟲ Homoeopathic Treatment

There are women who don't like to drink tea and would much prefer to take a homoeopathic remedy. In the case of true lochia insufficiency, the midwife will prescribe *Bellis perennis*. *Pulsatilla* and *Sepia* are also substances administered to women with insufficient postnatal bleeding accompanied by delayed involution of the uterus. Bellis perennis, the daisy, is one of the homoeopathic remedies most frequently used during the postnatal period …

… a farmers' wife took advantage of postnatal care by a midwife for the first time after the birth of her third child. I supported her in her wish to discontinue her intake of a medicine called Methergine®, because she herself had read on the package insert about its undesirable side effects. This is the only remedy offered by mainstream medicine against insufficient involution of the uterus. As had been the case with her first two children, she had to supplement the breast milk with infant formula and, what is more, the newborn had been suffering from massive flatulence for a few days already. The woman told me she had received two shots a day until her discharge from the hospital and was now supposed to take the abovementioned drops. When I examined the position of the uterus, I was astonished: on the seventh day, it was still only two fingerbreadths below the navel. I advised the woman to take Bellis perennis in the form of homoeopathic globuli at least once every two hours. Her uterus had already contracted considerably by the next day and the flow of lochia was stronger. The involution made slow but steady progress and there were no further complications. Three days after she stopped taking the Methergine, the milk began to flow and the problem with wind was better. When I paid her my last house call, I explained to her that the next time she gave birth she should tell the doctor and midwife in attendance that they should expect the involution process to be slower than average, that in this respect she simply did not meet the norm, that she shouldn't allow herself to be alarmed by their reactions, and that she should take the daisy globuli with her when she went to the hospital. When she heard the word "daisy", she laughed and told me: "Now I know why my grandfather used to send us out to pick daisies when a cow had just calved. Why shouldn't it also help people?"

⟲ Aroma Therapy

I have frequently also had good experience with abdominal massages in conjunction with the product *Ut-Öl/Uterus Tonic 𝒟®*. I take this blend of verbena, cloves, cinnamon and ginger on a fatty oil basis with me to every postnatal house call. Initially the midwife will carry out the massage, but soon the mother can take over this task herself. With the massage methods taught her by the midwife, she will regularly apply the oil to her lower abdomen, preferably before breastfeeding, in order to achieve increased afterpains. Uterus Tonic is likewise effective in combination with a hot compress or as a bath supplement. Even before the massage is over, many astonished women tell me that they could feel that the bleeding had started. I had my most memorable experience in this context with Mrs. M. …

… after giving birth by caesarean section she asked me to pay her a call to help her with her breast-feeding problems. Out of habit, I happened to ask her about her bleeding. She looked at me, puzzled: "What bleeding? I haven't had any bleeding for the entire two weeks, just a sticky brownish discharge." When I determined the position of the uterus, my suspicion was confirmed: not only the milk, but also the lochia were not flowing properly. I taught the woman the uterus massage and recommended that she carry it out herself as often as possible. The next day she happily reported: "My breasts are better and, just think, I'm bleeding! Last night, shortly after the massage, I began bleeding as strongly as when I have my period. It kept stopping after a while but then started again after every massage." The treatment I had recommended worked so well that I was astonished myself, and the involution of the uterus had also made considerable progress.

A delayed involution of the uterus nearly always goes hand in hand with conspicuous problems with the lochia. Don't hesitate to describe your observations to your midwife, and don't be surprised if she checks the position of the uterus at every visit and asks you detailed questions about your bleeding.

Rapid Involution of the Uterus

If the involution of the uterus progresses much faster than average, there is never anything to worry about – quite the contrary, you can thank your lucky stars. Obviously, in this situation, the lochia will slow down and take on a brownish colour sooner.

Retention of the Lochia

Retention of the lochia – also called lochiostasis – seldom happens if the woman is examined regularly, because it is almost always preceded by conspicuous postnatal bleeding disorders or delayed involution of the uterus.

Either the woman speaks up of her own accord during a postnatal care visit because she has noticed something unusual, or the symptoms are discovered in the course of a house call during which she complains of a headache in the area of the forehead. When asked about the lochia, women afflicted with this disorder tend to report happily that they haven't had any bleeding yet all day. When we hear this during the early postnatal period, we midwives perk up our ears and the first thing we do is check the position of the uterus, which is usually not as it should be. In this acute situation, I recommend prescribing *Rückbildungstee/Involution Tea* and, if the woman agrees to it, a suitable homoeopathic remedy. An abdominal massage of the uterus with *Ut-Öl/Uterus Tonic D*® is another sensible measure, and the woman should carry it out regularly and frequently until the bleeding has resumed.

Constipation

The problem of delayed involution can also very often be solved by administering an enema. In situations of this kind, the midwife naturally has to ask about the various bodily functions. It is quite astonishing how many women in the postnatal period have digestion problems and are still constipated after six days in the hospital. Women often report that they have already received medicine or shots in the maternity ward because the involution of the uterus was not proceeding at the normal rate. When I ask a woman whether the hospital personnel were aware that she had not been able to empty her bowels properly since the birth, the answer is often negative: the woman has kept her condition a secret so as not to have to take a laxative. I urge you not to take this approach, because, as you see, it can lead to complications. As I mentioned previously, an enema can be very effective.

Retroflexion of the Uterus

It can happen, though, that the uterus appears to have returned to its normal size, the bladder is not full, the bowels have been emptied and the mother nevertheless complains about the particular form of headache which accompanies retention of the lochia. There are also cases in which the bleeding suddenly stops, even though it had been plentiful until the previous day. In these situations, it is often helpful for the midwife to ask the mother whether she has pains in the lower back, which is almost always the case. Usually the woman says: "Yes but what do back pains have to do with my headache and the fact that the lochia have stopped? I was up a lot today and my back is hurting as a result." Usually, however, my suspicion that the woman has a retroflexed uterus (i.e. that it is tilted backward) – already detected by the doctor before pregnancy – is confirmed. But many other mothers have never even heard that a uterus can be tilted backward towards the sacrum. Your midwife will explain to you that, since the uterine ligaments have been overstretched, the uterus is now more or less tumbling around in the abdominal cavity with nothing to hold it in place. If the primipara gets up too soon after childbirth or stays up too long, it can happen that the uterus buckles in the area of the cervix and slips down into the pelvis minor. As a result, the lochia can no longer flow out, they fill up the uterine cavity and cause pains in the lower back. If this situation goes unnoticed too long, a dangerous uterine infection can come about, the first sign of which is fever.

In the case of a retroflexed uterus accompanied by retention of the lochia, in addition to the above-described methods it is absolutely essential that the primipara assume the *all-fours position* or *lie on her stomach* for as long as she can and as often as she has time, and carry out energetic abdominal muscle exercises until everything starts flowing again. She should also have someone massage her lower back vigorously with *Ut-Öl/Uterus Tonic D*® and also apply a hot-water bottle alternately to the sacrum and the abdomen. If she already has a fever, the proper homoeopathic remedy must be found as quickly as possible. If the bleeding doesn't set in and the woman's temperature doesn't drop again soon, the doctor will probably have to have her admitted to the hospital. But usually, this palette of naturopathic treatments and the newborn baby – which should be breastfed as frequently as possible –, activate the body's self-help mechanisms to such an extent that hospitalization is not necessary.

⑤ Homoeopathic Treatment

Homoeopathic medication can undoubtedly be used to treat retention of the lochia successfully, but only if the postnatal situation is considered holistically. Once again, what this means is to perceive the current postnatal situation and recognize what is "blocked" in the family. I would like to point out just a few of the substances that might come under consideration, because any midwife or doctor with knowledge of homoeopathy will know that a great number of remedies resemble the combination of symptoms and that it is an art to find the one that is really the most similar. Perhaps *Aconitum, Belladonna, Pulsatilla, Sepia, Natrium Muriaticum, Kalium carbonicum* or *Nux vomica* will turn out to be the right choice.

Here I would like to recount one of my most memorable experiences with Natrium muriaticum …

… Ms. S. asked me to attend to her during the postpartum period. This time she had come home from the hospital two days earlier because her older daughter needed her. When I arrived for my first visit, she greeted me with a friendly smile and immediately asked me if her roommate from the maternity ward had contacted me because she was urgently in need of a midwife's postnatal care. When we entered the living room, she quickly cleaned up the toys that were strewn across the floor and apologized for the untidiness. I carried out my usual examination routine, and was very surprised to discover a large, poorly contracted uterus. With a strange, seemingly carefree smile she assured me that she wasn't bleeding right at the moment but was sure to start again soon. I managed to persuade her to drink Rückbildungstee/Involution Tea. I left the house with an uneasy feeling and decided that I would have all my antennas out the next day. Again, Ms. S. opened the door with a smile that seemed even more forced than the day before. She told me that her husband wasn't there, but that she would be fine. She described to me how grown-up and intelligent her older daughter was and didn't show any signs of jealousy, was even very cooperative about being taken to Grandma's house and letting Daddy put her to bed. Her worries had all been for nought, but she was happy because she loved her older daughter more than anything. When I cautiously asked whether it wasn't a bit painful for her to see how well her daughter coped without her, she broke into tears. And then she spilled out her whole unhappy story – about her unloving, enterprising and constantly busy mother, her fear of being the mother of two, even her recurring depressions, which she had been keeping concealed from her husband for

years. As she made this last confession, she couldn't even look me in the eye. It was clear to me that she couldn't accept consolation and I noticed her dry lips with a large cold sore on them. There was no doubt in my mind: this woman needed Natrium muriaticum. When she was finished talking, she shyly asked me for help: "Please excuse me for taking up so much of your time, but I just had to tell you that. Maybe you know of some homoeopathic remedy; I really am often afraid that I won't be able to cope with all of these demands. But please, don't tell my husband, alright?" I promised to bring Natrium muriaticum with me the next day – I don't think I had ever been so sure that it was the right choice – in an LM potency, because in such a critical situation I didn't want to risk the initial negative reaction often brought about by homoeopathic substances. (In homoeopathic treatment, the choice of potency is decisive for avoiding the so-called initial aggravation of the symptoms – which is often very brief but can also be quite unpleasant). Even before we had finished talking, the lochia began to flow again. All blocks had dissolved in the flow of tears and words. Ms. S. called me a week later, as we had arranged during my last house call and told me that she had been relatively stable since our talk and the intake of the remedy, and not had any severe depressions. She was even considering going into therapy, as I had advised her to do.

My intention in telling you this story is to point out once again that, for homoeopathic treatment, it is necessary to observe the circumstances without judging them in any way, and gain an overview of the symptoms – i.e. not merely look at the uterus, but at the woman in her overall emotional and physical state. This is essential if the choice of remedies is to prove successful.

Inflammation of Varicose Veins

Disorders of the uterine involution process or the lochia are not the only situation that will cause a midwife to pay the woman a postnatal visit immediately and then remain in contact with her until further notice. Thrombophlebitis (clotting and acute tender inflammation of varicose veins) can also rob a midwife of her composure and confidence, at least that's what happened to me in the early years of my self-employment. Thanks to naturopathy and preventive measures, such worries can be kept at bay, and if worse comes to worst, there is always Heparin (an anticoagulant produced by the body) to fall back on. Throughout my entire period as an independent midwife, I cared for only one woman who accepted the doctor's offer and had the prescription filled. Women with varicose veins already get elastic stockings put on them by the midwife right after birth, as is likewise the case when the birth takes place in the hospital. The new mother receives daily instruction in exercises that take the pressure off the veins, and has to promise to do these exercises frequently, keep her legs elevated and get up regularly for a few minutes at a time. Thanks to *Arnica*, there are seldom major problems.

If the veins should become inflamed despite all of these preventive measures, good old elastic bandages are a big help, and the midwife should not shy away from bandaging the woman's afflicted leg.

☺ Aroma Therapy

The sensitive, reddened zone can be treated either with healing earth ("Heilerde") or quark, both of which have a cooling effect, or these two remedies alternately, mixed with *Lavendel-Zypressen-Öl/Lavender-Cypress Oil 𝒟*®, containing the essential oils lavender, lemongrass, myrtle, yarrow, juniper and cypress. *Retterspitz External* is likewise a very valuable aid.

☺ Homoeopathic Treatment

Internally, a homoeopathic remedy such as *Calendula, Hamamelis, Lachesis, Lycopodium* or *Pulsatilla* can be employed.

As a young mother, you will have noticed as you read these pages that I often address the midwife. I hope I have managed to make the reason for this clear: you must never treat pathological conditions of the kind I am describing on your own, without a midwife or doctor. Please consult a midwife; she knows what will help you best.

The Pelvic Floor

Perineal Care

Childbirth subjects the pelvic tissue to a maximum of stress, immense stretching and almost always abrasions or lacerations of greater or lesser severity – often sensed by the woman as injuries not only to the body but also the soul. The muscles have been prepared for these circumstances during pregnancy – hormonally as well as by means of physical exercise and naturopathic applications. During the early postnatal period, what this part of the body needs most is relief, rest and recovery. During the late postnatal period, these muscles will gradually firm up again. The entire postpartum process is hormonally controlled and can, like pregnancy and childbirth, likewise be supported by means of gymnastic exercises and naturopathic applications.

Sensations and Feelings

It is very important to me to communicate to all women that the genital zone will by all means return to normal, even if it feels a bit strange initially. Expectant and new mothers alike very often signal to me, between the lines, feelings of fear, uncertainty and worry about the appearance, condition and sensitivity of their sexual organs. And undoubtedly, many a young father will also wonder about "afterwards". (For a discussion of sexuality after birth, see the section on "The Late Postnatal Period", p. 427 f.)

I can assure you that the vagina will soon look and feel like normal. In the first hours following birth, the labia will be more or less swollen, but will close the vagina in the proper manner. A person who didn't know would never be able to tell that "Aha, this woman has just delivered a baby" just by the sight of the woman's genitals. It is only at the very end of the birth process that nature opens the door to the world and closes it again as soon as the baby has passed through.

During the first few days after birth, the pelvic floor always feels strange. There is no sensation of tension, stretching, or weight; everything is somehow numb but sore at the same time. Here in Allgaeu, we say it feels "pelzig" – "furry". Women who have not had an episiotomy are often surprised by this unpleasant feeling. But if you think about it, the birth of a child can't just be over and done with and forgotten an hour later; there are also "afterpains" in the physical sensations. Many women try to find words to describe what they feel and say something like: "It all feels a bit swollen. My vagina feels like it's been overstretched. It's as though I had been to the dentist, but with my behind. It's like sitting on raw eggs. It feels sensitive and sore." These feelings last about two or, at the most, three days. Then the vaginal zone gets back to feeling the way it always did, provided there are no more major injuries.

The Appearance of the Pelvic Floor

One thing that will help you come to terms with the feelings and sensations in your intimate zone is to look at yourself in a mirror as soon as possible. Feeling yourself with your fingers is undoubtedly also good, but due to the soreness and/or injuries of the tissue, it might leave you with a somewhat distorted impression. Moreover, for that very reason, women are often shy about touching themselves there.

Naturally, you yourself should decide when you have the desire and feel prepared to look at yourself. Perhaps you want to do it entirely on your own, or perhaps with your midwife or your partner. Here I would like to urge everyone – men and midwives alike – not just to surprise the new mother with a mirror or force her to look at herself without asking her. This would be paramount to emotional rape. Those of us in attendance must be aware of the fact that the woman has the feeling of having been injured in her most intimate sphere by the birth, and has to sort out her own feelings with regard to herself. And that takes time. During our house calls, we midwives must likewise protect the woman's intimate sphere and allow her to decide when and where she will allow us to gain an impression of how the birth injuries are healing. When we are attending to a young mother at home, we should communicate to her that she is free to develop her natural feelings of shame again.

When you, as a first-time mum, have reached the point where you would like to venture a look at your vagina, the mirror will also help you learn to touch yourself again and to recognize that the child has not changed you. It is possible that, if you have had a perineal suture, you might be a tiny bit shocked at first at the size and appearance of the wound. But if you take a look once a day, you will be able to observe how the healing process progresses. During my house calls I have experienced again and again that most women in the postnatal period are pleasantly surprised by their appearance. So take heart and look at your vagina. It is important for you to find and like yourself again.

Protection of the Pelvic Floor

I know from experience that it is important for me to urge all new mothers to go easy on their pelvic floor, in other words to lie down as much as possible. The contracted uterus is very heavy and, when the woman stands, puts a huge burden on the over-expanded pelvic floor. Due to the above mentioned numbness, this pressure often goes unnoticed. Actually, this advice not to burden the vaginal and perineal muscles unnecessarily is only important for women whose perineum was not injured during birth, because women who have undergone an episiotomy or laceration of the perineum will want to stay in bed anyway, due to the pain of the wound.

Injuries to the Pelvic Floor

Perineal Tears

Women who have suffered a perineal tear which was not sutured following the birth of the child are hereby strongly urged to avoid spreading their legs at all costs. In the home birth context, we prefer not to suture small tears if possible. In these cases the women have to promise not to sit and not to spread their legs for a few days – although normally there is nothing the primipara will want to do less. Generally, a woman who has suffered a perineal tear cannot sit cross-legged again for several days. Incidentally, my experience with the healing process of "untreated" perineal lacerations has always been very positive. Every tear, even the more severe ones, healed excellently. When I have later contact with a woman I have cared for during the post-natal period, I take advantage of the opportunity to ask whether she has had any problems with her perineum. Until now, the answer has always been no. On the contrary ...

... Simone said: "I'm so glad we didn't suture the tear. You were right; I can feel that my anatomy in the area of the vagina is back to its normal state. After the birth of my previous child, due to my sutured episiotomy, that wasn't the case for ages."

So please don't worry about it if a small tear has not been sutured; all you have to do is take care not to put any weight on the injury or stretch it by spreading your legs.

Lacerations of the Labia

The same applies to lacerations of the labia. When the perineum remains intact, the labia are often injured. These tears are sometimes sutured in the hospital, but just as frequently left to heal on their own, as in the home birth context. Here again, I can reassure all women that the tear will certainly heal well. Injuries to the mucous membranes – and that's what these are – always heal well and quickly.

Episiotomy

If you have had an episiotomy – a surgical incision of the perineum undertaken to facilitate childbirth – the pain will naturally last longer. As in the case of all lacerations, it will depend on the length and depth of the cut. The incision may have been carried out in a straight line in the direction of the constrictor (anal muscle), or diagonally from the centre of the perineum towards the gluteal muscle. The length can vary from two to as many as eight centimetres/three quarters of an inch to three inches. Not only the size and depth, but also the method of suture and the body's natural healing process will be decisive for how much pain you suffer. During the first few days, the local pain will be covered up by a general feeling of exhaustion, and only become discernible as incision pain on the second to third day after the birth. Usually the pain culminates on the fourth and fifth days, since the suture thread swells up and causes additional tension. The suture material presently in use unfortunately only dissolves after as many as three weeks. For this reason, incidentally, it is quite advisable just to remove them with a pair of scissors and a pair of tweezers, provided the healing process has made good progress. I recommend to midwives and mothers alike that they begin with the partial removal of the threads beginning on the fourth day, because on the one hand it is rarely painful and on the other hand it often brings relief. "But they will be absorbed by the body; they don't have to be removed", is often the reaction. Experience shows, however, that this is not a generally applicable approach: whereas one woman may still clearly need the support offered by the stitches on the fifth day, in another case the injury may be almost completely healed by that time. As we have already seen in numerous other contexts, an individual decision must be made, tailored to the situation, and not on the basis of the quality and brand name of the thread. Again and again, I have observed that, already after a few days, the threads are nothing but a painful nuisance and that the tissue is sensitive and inflamed at every puncture. This phenomenon can perhaps best be explained by the "splinter principle": when a splinter has dug its way into the skin and is not removed, after a few days the body begins attempting to reject it. It is often my impression that the same is true of the perineal suture threads. The timely removal of the stitches is a helpful and pleasant measure for the mother, because it relieves her of the pinching and pulling. In the case of subcuticular sutures (i.e. beneath the skin) it can be a big help at least to loosen one of the knots on the outside – again, to relieve the unpleasant feeling of pulling. In my experience, subcuticular stitches initially heal faster and cause less discomfort, but then cause the woman quite a number of problems after all before they are finally completely absorbed by the body. Here I must admit that I didn't really understand what it means to have a perineal suture, with all of the accompanying pain and discomfort, until I went through it myself. As a young midwife I simply repeated what the doctors always say: "It can't hurt; the suture looks fine." But every gynaecologist and every midwife should go through an incision and a suture on their genitals before they are allowed to pass judgement! As a midwife I am aware that some episiotomies cannot be avoided, but then all obstetricians and the women's partners should show the woman understanding for her in her pain and in-disposition. It makes my hair stand on end when I hear men end a report on child-birth with the casual remark: "They just had to cut a little." It seems to me that this wording and lack of sensitivity may well have been inspired by something the doctor has said. When will men stop referring to our episiotomies – which are carried out much too often – as trifles? Gisela speaks for many women: "I can well remember the peaceful-sounding words of the doctor when he said to the midwife: 'Let's provide her a bit of relief.' That 'relief' bothered me for months afterwards!" Again and again, women complain to me about the fact that, even after a year or longer, they are still having trouble with the "relief" incision.

When a woman has already has already had an incision – which, particularly in the case of operative deliveries, naturally cannot always be avoided – we, the midwives, doctors and partners, should do everything in our power to help the wound heal as well and quickly as possible.

Helpful Measures in Cases of Birth Injuries

- *Rule Number 1:* During the first few days, the most important rule to be observed by every woman who has suffered an episiotomy or perineal tear is to lie down as much as possible and avoid all sitting, standing or walking.
- *Lying:* You can obtain additional relief by lying on your stomach as often as possi-ble, with a small cushion to provide support. When you lie on your side, try to lie on both sides alternately, despite the pain of your wounds, to avoid assuming a relieving posture and the muscle pain often associated with it.
- *Getting into and out of bed:* If you are in the hospital, have the nurse bring you a stool so that you don't have to spread your legs – and your perineum in the pro-cess – too far. The height of hospital beds is undoubtedly one reason why many a tear has to be sutured to ensure that it heals well. At home the beds are fortunately not as high. The best thing the new mother can do is literally crawl into bed. Climb onto your bed with your hands and bent knees and then lie down with a turning movement. When you get up, you can overcome the obstacle presented by the edge of the bed without causing yourself all too much pain by crawling out of bed backwards on all fours.
- *Sitting:* You should avoid sitting as long as possible, and when you do sit, it will initially be possible only with an aid: I advise all partners of women with major injuries to the perineum and/or vagina, whether in the hospital or at home, to get a doughnut-shaped 'sitting ring'. In a pinch, you can fashion one yourself by cut-

ting a hole into a thick piece of foam rubber or, more simply still, firmly rolling up a large towel and forming a ring with it.

- *Standing:* With birth wounds, standing is also sure to be unpleasant, but if it cannot be avoided, it will be more bearable if you can brace your upper body, e.g. on a table or the back of a chair, thereby taking a load off the pelvic floor.
- *Walking:* Walking will still be the most pleasant alternative to lying, but if pain is to be avoided then you will probably have to take very small steps. By the way, during the postnatal period, you can wear shoes with heels, because they also serve to take pressure off the perineum.

The amount of time it will take until you can walk, sit and stand painlessly for a longer stretch of time will vary from one woman to the next, and depends to some extent on the above-discussed factors regarding the healing process. What is important is that neither the partner nor the woman herself undertake comparisons with other women in the postnatal period who may be back on their feet sooner. This can lead to unnecessary pressure to perform or even cause feelings of inferiority.

Physical Applications

- *Cold applications:* Immediately after the birth and on the first day of the postnatal period, newly delivered mothers find it very pleasant – and a good means of relieving pain – to apply an ice wrap to the birth wounds. So-called cold packs are available in most maternity wards, so ask for one. At home I very much like to use arnica or calendula ice cubes. These can be made by the parents beforehand; they are wrapped up in a gauze swab or pad and applied to the birth injury. Arnica ice cubes are a good means of treating haematomas and haemorrhoids. A haematoma – a swelling filled with blood resulting from a break in a blood vessel/a bruise – can easily develop on the perineal or caesarean incision, but if ice is applied immediately it will subside very quickly. The same applies to haemorrhoids which have been pushed outward during the birth. In cases like these it is helpful to brush the ice cube with the *Original 𝒟® Aroma Blend Hamamelis-Myrte-Balsam/ Witch-Hazel-Myrtle Balsam 𝒟®* or another haemorrhoid ointment before wrapping it up in a compress. With this treatment the woman in the postnatal period will soon be relieved of her suffering since the blood clots quickly shrink and allow themselves to be pushed back. Calendula ice cubes can be used in a compress in cases of perineal lacerations or a vulval oedema (swelling of the vagina). But please wrap them up in at least three gauze swabs! The new mother will thus be able to bear the cold quite well during the first few hours. As soon as it feels icy, however, it is time to stop the application. As always, you can rely on your body to give you the right signals.
- *Rinse:* A regular rinse, as described in the section on "The Lochia" (p. ■f) is pleasant and promotes the healing process into the bargain.
- *Air and sunlight:* A time-tested method of treating wounds and supporting the heal-

ing process is exposure to air and sunlight. Remove the maternity pad/sanitary towel as often as possible and allow the air to circulate around the wounds. I am aware that this isn't so simple in the hospital, but at least you can do it under the cover of your blanket, and then at home after you have been discharged. In cases of perineal wounds that heal poorly, it proves very helpful to expose the wound to air after passing water or taking a sitz bath. Naturally, infrared light radiation is an extremely effective aid to the healing process. You will not be able to tolerate this intense warmth until several days after the birth, however.

- *Sitz Bath:* The most successful as well as the most pleasant method of promoting the healing process during the postnatal period is the sitz bath. Sitz bath therapy is handled very differently from one maternity ward to the next: whereas the one hospital recommends one to several sitz baths a day from the first day on, the other rejects the mere idea of a sitz bath. When and where the sitz bath is taken naturally depends on the way the particular hospital is set up. At home you can decide for yourself when you would like to start treating yourself to sitz baths and what you would like to supplement them with. As a midwife I can only recommend that you get into the prepared basin or tub as soon as you possibly can. Regardless of whether your perineum is intact, abraded, torn or cut or you have other injuries of the labia or vaginal wall, you can enjoy a sitz bath from the second day onward. One thing you must observe, though, is the proper water temperature. On the first day, I recommend cool to slightly lukewarm water (28° C/82.5° F), on the second and third day lukewarm (approx. 32° C/89° F) and, when the pain of the wound subsides, the water can be body temperature.

Herbal Medicine

Oak bark is a good choice of sitz bath additives, since it contains tanning agents, which have an astringent and antiseptic effect. *Chamomile* is probably the most well-known sitz bath supplement in this context. During the late postnatal period it can be used to promote the healing process, but should not be added to your sitz bath during the first few days. During my early years of self-employment I often witnessed that, if chamomile was used too early for an open injury to the mucous membranes, the wound would heal superficially quite rapidly (presumably because of the azulene content) but then irritations and reddening would occur, sometimes even to the point where the wound would open again. Perineal tears and incisions should heal from the inside out, so to speak, which is why I stopped recommending chamomile rinses and sitz baths during the early postnatal period.

Aroma Therapy

Since I have had so much good experience with essential oils, the possibility of using them for sitz baths seemed obvious. Because of its antiseptic, cleansing and immuno-logical effect, Dead Sea Salt presented itself as an emulsifier for the essences. This salt also has the property of drying out the skin, which is desirable in the case of birth wounds. A fragrant sitz bath with essential oils is a wonderful boon for any woman going through the postnatal period. In the *Original $\mathcal{D}^*$ Aroma Blend Sitzbad/Sitz Bath $\mathcal{D}^*$* the following essential oils are added to the Dead Sea Salt: chamomile blue, lavender, rose, rose geranium and yarrow. (You can read more about the effects of the individual oils in my book *Time-Tested Aroma Blends*.)

I can no longer imagine the postnatal period or the treatment of wounds without my *Sitzbad/Sitz Bath $\mathcal{D}^*$*. I could write a whole book just on wound healing processes with this wonderful bath salt and its essential oils. Even for me, it seems incredible that essential oils possess such healing powers. I have used them for such a range of wounds – including deep, infected episiotomies left open to heal on their own, poorly healing caesarean sutures, severely sore mamillae (nipples) and babies' "nappy zones", even deep flesh wounds in children. And for many years, I have also been receiving innumerable reports: from fellow midwives who have managed to have this wonderful healing salt employed in hospitals, from other colleagues who have succeeded in healing open leg ulcers with it, even from a family which was able to heal its badly injured – and severely weakened – broodmare with it, thus saving the valuable animal's life. With each success, my desire to share the effects of essential oils with others has grown.

⑤ Ointment Compresses with Herbal Products

Unfortunately, it can happen that an episiotomy heals poorly or even opens again partially due to an infection. Interestingly, I can't remember this ever being the case in women who have spent the early postnatal period at home. Are the preventive measures and the care perhaps really better at home? Here I would like to pass on a number of pointers on the employment of compresses. Many of my readers will be familiar with other good healing methods; after all, other people have other experiences. With my suggestions, I would particularly like to help inexperienced mothers and provide young midwives starting out in self-employment with a range of naturopathic treatment methods.

In cases where the wounds heal slowly and poorly, I recommend taking an air and/ or sun bath following the sitz bath or blow-drying the wound. In addition, a sage compress can be applied twice a day. In the case of reddened, slightly open wounds, *Ringelblumensalbe/Calendula Ointment $\mathcal{D}^*$* – an *Original $\mathcal{D}^*$ Aroma Blend* on a lanolin basis, further containing propolis tincture and beeswax – is very effective.

Beinwellsalbe/Comfrey Ointment $\mathcal{D}^*$ is extremely suitable in cases of deep, open perineal wounds. The reason comfrey helps to heal deep wounds so outstandingly is that it strongly supports cell renewal. With regard to the healing of wounds, the comfrey root possesses phenomenal qualities. It is essential, however, that the comfrey you use is free of pyrrolizidine alkaloids ("PA-free"). The ointment basis of *Beinwellsalbe/Comfrey Ointment $\mathcal{D}^*$* likewise consists of propolis tincture and pesticide-free lanolin as well as St.-John's wort and calendula oil.

Another remedy I have had excellent experience with in treating poorly healing, infected perineal wounds is *Rose-Teebaum-Balsam/Rose-Tea-Tree Balsam 𝒟®*. The essential oils contained in this product speed up the healing process immensely.

Yet another healing ointment is *Traumeel®S Ointment*. All of the other Traumeel®S products exhibit the same properties. For women in the postnatal period, Traumeel®S drops are highly recommendable as a healing and anti-inflammatory complex homoeopathic remedy.

⑤ Calendula Essence

A so-called secondary wound healing with delayed re-epithelialization and contraction, i.e. an extremely poorly healing and/or infected perineal suture, can likewise be treated with a rinse or compress using *calendula essence*. The good healing properties of calendula have been known to woman since time immemorial and have proven their value over and over again in cases of infected birth wounds. The parents also learn from the midwife that they can use whatever is left of the essence to treat infected wounds in the family later on. Once a grandfather overheard me talking to a woman about the application of this essence during the postnatal period …

… I noticed him becoming more and more interested in my explanations and finally his curiosity got the better of him and, in heavy Allgaeu dialect, he asked: "Maybe the midwife knows something for me as well, doesn't she? For a whole week now, I've been running to the doctor, but it's no use. A cow kicked me here on my arm and the wound just refuses to heal. Can I use the calendula for this too?" I said of course he could and explained how his wound should be treated. A mere two days later, when I paid my next house call, he told me the wound was healing so well he could almost watch it happening. A week later, his wife brought me a big bunch of flowers from her garden as a token of thanks. She was so grateful that her husband, who had been so grumpy since the injury, was in such a good mood again because he no longer had to go into the village every day to see the doctor, but could be cared for at home, and the wound was now almost completely healed.

Experiences of this kind add a lot of spice to the daily routine of a self-employed midwife and provide good insight into what it used to mean to work as a midwife in rural areas. It is always particularly satisfying – and the best token of recognition – to be acknowledged by older members of the family. In these situations I am very often told stories about the things "our old midwife" did. I think it's wonderful that the job description of the "old midwife" hasn't disappeared entirely.

Breast Milk Applications

Another successful method is the application of breast milk, a true all-round remedy! Breast milk contains natural, individually tailored antibodies (precisely the kind that cannot be pharmaceutically produced) which support every healing process. Any mother who is open to this method can press milk out of her breast onto a compress or catch the excess milk that continues after the baby has finished suckling, and apply it to her perineal incision. Women who have a lot of excess milk can even use it as a sitz bath additive.

The Father during the Postnatal Period

As I have mentioned frequently, the birth of a child crowns the parents' love for one another. The postnatal process is accordingly the coronation ceremony, which means that the new father is just as much a part of the picture as the mother and the baby. Unfortunately, our society often sees things differently. Men often encounter remarks like: "Just because his wife had a baby, he's taking leave from work for three weeks and he's not even coming to our weekly pub get-togethers." It would be great if the event of becoming a father were not always celebrated just with alcohol but also with understanding.

There is no doubt in my mind that many men likewise experience something like the postnatal process and the vacillating moods that accompany it, because otherwise there wouldn't be such a great need to pour alcohol over everything. To be a father means to take responsibility, to care and provide for the mother and child. The man undergoes a reorientation: what's my position in the relationship now? Does the child always come first? Are cuddling, affection and lovemaking things of the past? Will the baby lie in the middle from now on? To some extent, this phase is surely also accompanied by feelings of jealousy.

Days One and Two

For many a new father, sobering thoughts about his own helplessness during the birth come up in the days that follow. This is particularly the case when he has imagined himself accompanying his wife and providing a lot of major assistance during labour, and never realized that all he could really do was stand by her, and just be there. Often the consequence is that the father reacts with the stomach flu and has to stay in bed at home while the mother spends the postnatal period in the hospital. In many cases this is surely the man's physical reaction to the fact that he feels terrible about being separated from his child and his wife because, interestingly enough, I do not hear of or observe these phenomena after home births.

Fathers who have the opportunity to care for the freshly delivered mum and the newborn at home make the impression of being "on Cloud Nine" during the first few days. They bustle about, attentive and affectionate, caring and protective all at the same time. Like a Good Fairy they whiz through the house on quiet feet and, like an experienced manager, see to it that the baby is warm enough, the food is on the stove, the washing machine is running, the phone ringer volume is turned down, visitors are greeted or asked to come back another day. When I come to pay a house call, the father sits down with his wife and me as calm as can be, even though the dirty dishes are waiting in the sink. It is wonderful to experience family situations such as these.

Day Three/The Baby Blues

On the third day, though, the childbed manager starts showing signs of stress because the phone is ringing more and more often, there are official obligations to attend to and the noodles are already way beyond "al dente" again. I recommend falling back on a "TV dinner" or asking Grandma or a friend to come and help – they've been waiting to be asked for what seems to them like ages anyway – and young parents generally regard these suggestions to be excellent ideas. By the third day at the latest, many a father realizes that it would have been quite practical to hire a housekeeper temporarily. But all of these matters are really only very minor for the man, because as soon as he is holding his baby again he's the proud, tender, affectionate father from head to toe.

One thing the partner can't always cope with so masterfully is his wife's hormone-induced emotional ups and downs, which usually reach their lowest on Day Three. I frequently have to request understanding for the woman and explain to the man that she would really rather be hugged than see him zipping around with the Hoover again. Business calls also often give rise to a crying fit on the part of the woman. The man simply cannot understand it because, after all, he's taken care of all the necessary housework and merely needs to clear up this one business matter. It is undoubtedly very difficult for a man to understand why his wife constantly has tears rolling down her cheeks although she has already recovered quite well physically, the baby is healthy and the breast milk is beginning to flow. Again and again, I have the impression that it is necessary to explain to the man that the slightest incident suffices to make her lose her composure. She is in the postnatal period, she has given birth to a baby, and has a feeling of emptiness and having nothing to hold onto. She seeks protection and needs a feeling of security more than anything else; from her point of view, a well-organized household and a three-course menu are matters of very minor importance at the moment. Women who spend the postnatal period in the hospital go through exactly the same thing – often even more intensely. It's just that you, the man, only witness the tip of the iceberg; the tears continue to roll in the evening, under the blanket, while you're at home or out celebrating.

The woman's hormone system has never been more seriously shaken up. After childbirth, the one hormone level drops to rock bottom; the other one rises steeply and suddenly in conjunction with the lactation process. The hormonal (and thus the emotional) ups and downs are a regular roller-coaster ride. And this "emotional fun-fair" has to be endured after a cumbersome pregnancy and a strenuous birth.

In your role as the woman's partner, try to be tolerant even if you don't understand. Stay with her, lie down with her, hold her. And, by the way, a little pointer from a member of the female sex: women in the postnatal period are delighted by a little token of love. One father I encountered had a beautiful idea. In celebration of the birth of their daughter he gave his wife an opal pendant, saying: "Our little girl can wear this when she's big enough!"

Days Four and Five

The fourth and fifth days of the postnatal period are often ones of rest and recovery; the parents either let the dirty dishes be dirty dishes or get someone to help them. When I come for my house call in the morning, I'm glad to see the father leaving the postnatal bedroom with a mattress under his arm and disappearing into the bathroom for a shower. Other men just take pleasure in staying in bed, enjoy their child fast asleep on their tummy, and proudly announce to me: "You know, I finally got the baby to sleep and now I'm just going to stay in bed myself – after all, it was a loooooong night!" I often find the father explaining the nappy-changing procedures to the mother, after having been the sole nappy-changer during the first few days.

Days Six, Seven, etc.

Beginning on the sixth day, the man is glad that his partner feels up to sorting the laundry or reading a go-to-bed story to the older child. And it's no longer such a problem for the woman if it takes him a bit longer to do the shopping.

The End of the Early Postnatal Period

Towards the end of the early postnatal period the families try to reorganize the daily routine, but find that it is still difficult to stick to any kind of schedule with a newborn in the house – every day brings new surprises.

The Phase Following the Early Postnatal Period in the Hospital

If the woman has stayed in the hospital during the early postnatal period, fatherhood doesn't start in earnest until she and the baby come home. The father unfortunately often has to wait until then to have time to enjoy his child. A week after childbirth, he finally has the opportunity to see what the baby looks like naked and kiss its tender skin. He will find that he has a lot of quick catching up to do as regards nappy-changing techniques.

Often when I come for my first postnatal house call, I am greeted by the father holding the one-week-old child in his arms…

… "I sure am glad to see you! Yesterday before we left the hospital everything was fine. Now my wife is lying in bed and crying, the baby has been screaming since last night and refuses to go to sleep again, and also I'm afraid it's got diarrhoea –when I changed its nappies the faeces were extremely watery." This is when my work as a postpartum midwife begins: I take the screaming bundle off the father's hands and soothe it by letting it suck my finger. At the mother's bedside I learn that he should please just stay home now and not go looking for something in some shopping centre. To which he replies:

"Yes, but yesterday you said yourself that you were fine and I could run this errand." "Yes, but now …"
(mother starts crying again). The newborn no longer contents itself with my finger and suddenly starts
yelling again. When I ask cautiously whether the mother would like to nurse her child now, she wails:
"I don't have any milk, my breasts are completely soft, and anyway, it was drinking all night." At this
point I send the father to the kitchen to heat water for tea and a hot-water bottle. Of course it takes
him a while to find the latter. I take the opportunity to get a more complete report from the mother on
the nocturnal breastfeeding. We come to the conclusion that she has to put the baby to her breast one
more time, then the father and I will change its nappies and we'll put it to bed in its cradle with a hot-
water bottle. As she breastfeeds, I show her that there are still large stores of milk to be felt in her
breasts and point out to her that she should listen to how the baby swallows. During the subsequent
nappy-changing session, I explain to the father that this "diarrhoea" is entirely normal for a child be-
ing breastfed. The mother and father breathe a sigh of relief, give each other a hug and a kiss and
laugh: "Becoming a father is easy, it's being a parent that throws you for a loop!" At the end of my
house call the baby is naturally not lying in its cradle after all, but in mum's bed, since we talked about
the fact that letting it do that is not spoiling it. We arrange that I will come back the next day. The fa-
ther shows me to the door and confesses: "I should have taken the advice you gave us during the ante-
natal class more seriously: I thought that was all just girl talk. Being a father really is a learning pro-
cess. But I wouldn't have wanted to miss it for the world."

The fathers among my readers will naturally be thinking: "In our case it was completely different." Or you will resolve: "We will be very well prepared for the period
immediately following the birth; those things won't happen to us." You are no doubt
right – there are thousands of different courses the postnatal period can take, but
please remember:

> *First of all, things don't always happen*
> *Second of all, the way you expect, but*
> *Third of all, the way the baby thinks they should!*

It is my sincere hope that no man withdraw from participation in the postnatal process. It is a beautiful phase that you would miss out on. You can't make up for it when
the next child comes, because that will be a different child. Don't look for career-re-
lated excuses. If you were undergoing the postnatal process yourself, the company
would have to function without you, and your wife would surely take care of you just
as affectionately as you will now do for her. If possible, take leave from work for two
or three weeks. It will do the family good, as well as you yourself – after the first ten
days, you will likewise be in need of some rest and recovery. You'll see; you'll look
forward to going back to work. During my final house call, men often tell me: "I really
admire your husband for being a househusband; I couldn't handle that." Others ask
me how things work in our house with our exchange of roles. They realize it's not really so bad, taking care of the family. It's interesting how different people can be in this
respect as well.

There is one thing I find it important to urge you, the father, to consider: you have undoubtedly had a lot of new experiences in the past weeks, and sometimes you would have been grateful to hear about what is in store for a young father sooner. Maybe you would have liked to communicate with another man about your feelings. Now you yourself have a number of new experiences under your belt – please don't keep them to yourself, but go to a "pregnant fathers'" meeting. If it hadn't been for countless woman-to-woman talks, this book would never have been written. So why not have talks from man to man? As a midwife I am aware of an information deficit, but as a woman I can't speak men's language or tell about life in the father's world.

THE NEWBORN

From the Womb to the World

The newborn child comes out of a protected environment in which it enjoyed a constant cosy body temperature. It was gently bedded in water for months, though it could hardly move any longer during the final weeks.

On its way through the bony but well-cushioned birth canal to the outside world, the baby is now pushed, now pressed, now tries to wind its way around a curve on its own. Squeezing through a pliant, but very tight slit, it finally succeeds in seeing the bright light of day.

The newborn is greeted by loud voices, touched by hands gloved in rubber, wrapped in hard cloth, and the first breath of air it takes is so cold it cries with pain. As if that were not enough, the amniotic fluid is vacuumed out of its mouth, perhaps even its stomach, with a plastic tube. Under certain circumstances a cold, hard stethoscope is put to its heart and a strange black something constantly blows oxygen into its nose and mouth, although it would much rather breathe on its own. It tries to prevent the cutting of the umbilical cord which has been its lifeline, but it's too late.

What kind of impression will the child have of our world if this is its "welcoming ceremony", as is unfortunately still par for the course in many hospitals?

How wonderful that so many parents and midwives are aware of these torments and try to make the baby's transition into this world as gentle and smooth as possible. They bid it welcome with a subdued reddish glow of light and a pleasantly warm room, and wrap it in soft, warm towels. After the first draughts of breath, the mother's heartbeat and the tender whispers of the persons present are the only sounds the baby hears.

The Exertion of Birth

Many still unborn children are already so stressed shortly before reaching their destination that they simply give up in the last curve of the birth canal. They are then yanked into the light of the world with the aid of a vacuum extractor, forceps or a caesarean section. Many newborns are so indignant about these procedures that they scream out loud, to the joy of all who have witnessed the birth hoping and praying, their sleeves rolled up. Other babies are in such a state of shock about being born that the oxygen mask is the only means of bridging the gap until they manage sufficient respiration on their own. Many human beings are robust and have a will to live from the moment of birth onward – just a few minutes later, these very children stiffen in loud yells of protest about the treatment they are being subjected to – to the joy and relief of everyone present. The baby is screaming!

Particularly children who have been delivered with the help of a suction cup (also called a ventouse delivery) cause their parents concern about their appearance. They usually have a so-called caput on their heads, so-called because it is slightly reminiscent of a purple bishop's cap. This perfectly round blue mark measuring some six centimetres in diameter has been caused by the vacuum pressure of 5 atmosphere gauge applied by the extractor. It looks quite horrible on children with bald heads, but let me assure you that it will disappear very rapidly. Already the next day, people who don't know it's there won't notice it. For the baby, the ventouse is surely very disagreeable and its head is presumably aching from the procedure. For this reason, it is important to be extremely careful with the baby's head during the first few days. I highly recommend giving these children a homoeopathic dose of *Arnica C 30* in the pouch of the cheek. In out-patient cases I have applied Arnica compresses to the baby's head to achieve the rapid regression of the haematoma. Incidentally, in the course of the next several months, you will notice that the baby frequently presses itself head-first into a corner of its cot and tries to push itself "through". Presumably it is attempting to reproduce the birth situation. Please don't try to prevent this; it may be the baby's way of processing the experience emotionally. The same behaviour can naturally also be observed in children whose deliveries proceeded normally.

Parents whose children were born by means of a vacuum extractor/ventouse, forceps or caesarean frequently report that those children have restless sleeping phases for a long time afterward. It may well be that they try to relive their births in their sleep. In these nocturnal situations it often helps to take the child into your arms in a tight embrace, in other words to give it the confinement it has perhaps just been dreaming about, and then to release it gradually and gently into the expanse of the bed (the world of being born).

The First Cry

Amazingly enough, parents always wait for the classic sign of life – the first cry – and are initially very disconcerted if all their baby does after birth is take a quick look around and then go back to sleep. There really are children who virtually sleep through their own births. But if it has been determined that the umbilical cord is pulsating, and the lungs and heart are functioning properly, and if the baby's skin takes on a rosy hue, everyone present will be convinced that it's really just sleeping.

The First Minutes of Life

Appearance/Pulsation of the Umbilical Cord/Breathing

In the first few minutes of life, the baby doesn't look rosy at all, but rather a shade somewhere between pale white and greyish blue. It is only when respiration sets in that the child will take on its baby-typical delicate pink complexion starting on the torso, then spreading to the head, and later to the arms and legs.

It is interesting to observe that the development of the rosy hue goes hand in hand with the decreasing pulsation of the umbilical cord. By the time this pulsation stops entirely, nearly all children begin screaming loudly. Perhaps there is a much closer connection between the umbilical cord functions and spontaneous respiration than has hitherto been assumed by the science of obstetrics. Again and again, I have witnessed that there is no cause for concern as long as the umbilical cord is still pulsating. Nevertheless, the first few minutes of life are accompanied by fears, hopes and prayers as to the child's well-being – as to whether or not it is breathing.

If the first breaths the baby takes are in any way worrying, very effective help is provided by Dr. Bach's *Rescue Remedy* and/or the homoeopathic medication *Aconitum C 30*. Ideally, the Bach Flower drops are administered directly to the baby's fontanel ("soft spot") or dissolved in water. Naturally, I never would have wanted to be without my oxygen mask and tank, but usually the latter remained packed up in its case.

An old home-birth midwife allayed my fears when I was just starting out accompanying home births, saying: "Don't be so scared; in the old days we midwives had no doctors, no medicine, no oxygen, and the nearest hospital couldn't be reached in the wintertime. Often my only means of transportation to the woman in labour were skis and a knapsack. But no baby ever died on me; I brought every single one of them through, even if your young doctors don't believe it. As long as the umbilical cord is still active, there's no reason to be disconcerted. But if the cord isn't doing anything anymore, get the baby to cry by whatever means you can. As soon as the umbilical cord turns pale and limp, you've got no more time to lose. We used cold water and our hands; you young women have oxygen with you. No matter how you do it, get the child to start breathing!" I always listened very carefully to what this old and very experienced midwife told me, and to this day I am grateful for the advice and encouragement I received from her. It's a shame that older colleagues don't pass on more of their experience because they think the present generation is much better trained than they were. In reality, however, midwives had a great wealth of knowledge and experience at their disposal, even though there weren't any books like those by Frederick Leboyer, Sheila Kitzinger and Ina May Gaskin. The midwives of the present have the benefit of the most recent scientific findings, but the extremely valuable wisdom of the past has been lost and we must painstakingly try to reconstruct it. One such bit of time-tested wisdom was the warm bath. This is a method whose value and effectiveness I can only confirm. When the newborn has difficulties adapting, it quickly recovers in warm water, into which it is laid immediately after birth.

The adjustment phase is accordingly uncomplicated for children delivered under water, because they are in the element water to begin with. The baby is lying in its mother's arms, but she can immediately slip it back into the water part way if need be. If the baby is above the surface of the water, it is likewise covered with warm towels.

Cyanosis Due to Congestion

Many babies are born with a dark blue head, referred to as cyanosis due to congestion. With great effort, the baby has fought its way through the birth canal with its large head, and it takes another contraction before the broad shoulders are born. In the intervening time, the head is subjected to enormous pressure, and the reflux of the blood is partially prevented – the blood accumulates in the head. This causes the blue colouration, which gives the parents a shock while for the midwife it represents no particular cause for concern. We attempt to console the parents by telling them that this bluish hue will disappear again very quickly. At the beginning it does look quite strange – a rosy baby with a blue head. The big brother of an infant girl born with a congested head remarked flatly: "I don't want a baby with such a dark face."

The cheeks already take on a rosy colour within the first hour of life and by the next day, the head looks like that of any other newborn. Upon closer examination, tiny blue spots can be detected, like little granules. The latter are no longer discernible after forty-eight hours. Newborns with this type of cyanosis should by all means be given a dose of *Arnica C 30*. This is very likely to speed up the disappearance of the blue colouration.

The Gaze of the Newborn

It is extremely interesting to observe what the baby does with its eyes during the first few instants of life. Often they already look at the world around them with wide-open eyes during the very first minute. It is as if the baby has just reached the end of a long journey and is bursting with all the adventures it had along the way. The facial expression, the gestures and the eyes often don't seem to be responding to a new and strange world at all, but rather to be informed by knowledge of what life is. The midwife is often the first person who has the good fortune to see this gaze when the newborn is still lying in her lap while the parents catch their breath, give each other a kiss and then seek initial contact with their child. I always have the feeling it's as though this little person has already experienced – and would like to tell me – all kinds of things. In this very moment, the eyes of the mother and father are within the baby's field of vision. They look into each other's eyes, and a deep feeling of love is born. The innocent, carefree, radiant gaze so typical of small children is not yet to be seen in the first few minutes of life; it only develops in the course of the coming weeks.

Gripping, Holding, Sucking

Another phenomenon to be observed during the first few minutes of life is the baby's ability to grip, hold and suck. With great determination, a large majority of babies quickly find their finger or fist and suck on it with a fervour that will rarely be witnessed again in the days that follow. The newborn grips its father's finger as though it would never let go again, seeking some kind of anchor in this strange world. As soon as the mother takes the baby into her arms, it usually starts looking for her breast immediately. The snapping movements it makes with its mouth fill the mother's heart with maternal love. Women still remember this years later. Only very few children make an exception to the rule and initially prefer their own fingers to the mother's nipple.

Bodily Waste

In the midst of the childbirth atmosphere, it is always quite comical when the newborn "wee-wees" onto the hands of the midwife or its mother in the first minutes of life. Often a child reacts to its start in life by eliminating a whole load of meconium – dark green faecal material that accumulates in its intestines while it is still in the womb. This is a true rite of initiation into parenthood. Already in the first few minutes, the baby signals to its father and mother that it is not there just to be cuddled with but also to be fed, cleaned and taken care of.

The Hour That Follows

For the newborn, the phase of transition from the birth to the postnatal period it will share with its mother is associated with a number of further discomforts and inconveniences. Many babies are born so clean that we decide not to bathe them. If a bath is necessary or part of the hospital routine, the father can take over this job with a bit of professional guidance. Most children enjoy the bath. I would like to encourage you – the father – to venture this task; after all, it's your baby! Many men proudly recount this first bath for a long time afterwards. At home, we often add one or two drops of the costly *Rose Oil 10% in Jojoba Wax*. Bathing a rosy baby in the fragrance of roses is a wonderful way of concluding the birth. In age-old fairy tales and tales of childbirth you read: "And she bathed the child in rose leaves." Then the unpleasant side of life begins for the baby: despite the warmth offered by a heat lamp or the like, being dried off, having its navel attended to, being measured, weighed and dressed is only halfway bearable for the baby if it can suck on Dad's finger in the process. Otherwise loud protests are almost always to be heard.

Usually the midwife or doctor will take this opportunity to carry out the baby's first check-up. After the baby's weight, length and head circumference have been determined, its heart and lungs will be listened to, its inner organs palpated and its genitals examined. Its reflexes and joints will be tested. And then the parents will already have to make the first decisions concerning their child: they are faced with the question as to whether the baby should be given the eye prophylaxis and vitamin K. Of course, it is helpful if the parents have informed themselves on these subjects during the pregnancy and cleared up these questions with the obstetrics team before the birth, so they are not suddenly caught by surprise with having to make a decision – and above all so they can protect themselves from being abruptly yanked out of the wonderful postnatal mood.

The eye prophylaxis has no longer been carried out routinely for many years. It used to be conducted in order to prevent the child from becoming blind as a consequence of an undetected gonorrhoea infection in the mother. The silver nitrate employed for that purpose is no longer common. But due to the frequency of chlamydia infections in the mother's vaginal area, many hospitals recommend a preventive antibiotic treatment of children's eyes. If there are no pathogens to be found in the mother, however, it is not necessary to subject the child's eyes to this antibiotic therapy.

In Germany, vitamin K is administered to the child three times during the first four weeks of life in the form of drops to prevent bleeding especially in the brain. Vitamin K has never been observed to have a negative effect. On the other hand, however, it has not proven possible to rule out life-threatening cerebral haemorrhaging among infants entirely by means of this preventive measure. It is important for you to know that only four in every hundred thousand children suffer from such haemorrhaging. Vitamin K was formerly recommended only after traumatic births; today it is administered to almost every child. The parents are free to make their own decision for or against this or any other prophylactic measures. Children who are breastfed provably have less vitamin K; bottle-fed children receive it as an additive in the formula.

In connection with the administration of vitamin K, it should also be remembered that the so-called colostrum or foremilk secreted before the production of true milk has a very high vitamin K content. It should really be our duty to see to it that every newborn child gets these invaluable first drops of breast milk, because only a very short time later, nature no longer deems increased vitamin K content necessary.

Vitamin K is stored in the liver and administering an extra dose of it therefore may put a strain on the immature infant liver. An overdose is even suspected by some of being carcinogenic. The extent to which this therapy can bring about an increased chance of contracting neonatal jaundice is not yet known; as a matter of fact, no long-term studies whatsoever have yet been carried out on this still relatively new form of prophylaxis. If the child is premature, traumatized or has already been treated with antibiotics, it is sensible to decide in favour of vitamin K prophylaxis. If this preventive measure is not carried out, premature and traumatized babies should by all means be given *Armica C 30* or *C 200*.

Once the first check-up has been conducted and the baby is nestled in its mother's arms, warmly bundled up, it will usually fall into a deep and restful sleep. In the case of an early discharge it will be bedded in a pre-warmed baby car seat or the like and is allowed to go home with its new parents. If the newborn remains in the hospital, it will either be moved into a room it can share with its mother, or into the babies' room. About two or three hours after the birth, the mother and child will either be transferred to the maternity ward, discharged or, in the case of a home birth, the midwife will take her leave, giving the new parents final instructions for coping until she comes for her first postnatal house call.

The First Hours, Days and Weeks of Life

In the following sections I will attempt to describe the initial phase in the life of a child. As in the previous sections on the postnatal period, I will limit myself to the depiction of the "normal" course of events. Naturally, every child will display its own individual way of living, even in the very first stage.

Everyone who has contact with and cares for the newborn during the first hours, days and weeks should be aware of what the child experienced before and immediately after its birth. In my opinion, during the first few weeks, it is our obligation to allow the baby a start in life that is as gentle, careful and pleasant as possible. The best place for this is the mother's bed. The baby is a newborn for eight weeks, approximately the length of time it takes for the mother's hormone system to readjust. This new little person will be able to adapt to this hard world best if we continue to offer it a lot of warmth, safety, closeness and a cosy nest. Noise and disturbing sounds should reach its ears as muted as possible – the way it perceived them while it was still in the womb. It should likewise initially be protected from strong light. The newborn should be able to decide for itself when it wants to be fed; after all, in the womb no one prevented it from sucking its thumb or drinking amniotic fluid whenever it wanted to. The same applies to its sleeping phases. I don't know of any mother who ever woke her child during pregnancy. On the contrary, she was happy when peace and quiet reigned in the womb for a while. We can't give the baby this watery environment back again; after all, it's a human being. As we know, the amount of amniotic fluid decreases towards the end of pregnancy – in other words, nature wants the baby to take leave of this element. But with carefully chosen clothing it will adapt more quickly to cloth and air. The same is true of skin care: natural products, free of irritants and synthetic aromas, are absorbed best by the baby's skin.

The Postnatal Period at Home

Here, once again, my aim is to describe the course of the postnatal period in the home, because all women who have given birth at home or been discharged from the hospital or independent birth centre soon after childbirth will spend the postnatal period within their own four walls. It is entirely natural for a healthy newborn to get accustomed to life on earth in the intimate circle of the family.

The Maternity Ward

Naturally, I would also like to incorporate brief remarks of relevance for the many women who remain in the hospital for a while with their babies. This is not an easy task for me, however, because on the one hand I am an independent midwife, and on the other hand, in every maternity or obstetrics ward there are certain structures and habits specific to that particular ward, so it is impossible to make generally applicable statements. This said, I believe that every mother will find advice, help and explanations on her baby's well-being in this book. I would like to remind and encourage all mothers who spend the first few days in the hospital to defend their baby's needs and interests; for that it's never too early to start. Don't just leave the baby's care to the hospital staff, but specify your wishes clearly.

In most hospitals, nursery nurses are responsible for the newborns. In smaller maternity wards and in a few larger hospitals, there are self-employed midwives who maintain an affiliation with the respective hospital. In this set-up, the midwife pays daily postnatal visits during which she gives the mother advice, examines her as well as the baby and teaches her to bathe and breastfeed her child.

Midwives and nurses have no way of knowing what relationship you have already developed with your child. There are still women who would rather go and smoke a cigarette while the hospital staff takes care of their babies. How is a nurse supposed to tell whether you're the type of mother who wants to sleep at night and complain if they are awakened for breastfeeding? Not every mother is convinced of the benefits of rooming-in; you have to speak up if you want to have your baby with you in your room as soon as possible or would like to be put into a mother-child unit. There are nice, pleasant maternity wards in which every effort is made not to disturb the "mother-child unit". And this book also provides you with a means of gathering information in advance. Now it is up to you to see to it that you have a restful, pleasant postnatal period which you can enjoy.

Take responsibility for yourself and your child from the first day on. Remember that, beginning on the day you are discharged, at the latest, you will have to cope with the care of the baby, and all problems that arise in that context, on your own. Ask the nurses for advice and don't allow yourself to be disconcerted by a roommate who is already more confident in handling her baby: she may be no more than a few days ahead of you. Don't complain after going home, but communicate with the personnel while you're still there; many a misunderstanding is easily cleared up. Don't blame the staff for the way the rooms and the hospital routine are set up, but do what you can to support the nurses in their efforts to improve their working conditions; communicate whatever shortcomings you experience to the hospital administration in brief, precise messages.

The First Sleep

After suckling for the first time, being given its first bath and wrapped up in its first nappies, the baby understandably falls into its first sleep. In view of the strenuous birth and the activities that follow, this sleep often lasts several hours. It is amazing how Mother Nature sees to it that the mother and child can rest and recuperate. The mother is exhausted, the Dad usually tired, but as a rule, neither one of them falls into a deep sleep. Rather, they doze, lying arm in arm with their baby between them, always keeping one ear on the newborn's breathing. I once heard a paediatrician say: "Parents are the best intensive-care nurses! Nobody observes and senses the newborn's condition – without a single monitoring device – better than brand new parents." He didn't see any problem in letting the child go home with its parents a few hours after birth. This approval was balm for my midwife's soul, because I had finally found confirmation for something I had been observing for years. Unfortunately, doctors often hold precisely the opposite view, namely that the maternity ward is the best conceivable place for a newborn because the baby nurses are well trained to keep an eye on the child. The fact that the nurse has umpteen other children to tend to, is often alone on the night shift and responsible for twenty babies, is all too often forgotten. In my opinion, "experts" should leave it to the parents to decide whether they would like to have their babies in bed with them or in the babies' room. Just as different doctors and midwives have different views, parents have different needs. In many places, the advocates of bed sharing for mother, father and child still represent a small minority, but that's no reason to treat these parents – and their midwives – as outsiders. I have never once experienced parents who weren't capable of taking care of their newborns the first night, by themselves, at home, or seen a child who was inadequately attended to.

Day One

Many of the following pointers are relevant for the first several weeks and you can refer to them frequently in the course of that time. Don't allow yourself to be confused by the headings pertaining to such-and-such a day, because for many parents the "first day" is the day of or after being discharged from the hospital, which could be the sixth day of the baby's life if the early postnatal period has been spent in the hospital or, in the case of a premature birth, the twenty-eighth day or more.

Need for Warmth

In the first twenty-four hours following birth, the baby is content if it is warmly clothed and lying in its cradle or parents' bed with a hot-water bottle. Constant warmth is probably the most important factor for maintaining all of the bodily functions optimally. During the first few weeks of life, infants are not capable of regulating their body temperature on their own. They become cold very quickly, even entering the hypothermic zone. If they are too warmly bundled up, however, precisely the opposite is the case: their body temperature rises; the baby is hot and develops a fever. Regardless of which extreme occurs, the babies usually just peacefully abandon themselves to their fate. This is why the first thing the midwife does when she comes for a house call is to look at the colour of the sleeping baby's skin. If its cheeks and hands are rosy, she knows immediately that it is faring well. Its hands are allowed to be slightly paler than its face. If its head is glowing red, on the other hand, its temperature must be taken. In this case the midwife will undress the baby, take a look at its clothing – with the parents, of course, so that they take an active part in figuring out how much warmth the baby needs and how they can determine its temperature themselves without constantly having to reach for the thermometer. During all my years of making house calls – of which the first takes place a few hours after a home birth or discharge from the hospital – I rarely encountered a baby in a condition of hypo- or hyperthermia. In principle, newborns who have been carried to term will exhibit less of a tendency to become cold than those born prematurely. The rule of thumb here is that the baby's temperature balance will stabilize as it gains weight. In general, therefore, the more mature, heavier and older a newborn is, the more stable its body temperature.

During her first look at the child, the midwife also slips her hand under the blanket – carefully, so as not to disturb its sleep – to check the temperature of its tummy and feet. The parents should follow suit so that they learn to judge whether the temperature in the cot is normal body temperature (37 °C/98.6 °F) or not. If the child is lying in the mother's bed, there is no reason to worry that it is being exposed to the wrong temperature either way, because women in the postnatal period are very sensitive to body temperature and recognize on their own if they're too warm or cold. Human beings are the best hot-water bottles, by the way, a rule of thumb of which babies are presumably already aware, because they love to sleep in their parents' bed from the first day on. Then suddenly there's no whimpering and whining; almost all babies slumber quite peacefully there, listening to the familiar heartbeat and dreaming of the "old days" in the womb. Suitable places for checking the body temperature are the baby's forehead and neck. If the skin there feels as warm as your hand, then your baby is properly dressed and covered. If its forehead, neck, feet or tummy is colder, the newborn needs additional warmth. During the first year, don't allow yourself to be disconcerted by cold hands, because a baby's hands are cool almost throughout that first year of its life. On the contrary, warm hands, especially if accompanied (as mentioned above) by a flushed head are reason enough to remove a layer of clothing. Feeling the baby's tummy with your hand is a good, quick way of determining whether it is too warm.

Feeding

During the first twenty-four hours, the newborn often only wants to be breastfed two or three times – in between those times it is content to suck on its own finger or that of its mother. Naturally, there are babies who want to suckle at their mother's breast more often. The parents can decide for themselves whether they would like to give the baby a few sips of tea to satisfy its sucking instinct. If the newborn shows massive signs of being postterm, the midwife will encourage the parents to offer it tea, plentifully and frequently. On the other hand, I have often observed that mothers of postterm children already have plenty of colostrum and the child therefore receives sufficient fluid. Mother Nature knows what she has to offer a human being right after birth. In general, parents are increasingly being advised not to give their newborns tea during the first twenty-four hours after birth because the mother produces enough colostrum. Very many babies spit up the mixture of tea and breast milk – a phenomenon considered entirely normal by professionals in our field. For many parents, however, a gagging, spitting newborn is a bit more than they can handle. It undoubtedly costs the child quite a bit of energy and thus also represents a burden for the child. Is it really necessary to get the parents all worried just because we're afraid of the lab test results? I am quite certain that midwives used to know why the child didn't take in any fluid during the first twenty-four hours. This is another instance where we are called upon to regain our faith in the natural course of events. A newborn won't starve to death during the first few hours of life, but being awakened and having its nappies changed constantly might cause it quite some stress.

Contrary to widespread opinion among doctors and midwives, there really are lots of newborns who get through the first twenty-four hours without tea and without being breastfed particularly often. And they get through these hours without the slightest damage to their health or too great a loss of fluid, which would be evident in their excretions, their skin and/or their body temperature. I simply refuse to put all newborns in the same category or follow any general rule to the effect that "the child must have fluid", as is unfortunately still par for the course in many maternity wards. As a matter of fact, the baby's kidneys are not capable of metabolizing large amounts of fluid yet. Its organs are still in the process of getting used to life "outside". Once again, an individual decision should be made, based on the baby's vital functions, skin, excretions and sucking behaviour. In the hospital, this task will be performed by a midwife or baby nurse. We midwives are trained to oversee these matters!

Changing and Dressing a Newborn

The newborn is usually changed only twice during the first twenty-four hours. The first time is when the midwife makes her first house call after the birth. The parents are glad to have this chance to refresh their memories. Naturally, they can change their baby themselves if they would like to. As regards the amount the baby excretes, two nappy changes are entirely adequate. Putting it through the process more often would only cause the child unnecessary loss of warmth and expenditure of energy. For the baby's skin, more frequent nappy-changing presumably represents nothing more than additional exposure to laundry detergent residue.

What I most like to recommend, at least during the first few days, is dressing the baby in a soft cloth known as a swaddling blanket. This means that the baby does not wear a romper/baby suit at all, but is wrapped in a large, white, fluffy cotton cloth or in a warm nappy sack of the kind currently offered by manufacturers of natural textiles. Some mothers may be acquainted with this method from the antenatal or infant care class. It ensures that the baby's feet are warm while at the same time allowing it to feel the familiar nakedness, at least on its feet. Parents are readily convinced that a "bundle" of this kind is warmer than a bodysuit. It's like the difference between a mitten and a glove – the former warms the fingers much more effectively than the latter. Playsuits/rompers are cute to look at, but cold for the feet. Naturally, it is for the parents to decide whether to wrap the baby in the swaddling blanket only during the first few days or for several weeks. If they decide against using it altogether, they should put woollen booties on the baby's feet over the playsuit feet – as used to be common practice – or, better still, the booties <u>under</u> the romper, so they don't keep falling off.

There are also families where the baby lies in bed in a bodysuit and without a cap. The decision as to the care, clothing, nutrition and general handling of the child is always for the parents to make. As a midwife, all I can do is stand by you in an advisory capacity. As long as the baby thrives and is clearly not suffering from want of anything important, we midwives will accept the measures taken by the parents. The same applies to the nappy-changing method.

I will always recommend something in the category of cloth nappies and cotton nappy panties because, no matter how you look at it – from the perspective of the environment, cost, practicality or whatever else – cloth will always be the better choice. And in any case, it is more pleasant for the baby than plastic, even if the advertisements would have us believe how incredibly absorbent, breathable, etc. disposable nappies are. I don't know a single adult who would be willing to exchange his or her silk or cotton panties for a pair of plastic ones. Adults who are forced to wear disposable incontinence pants would be only too glad to get rid of their "sweat packages".

Protecting the Baby's Head

After the baby has been changed, the cap it has been wearing since birth will naturally be returned to its head to protect its sensitive ears from loud voices and noises. Even more importantly, the cap helps avoid any loss of warmth, which is otherwise considerable, because both the baby's head and the fontanel are still quite large in relation to the rest of its body. Since the head is not sealed by a bone, for an infant it's what going around in winter with a naked, uncovered tummy would be for an adult. This is precisely the part of the body most of us instinctively attempt to protect from getting a chill, because the latter can lead to very disagreeable and/or serious problems. That is how a baby feels during the first few weeks with its uncovered fontanel: it is subjected to all fluctuations in temperature and feels vulnerable. It's up to the parents to decide how long they want to put a cap on their baby's head, but the "newborn phase" lasts eight weeks, and the cap is highly advisable for at least that length of time. In the summertime, it is sensible to use a silk or very thin cotton cap with a visor in order to keep the head from getting too warm. Actually, all parents understand why infants and toddlers almost always require a head covering out of doors. In places protected from the wind and the sun, the cap can be taken off on hot days. One important thing is to protect the ears, especially from cold drafts or wind. If the ears take a chill very early in life, they often remain vulnerable to infection the person's whole life long. Unfortunately, more and more people are of the opinion that a cap represents a danger of the baby's becoming overheated. I can only contradict this view with vehemence. The arguments cited above all speak in favour of using a cap; next, the material chosen for the cap must be considered. The fact that silk or thin cotton is the best choice during the summer months, and that, under certain circumstances, the baby can go "capless" on hot days, has already been discussed above. It is an individual decision, based on a number of factors, whether or not the baby wears a cap and, if it does, what kind, depending on the outdoor temperature and the child's age – is it just a few days old or already a few months? Moreover, it is important to realize that some children have a stronger need for warmth and protection than others.

Skin Care

On the first day, the care of the baby's skin in the nappy zone will consist solely of washing off the sticky meconium with warm water, and if necessary, a bit of soap. Afterwards, a first-cold-pressed fatty plant oil is rubbed into the baby's skin with slightly dampened hands (a bowl of water at a temperature of approximately 43 °C/ 109 °F has been placed on the changing table beforehand). For this purpose you can use the *Original D® Aroma Blend Babyöl empfindliche Haut/Baby Oil Sensitive Skin D®*, which has a delicate rosy scent. The application of the oil must be carried out with extreme care, because the surface of the skin is tense and sensitive due to contact to air and clothing as well as the loss of warmth. The parents must try to imagine that the baby feels the way we adults feel in our skin after the first sunbath of the season, which is often too long. When the oiling process begins, most babies scream, but when the amount of moisture on the skin increases, they calm down, relax and enjoy the treatment. Extreme care must likewise be taken when using water in conjunction with the oil, because as soon as the water is too cold, the child's body temperature can sink rapidly due to the relatively large amount of liquid. This massage should accordingly be carried out in a well-heated room or, better still, beneath a heat lamp/quartz radiator.

Particularly postterm infants benefit from the water-oil massage – due to the loss of fluid they have suffered, their skin tends to dry out rapidly and become cracked. When a baby is carried past term, its skin loses the protective layer of vernix caseosa, becomes sensitive and wrinkles easily. As a matter of fact, in cases of children born much later than the due date, it can even be observed that bits of skin flake off of the hands and feet. Skin care is therefore an especially important issue if the baby is postterm. I have observed again and again that children who are restless but refuse to drink will quickly fall asleep – and sleep for quite a while – after this moist skin treatment. There is no doubt in my mind that these children simply no longer feel at ease in their skin and that's why they are so restless.

For me, the water-oil massage represents an optimal means of supplying the newborn's metabolism with fluid and at the same time countering the threat of infant jaundice.

Birthmarks

When the baby is lying on the changing table pleasurably kicking away under the quartz radiator for the first time or nestled on pre-warmed towels next to its mother in bed, the parents often have their first opportunity to see it naked. Sometimes they discover that it has a so-called Stork Bite, Angel's Kiss or Port-Wine Stain; the Latin term is naevus flammeus. With a colour anywhere from light to dark red, this mark appears on the forehead, the root of the nose or the neck – always somewhere on the central axis of the baby's body. It is caused by a widening of the vessels beneath the surface of the skin which disappears entirely of its own accord in the course of the first few years of life. It often shows itself again distinctly when the toddler has its first temper tantrums.

Now and then, a "Mongolian Blue Spot" can be found on an infant's back or in the area of the sacrum, with a diameter of as much as several centimetres. This "bruise" is a harmless accumulation of pigment, which will gradually disappear.

During the first weeks of life, a capillary haemangioma ("Strawberry Mark") can develop. This dark red, eminent, benign mark can appear anywhere on the body. It usually grows with the child for a few years and then disappears as suddenly as it appeared by the time school age is reached. It rarely has to be treated by a paediatrician. You, the parents, usually suffer more from it than the child does, and worry more about it than the health professionals do, because a Strawberry Mark is considered a blemish. I have attended to several children with this birthmark but have never once known it to become a problem.

Day Two

Need for Warmth, Fresh Air

On the second day, the newborn still requires a constant body temperature and, at best, surroundings likewise of a constant temperature. If it is bundled up well, snuggled up close to its mother's body or the sides of its cot/bassinette are lined with cloth, the baby can stand an airing of the postnatal bedroom. Fresh air is important for the mother and the child alike. The most important thing is, no matter what the season: avoid a draft and dress your baby according to the observation criteria described above.

When you change the nappies, it should in any case be nice and warm for the baby, at least 22 °C/72 °F, or preferably even warmer – you'll now be very glad you went to the trouble to install that quartz radiator. Particularly if you don't have a quartz radiator, however, it is advisable to warm the clothing you intend to dress the baby in. That will help you to protect the baby from taking a chill during the changing procedure.

Within the first twenty-four hours, however, the midwife will have to harass the baby a bit more, since it is common to take a blood sample to check the function of the thyroid and the metabolism by means of the so-called Guthrie test. We try to wait for a point in time during our house call when the baby is awake, has warm feet and is due to be breastfed anyway. Right before the child is put to the breast, the sample is taken by piercing its warm heel while the mother holds it in her lap in a vertical position. The mother can then console her baby and let it suckle at her breast, and it is spared a long crying bout. This blood sample is voluntary – very widespread, but not an absolute must. The midwife will explain its purpose to the parents and the latter will then decide for themselves whether they consider this examination necessary.

Feeding

The second day often begins with restlessness on the part of the newborn at the time of day when the contractions began in earnest, or when the birth took place. The baby will not perhaps make stronger use of its voice and usually craves more nourishment. After five minutes of hard suckling, however, it will fall asleep again, exhausted and satiated from the colostrum with its high protein and carbohydrate content. Incidentally, the breast milk will never again contain such a high percentage of protein as it does in the first few days of the baby's life. You can be sure that your child will have plenty of nourishment from this milk.

Tea as a Supplement?

If your child would like to drink pre-boiled water or warm *fennel or corn silk tea*, you can naturally give it some. Always make sure the tea is at body temperature – you can check this best by dripping a few drops on the inside of your wrist. The tea should only drip (not run) out of the rubber nipple and be light yellow in colour. When making the tea, make sure that it doesn't get too strong. A scanty quarter teaspoon of freshly crushed fennel seeds or half a teaspoon of corn silk to 100 ml/3.5 fl. oz. of boiling water is entirely adequate. There are babies who will take every kind of fluid, and others who won't drink a drop. In any case, the midwife will advise you as to whether your child really needs additional fluid or whether it will suffice to breastfeed it and satisfy its sucking instinct by another means.

I would now like to enlighten you a bit about fennel tea: a few years ago, the German Federal Institute for Consumer Health Protection and Veterinary Medicine (today called the Bundesinstitut für Risikobewertung – Federal Institute for Risk Assessment) issued a warning which caused great concern among consumers by advising against the regular consumption of fennel tea. I hope you also heard the rectifications which have been voiced by various experts in the meantime! The institute based its findings on experiments in the framework of which the estragole and methyleugenol contained in fennel oil had a damaging effect on mice and rats. These substances, however, had been observed in an isolated state, and not in the fennel oil in its entirety. Moreover, the results of such experiments cannot simply be applied to human beings. And it must also be taken into consideration that after the fennel has been made into tea, the amount of these substances still present in it is negligible. Fennel seed has been in use as a successful remedy for so many generations that it can truly be as regarded harmless, even for children. Even the above-mentioned institute confirmed that no specific risk for human health had yet been proven, a point the sensation-hungry media generally ignored.

Satisfying the Sucking Urge

Again and again, I witness that the sucking instinct has nothing to do with hunger, but is a habit left over from the time when the baby was in the womb. Maybe you can help it to find its thumb again, or offer it your finger or give it a dummy/pacifier. The dummy is a topic often already discussed in many families on the second day of the baby's life. I advise the mother to find a substitute of some kind rather than putting her newborn to her breast too frequently. The reason is that the skin of the nipples can quickly become irritated and sore. Moreover, the let-down reflex is stimulated to such an extent that the initial engorgement is very strong and will cause a lot of unnecessary discomfort. With her experience, the midwife will be able to determine whether the baby merely has a particularly strong sucking urge or really needs fluid, and will advise you accordingly. To this end she will check its sucking behaviour, the skin turgor (tension of the skin surface), the passing of urine and stool and the fullness of the epigastric region (upper abdomen). If it really is a baby with a particularly strong urge to suck – as is quite often the case –, then its father and mother should decide for themselves whether a dummy, thumb or silk doll (tied-cloth "pacifier") is the most suitable thing.

If you offer the newborn a dummy, make sure you get the proper size and also exercise patience. Understandably, most babies refuse it at first, because of the taste of rubber or silicon. The first time you try it out on your baby, it gags and spits it out, but only a few minutes later, when you make your second cautious attempt, it grabs hold of the dummy eagerly with its lips and suckles on it with obvious enjoyment. Thus even before their child is a week old, parents already learn that it only accepts their suggestions on the second try. In this context I would like to warn parents not to get into the widespread – and bad – habit of first putting the dummy into their own mouths to "clean" it before giving it to the newborn! Actually, this method doesn't clean the dummy at all, but, on the contrary, turns it into a conveyor for all kinds of germs, and significantly increases the risk of a fungal spore infection. And since newborns don't have any natural immunity during the first months of life, they are helplessly exposed to a fungal infection (oral candidiasis/"thrush"). In the early phase, please conscientiously sterilize the dummy in boiling water or clean it with salt or vinegar (rinsing it off with water afterwards) and keep it in a clean, airy place. The significantly older children in the family should likewise learn from the beginning that this is the baby's dummy and they should not put it into their own mouths.

A *silk doll* is another popular form of hygienic substitute for the mother's breast. It consists of a small square of silk dyed with natural textile dyes, in the middle of which a little "head", filled with wool, has been tied. Each of the four corners of the square is knotted. Silk is particularly suitable because it is extremely pliant (remember the silky surface of the placenta), easy to wash and quick to dry. What is more, on account of its natural protein fibres it wards off bacteria – unlike other materials against whose use doctors and other health professionals justifiably warn parents. I recommend having two such dolls at your disposal from the very beginning, in case you accidentally leave one somewhere, for example, and can't retrieve it for several days.

If the child is a *thumb-sucker*, it may be difficult to adapt it to a silk doll, but it is certainly worth a try. Incidentally, many newborns lose their inborn ability to suck their thumbs after just a few days of life. They won't have recourse to this comforting technique until after several weeks or months, when they find themselves in a situation in which there is nothing else to suck on. Dentists claim that thumb-sucking is much more damaging to the gums, and leads to worse malalignment of the teeth than dummies. At the age of four, it is presumably much more difficult to get a child to kick the habit of sucking its thumb than to get it off the dummy. Thumb-sucking has the supposed advantage that the baby can calm itself down at night and the parents don't have to look for the dummy and get the baby quiet again. But this should not be a prime factor in your process of deciding whether to teach the baby to suck its thumb or let it go on sucking it. After all, parents are also responsible for their babies at night. And furthermore, I would like to reassure you right now: sooner or later, the nocturnal disturbances will come to an end. If your baby is in the habit of sleeping with a dummy and needs only to have the same returned to its mouth before going back to sleep immediately, you will soon grow very tired of looking for it all the time: under the blanket? between the mattress and the bed? under the baby's tummy? or maybe by its feet? Please never give in to the temptation to tie the dummy to the bed – if the child strangled itself on the string, you would never forgive yourself! A much safer method is to stock up on dummies and always keep them in the same place. Then, at night, all you have to do is take one off the hook or out of the box you keep them in. It's worth your while to discipline yourself and the other members of the family in this regard. Every dummy that is found is automatically returned to the dummy collecting point! In the process, regularly replace the older dummies with new ones so the child doesn't become "stuck" on a particular one. Otherwise there is sure to be a major drama if that particular dummy gets left at Grandma's house a hundred kilometres away from your own home.

The father should also be involved in the decision re: dummy as breast substitute, and not just get around the whole matter by saying: "That's for my wife to decide." In several weeks, when the mother is out of the house the first time without the child, the father will very glad he is able to calm the baby down by this means. The parents should not wait several weeks before trying to use a dummy or tea to console the baby, because then their first experiment with one of these methods will presumably fail. Here I can report from experience, having had three children of my own. In the case of our third child, my husband attached great importance to being able to quiet the baby with another means aside from the breast. To this day, I am grateful to him for his insistence, because for me it was also as though some of my freedom had been restored to me, not to have to rush home with a guilty conscience. My experience in these matters – as a mother and as a midwife – does not confirm the widespread opinion that the baby will refuse the breast as soon as it has been given tea or some other substitute to satisfy its sucking urge – not in the least! This is a view which merely serves to create panic and an unnecessary interdependency between mother and child. What is more, people tend to forget in this context that there really are an increasing number of fathers who take over the primary care of the child even though their wives are still breastfeeding it, and likewise need a method of calming the baby down when the mother is out. So discuss this topic with one another early on, and without time pressure. The same applies to thumb-sucking: during pregnancy, everyone thinks it's very cute when the baby can be seen sucking its thumb on the ultrasound screen. But as soon as it's born, this habit is suddenly seen as something terrible: oh no, a thumb-sucker!

In my opinion we shouldn't get so upset, but simply understand that, all their lives, human beings harbour within themselves a longing to return to the womb, and suckling represents the simplest means of obtaining satisfaction for that longing.

Nappy-Changing and Physical Contact

Particularly when you have your first child, you will be happy if the nursery nurse (in the hospital) or the midwife (at home) takes over the job of changing the nappies again on Day Two. The first few changing rounds might well put your nerves through the wringer. The newborn, for its part, doesn't yet demand much in this respect on the second day, and only needs to be changed every five or six hours. In other words, there is plenty of time for a breather in between nappy-changing sessions. But however strenuous it may be, and however inexperienced you as the parents may feel in this pursuit, it is also something wonderful: you can touch your baby, caress it and kiss its tender skin. Getting to know and love one another is always associated with skin contact. But – also in relationships between adults – precisely the latter is rare and undertaken very cautiously at the beginning. Both of you, the mother and father of the child, also had to learn how to touch each other. It presumably didn't happen from one day to the next. So leave yourselves time; don't constantly be undressing the baby, but also don't let yourselves be robbed of the opportunity for physical contact. With its voice, your child will communicate clearly to you whether you are touching it too gently or too firmly. When you are applying oil to the baby's skin, its cries will convey clearly to you that you are still proceeding too gingerly, whereas when it coos and stretches with pleasure, you will know for sure that your child feels safe and well cared-for. When you touch, remember that the baby isn't fragile, that it was in your womb until just two days ago – where it hardly had any space to move any longer, and from which it was ultimately expelled with uterine contractions. The baby surely experienced these contractions like a firm, strong massage. Now you accordingly don't have to be afraid to knead your baby's skin exactly the same way. If your baby was born by previously planned caesarean – i.e. without contractions – it will not have had precisely this experience. It will have been conveyed into this world entirely unprepared. Now you have the opportunity to compensate by treating your child to these pleasant, repetitive massaging motions. It will relax and lie there peacefully. If you touch it too gently and superficially, it will be restless and cry. Try to remember how you react to limp handshakes. Do you feel safe in hands like that? Take your child into your arms, touch its little body in exactly the same way you love to be held and touched. Take your own needs with regard to physical contact as your orientation – that will never be the wrong approach when it comes to touching others. Even if the baby doesn't need or want to be massaged or changed, treat yourself and your child to as much contact as possible – carrying it on your body or letting it lie on your chest. The parent-child bonding is irreplaceable; it gives the child the sense of safety it needs and plants the seed of trust in the parents, the trust in the child which will grow more every day. Particularly in the coming weeks and months, you will not only enjoy carrying your baby, but come to appreciate it as a wonderful form of togetherness. Babies who are carried are moreover provably more balanced, calmer, and fare better in general. Many a crying bout thought to be caused by hunger can be stopped without breastfeeding, without a dummy, simply by carrying the child. Naturally, the baby sling is an excellent aid; it keeps your hands free for the household and your older children, and gives your youngest the intimacy and the rhythms of your movement it knows so well from its time in the womb.

Excretion

When you change the baby's nappies, you will again find the meconium. It will still be black to dark brown in colour, but already somewhat softer in consistency. It is equally possible that there will be no bowel movement on the second day if the baby eliminated quite a lot the day before. In any case, the midwife will inquire about the amount and consistency of the stool every day. The parents can rely on her to know whether everything is taking its normal course.

Women who have just become mothers for the first time are amazed at the amount of stool their babies produce. Those who have older children often remark with astonishment: "I've already had two children and it wasn't until now, with my third, that I really experienced what meconium is. When I think about all the things I never knew about in connection with the first two children because they were changed by the baby nurses! Now I realize that it's no wonder a newborn loses so much weight, considering the quantity of meconium in its nappies.

The amount of urine passed during the first two days, on the other hand, is scanty. Usually there are no more than a few little damp spots on the nappy. On the second day I warn the mothers not to be frightened if on this day or the following she discovers a pinkish spot on the nappy. This so-called "brick-dust urine" is passed by many newborns, though more frequently by little boys. It is an entirely normal process, and a sign that the baby has really eliminated the last urinary sediment and now requires somewhat more fluid very soon. I endeavour to explain to the parents that life begins with fasting and all organs have to be able to excrete properly for a start. Fasting means detoxification, a means of "tidying up" all of the metabolic functions. It is the little baby's way of ridding itself of all the toxins which have accumulated during the pregnancy. If this fasting and excretion process weren't necessary, nature surely would have seen to it that the mother could already offer the newborn abundant amounts of breast milk from the first day onward. But in view of the fact that lactation only starts later on, the newborn presumably needs this process as a means of stimulating its metabolism.

Skin Care/Baby Acne

In many cases, the elimination process apparently takes place by way of the skin. Many babies develop baby acne as early as the second or third day of life. It happens more frequently among children born with green/meconium stained amniotic fluid. The skin is strewn with yellow spots; the density can vary. To the mother's eye it looks worse than it presumably feels for the child. In particularly severe cases in which the spots often develop into pustules (pimples), we see to it that the baby wears clothing free of any form of irritant, cotton undergarments which can be washed in boiling water, or a silk undershirt. As much as I value the qualities of wool, for children with baby acne I recommend using cotton or silk instead. Don't allow yourself to be disconcerted by medical experts who tell you these spots have been caused by infected amniotic fluid and perhaps even suspect that the newborn has contracted a bacterial infection. The children are quite capable of coming to terms with these extreme skin reactions on their own. An excellent means of caring for this irritated skin is to add a few drops of *lavender extra* to the wash water or dab the spots with *Rose-Teebaum-Hydrolat/Rose-Tea-Tree Hydrolat* $\mathcal{D}^{®}$. Other than that, it is not necessary to subject the child to water or a body wash. In my opinion, everything which represents further stress for this sensitive baby skin should be omitted. Applying cold-pressed organic plant oil – e.g. almond or sunflower oil to which a bit of calendula has been added – on a daily basis suffices entirely. Incidentally, this condition can also develop as late as one or two weeks after childbirth. If the pustules spread out over the entire surface of the body, *Cistrosenöl für Kinder/Labdanum Oil for Children* $\mathcal{D}^{®}$ is a highly effective skin care product.

Day Three

Need for Warmth/Lamb or Sheepskin

It continues to be important to keep an eye on the child's body temperature, particularly in the case of newborns who have visibly or provably lost a lot of weight since childbirth. These children still require constant warmth from the outside, because their rolls of fat – small enough to begin with – are now even smaller. Children who weighed 3,800 to 4,000 g/8.5 to 9 lbs. at birth will now no longer turn a bluish colour and begin to freeze so quickly when they are undressed to have their nappies changed. Whether or not the child still needs a hot-water bottle when it is asleep will depend on the time of year. Newborns who sleep on a lamb or sheepskin maintain a constant body temperature, since natural skins have a temperature-balancing effect. These children accordingly don't lose as much of their initial weight, and they gain weight faster. It has become almost par for the course to bed newborns on sheepskins – even hospitals have started to practice this method, but if yours hasn't, you can bring your own with you. The skin makes such a soft, cuddly nest that most babies would rather be there than anywhere else. And this baby sheepskin often becomes a constant companion. As long as the baby has its beloved sheepskin, it feels at home everywhere and can sleep just as well in other places as it does at home.

When you purchase it, you should make sure that it is washable and tanned by an organic method which is both environmentally sound and represents no danger to human health. You can inquire with a company specialized in natural textiles for children. I advise strongly against putting a rubber mat under the sheepskin in the baby's cradle or bassinette. This custom has unfortunately become very widespread, but it only blocks the circulation of air – animal hides are "breathable" – and leads to precisely the accumulation of warmth you are trying to avoid. It is extremely important to air an animal skin regularly. Incidentally, if anyone in the family suffers badly from allergies, you should probably refrain from acquiring a sheepskin from the start.

As soon as some method has become established and proven its worth, it's not long until someone comes along and tries to prove the opposite. So it comes as no surprise to me that now, after two decades, the lambskin has found opponents. But it seems entirely inconceivable to me that lambskins could be one of the causes for SIDS (sudden infant death syndrome), as these persons argue. However sad and horrible it is that some children simply don't want to stay in this world, and however understandable it is that the causes are sought everywhere, it is an incontestable fact that we human beings must own up to our own helplessness. If the great majority of babies are put to bed on lambskins without any serious consequences, then the lambskins can't suddenly be branded the causes of death in the few cases where babies likewise lying on them have died. Don't allow yourself to be disconcerted by things you hear; rely on your own feelings and you'll recognize on your own whether your baby feels good lying on the skin or not. But also be aware: a child who does not want to live cannot be stopped from dying – regardless of whether or not you use a lambskin. The fact

that your concerns about the child are frequently associated with fears is entirely normal, because for you, a completely new and strange phase of life has begun, and you
are still in the process of learning to come to terms with it.

Feeding

In the great majority of cases, the newborn develops a ravenous appetite on the third
day. The calm and drowsy baby of the first two days is now suddenly an entirely different person. If it had its "druthers", it would be breastfed every two hours. Mothers
don't hold this against their children but, on the contrary, are very happy about it,
because the baby's newfound appetite almost always goes hand in hand with the initial engorgement of the breasts. Gulping audibly, the corners of its mouth moist with
milk, the child enjoys drinking its fill. Usually the breastfeeding procedure takes
about fifteen to twenty minutes per breast. Now there is milk in abundance; the fasting phase is over, and the newborn will refuse the fennel or corn silk tea from this day
on. It simply ignores the father who tries to pass the bottle of tea off on it and keeps
crying until it is put to the breast. This is something the father is not necessarily upset
about, because he is somewhat stressed as a househusband and now he has the opportunity to sleep through a meal at the mother's breast. The amount consumed will
differ to the same extent as the point in time the above-described transformation occurs. Many children are already capable of drinking their tummies full on the second
day, others not until the third. The midwife can tell by the nappy contents whether
the baby is really getting enough.

Nappy-Changing/Excretions/Transition to Normal Stool

Now it will be necessary to begin changing the baby's nappies regularly, approximately every four hours. The nappies will now be noticeably wetter, particularly if the
baby is still drinking tea in addition to breastfeeding. As the amount of breast milk it
consumes increases, the meconium will turn into transitional stool, which can exhibit a whole palette of different colours from brown to green. The consistency will
become more fluid. If there isn't much stool – often only a trace of it is visible in the
nappy – it is no cause for concern. But if the baby is already obtaining breast milk in
abundance, the nappy contents will be likewise plentiful.

Parents are often surprised when they suddenly find traces of blood in the nappy
or, during the changing process, see tiny traces of bloody discharge or drops of blood
coming out of their baby daughter's vagina. This is absolutely nothing to worry about
because it is completely normal for girls to discharge thick white mucus or have an
initial mini menstruation between the third and fifth day of life. This phenomenon is
caused by the fact that your daughter is drinking a lot of breast milk and thus receiving a large amount of female hormones, which cause this first menstrual bleeding.
You can see it as a sign that her reproductive organs are in proper working order. Boys
are also affected by the mother's hormonal readjustment, but the signs don't appear
until a day or two later.

When the midwife pays her house call on Day Three, the topic of the baby's genitalia frequently comes up, because the parents' observations are now more detailed. Maybe it also just takes awhile before they can find the words to express their initial impressions of the relatively well-developed genitals. The appearance of the boy's testes, for example, or the girl's large labia, can come as quite a surprise. Here again, the cause is the exposure to the maternal hormones. The scrotum is often a shade of dark red to dark brown and sometimes disproportionately large. One couple recalled how they felt during the postnatal phase with their first boy: "At the beginning we couldn't believe our eyes, such a gizmo! But during the first two years we had the impression every part of him was growing except his testicles, which seemed to be shrinking." Of course I could only confirm this impression; my reaction the first time I saw a male newborn had been exactly the same, particularly in view of the fact that, at the time, I didn't know that the proportions would change by the time the baby became a toddler. Incidentally, the vulvae of the girl are a telling sign of how mature she is: the longer she has remained in the womb, the greater the extent to which the labia are closed.

When changing the nappies, it is important to clean the stool and urine thoroughly from every crease and fold of the skin.

If you have a little girl, use one finger and a damp washcloth to clean the vulvae carefully from front to back. In order to avoid transporting germs from the anus to the vagina, it is just as important to wash your daughter in this direction as it is for your own intimate hygiene. With this cleaning motion in the direction of the anus, your finger only enters the baby's vagina as far as the labia minora, in order to clean that area of any bits of stool that might have made their way there. The thick whitish coating you will discover in the process, incidentally, is leftover vernix caseosa and should not be wiped away. Due to the danger of injury, please never use cotton buds/Q-tips to clean the female genitals.

In the case of a boy, it is very simple to clean under the scrotum by gently lifting it. Please dry this area well, because – particularly if the baby has very large testicles – this area of the skin can easily become irritated. Since it is quite difficult to clean the foreskin of the penis, you should leave it alone until your child is capable of pushing it back himself. And really not a day sooner! Even if you read something to the contrary or hear it from some health professional, you should refrain from "exercising" the foreskin by pushing it back regularly. It generally takes a year or two until your son is old enough to learn to clean his penis in the bathtub. If the foreskin proves to be very tight, it will be worth your while to encourage the child to retract it frequently to make it elastic and soft. A few drops of *Dammmassageöl/Perineum Massage Oil ℈®* will have an astonishing effect. You may be able to spare your son an expansion of the foreskin by medical – usually surgical – means. It is not at all uncommon for a piece of the foreskin to be removed or the child to be circumcised as a means of dealing with this problem. Find out before the operation exactly what the doctor intends to do; otherwise you may find that the foreskin has simply been removed altogether. But also be very careful with the stretching exercises and only carry them out in the warm bath water using the abovementioned oil. The latter is applied to the foreskin before the child gets into the water, and once he is there, the little boy should take over on pushing the skin back millimetre by millimetre himself.

Day Four

Need for Warmth/Sleeping Position

The baby's need for warmth has decreased somewhat but should not be underestimated. It is now necessary to dress the baby in pre-warmed clothing only after giving it a bath. The waking phases may already have increased in length, and afterwards, a hot-water bottle or the like at the baby's feet is certainly still a good idea; the same applies when the room is cold or the nights are cool. It is often sensible to pre-warm the baby's cradle or bassinette with a hot-water bottle at the head end and then, when you put the baby down to sleep, move the hot-water bottle to the foot end. This little trick will convince many a newborn that it can sleep fine in its own bed as well as in yours.

In cases where the parents can decide themselves on the baby's location and position when it is sleeping, the children usually rest almost exclusively in the parents' bed during the first few days. This way the parents have the opportunity to observe how the child wanders between two worlds, a state which often appears to us like superficial sleep and is reflected in its enchanted facial expression. On the first day it usually lies on its back, on Days Two and Three on its side. From the third or fourth day onward, however, the parents will want the child to be on its own more during its sleeping phases. In my opinion, it really needs to be left alone now while it is sleeping, and to that end it can lie in its own bed.

When the baby moves to its own cradle/bassinette/cot, the mother instinctively lays it on its tummy. If the child likes this position, then it is surely good for it. As regards the sleeping position, I explain to the parents that, just as in the case of other basic human needs, there is no norm. Some babies prefer to lie on their backs, others on their tummies, still others on their sides. In any case, if it is put in a position it finds uncomfortable, it will simply whine and complain until its mother or father turns it a different way. In response to the claim that a particular position is more or less dangerous with respect to SIDS, all I can do is shrug my shoulders and remark: "Typical statistics!" From the 1970s to the mid 1990s, all children had to lie on their tummies because the face-up position had supposedly been so hazardous in the previous decades. Now, since about 1992, there have been statistics aimed at proving that all children who died suddenly as infants had been lying on their tummies. I ask myself what other position they could possibly have died in, because no mother had put her baby to bed in any other position for fear of SIDS. It was inconceivable for a mother to be discharged from the hospital without being told to lay her child on its tummy – exclusively. You can already almost predict what the statistics are going to be proving to us in fifteen years, now that the tummy position is frowned upon and denounced by doctors and the media as being highly perilous. Incidentally, no other sleeping positions were even taken into account in the studies. And moreover, such criteria as premature birth, motherhood at a very young age, bottle-fed children and smoking during pregnancy represent equally high risk factors.

All I can do is appeal to every mother's common sense and say: "Put your child to bed in the position in which it likes to sleep and in which it sleeps well. Rely on your own maternal instincts and not on press reports and statistics. If the baby leaves this world, it is not your fault. Human beings are always looking for motives and someone to blame, because we no longer know now to deal with death and dying." As a mother and midwife, I refuse to believe that the death has been caused by something the mother did wrong in caring for the baby. Regardless of what age a mother is when she takes her baby to the grave, it is impossible for her to understand or accept the situation. Society has no right to make things even worse for these mothers with its accusations. To have to live in mourning for the child is already difficult enough.

Perhaps you are surprised or even appalled about the fact that I am discussing death here again, but it is a topic which is actually extremely appropriate in the period of the third to fourth day of life. It is in this period that most mothers reach an emotional low, which, among other things, is also associated with the question as to whether she will be able to cope with all of the burdens, worries and illnesses presented to her by life with this child. The memory of the birth is still so fresh in her mind, as is the feeling of having already experienced the boundary between life and death, and these emotional wounds have nowhere near healed yet. Such trivial sights as the baby's blue arm on which it was lying remind the mother that it isn't so very self-evident that her child is alive and well.

Another brief remark on the sleeping position: if your baby wants to sleep lying on its back, but you are worried that it will spit up and choke on the contents, put it down on its side in such a way that it can rest on one shoulder blade – but not on its upper arm, because the blood in its arm can become blocked. To stabilize the position, you can roll up a cloth or towel and brace the baby's back against it. This way you kill two birds with one stone because in addition to giving the child a secure lying position, you always have a cloth handy when it spits up, and don't have to go rummaging for one. Try to alternate sides as often as possible so that your child's head remains symmetrical.

The Birth Experience/Naming the Child

At this stage it does the mother good to talk about the events of labour, holding her child in her arms. It is often the baby's sleeping and waking rhythm which inspires the parents and midwife to talk about the childbirth experience. For everyone involved, it is important to find explanations, for example for the child's jumpy or restless behaviour. Both during childbirth and in the framework of the examinations often common or necessary in the hospital, it has had extremely formative experiences and sensations. For blood tests, for instance, the blood is usually taken from the baby's heel. It is possible that the baby hasn't completely "digested" the pain involved in that procedure, any more than it has the events of the actual birth. Our talks give us an opportunity to look for means of helping the baby come to terms with these experiences and showing it – as often as possible – that it can now feel safe and well protected.

On Day Four the topic of the child's name very often comes up again, because, interestingly enough, home-birth parents often take several days to decide on a name for their newborn. In Germany, the baby's birth has to be registered within a week, so parents do have a few days to think. Rest assured, therefore, that you're not the only parents who are taking their time and are still undecided on this matter. On the contrary, it is undoubtedly sensible to take the time you need to get to know the child a bit before deciding on the name. After all, the child will have to call itself by that name its whole life long, and the parents will have to justify why they chose this "stupid" name, of all names.

Feeding/Spitting Up

The newborn still drinks at relatively brief intervals of two to three hours. Its stomach is small and still can't digest such large amounts of fluid. Many children greedily drink as much milk as possible, then notice it was actually more than they can handle and, fortunately, spit up a fair amount of it again. Newborns have a kind of natural, healthy "excess flow valve". You needn't be the least bit worried. On the contrary, you can be glad, because the spitting up is a sign that your baby drinks enough milk. Take a look at the yellow spots produced in this context and imagine that, after a period of fasting you had to eat a portion of fatty meat – i.e. a food with a high protein and fat content. You would likewise be unable to keep down more than a few bites at a time. That's how the fatty breast milk is for the baby. Have faith that this is a natural process and let it take its course. During her house calls, the midwife will quickly recognize whether the amount that comes back up again is within bounds or not. If you are in the hospital, try to remain calm and not demand too much of the nurses' attention. They know that you have a completely normal newborn with equally normal drinking behaviour, even if you're both in the hospital – the place for sick people. But look for a competent woman who will take your questions seriously and advise you on everything you need to know. After all, what represents routine to the baby nurses, midwives and doctors are things that may very justifiably cause you uneasiness and concern, especially in view of the fact that – unlike those health professionals – you have a deep personal attachment to your child.

Weight Loss/Weight Gain

During the house call on the fourth day, the question often comes up as to whether the baby has already started gaining weight again or is still losing it. Very few midwives weigh the baby on a daily basis when the postnatal period is being spent at home. Instead, they judge the situation on the basis of their visual impressions and will also explain to the mother what to look out for. By the fourth day at the latest, the upper abdomen – which had initially been rather flat – becomes round and full. This is a sure sign of weight gain which is apparent to every mother and can keep her from having to be disconcerted by possible errors in the weighing procedure. For with great regularity, parents who like to weigh their children every day, or even after every meal, come to erroneous conclusions for one trivial reason or another. They then become uneasy and concerned, merely because the baby had one foot hanging over the edge of the scales or was crying so loud that the situation became hectic and the parents weren't able to take a proper reading and then, during the next weighing session, it looked as though the baby had lost a considerable amount of weight. I don't know of anything positive about constantly checking the baby's weight. On the contrary, it leads to uncertainty and worry on the part of the mother, who then torments her child by trying to get it to drink more than it wants to. Every time you breastfeed, remember that the baby senses very precisely whether you are going through the process with happy feelings or nagging, worried thoughts. The baby's instincts and senses of smelling and touching are extremely sensitive during this phase and help it to get its bearings during the first few weeks of life. It senses your fears, and is capable of smelling the change in the perspiration brought about by tension and excreted through the pores of the skin. Free yourself of everything that represents pressure to perform and uncertainty. The midwife should accordingly make it a point of never weighing the child before the fourth or – better still – the fifth day of life, so as to ensure that the news of the baby's weight is positive and encouraging for the mother. Of all the newborns I have attended to in the parents' home from the first day onward, not one of them has ever lost weight to a worrisome extent, and I have never had to recommend that the breast milk be supplemented with infant formula.

New mothers spending the first few days in the hospital will be told very clearly by the nurses: "Your child gained weight for the first time today." But if it's still losing weight she is often told, just as directly: "If this baby doesn't start gaining weight very soon, we'll have to give it infant formula!" In this situation the mother is subjected to enormous pressure to produce and perform. As a result, the baby is kept at the breast too long at every feeding session, and the danger of the nipples' becoming sore increases as a result. Now, thanks to this pressure, the entire "system" gets out of wack, the mother's nipples ache, the baby senses the mother's tension, even refuses the breast. Everything comes to a standstill – except the tears; everything escalates right when the postpartum down is at its worst. Many mothers then call me in a state of desperation and request the advice of an independent midwife. I begin by trying to console them and explaining that weight loss is a physiologically normal process for a newborn. After birth, a baby is allowed to lose as much as ten percent of its birth weight: if, for example, it weighed 3,300 g/7 lbs. (= 112 oz.) at birth, it can lose as much as 330 g/11 oz. I advise mothers to quote this formula to the baby nurses, because it is rare that a child really reaches the lowest tolerable weight. When the mother responds in this way, she shows that she is informed: "But newborns are allowed to lose weight; it's an entirely normal process. It hasn't reached the ten-percent limit yet. Tomorrow it will certainly have gained weight, and if not, we can talk about infant formula then." Mothers have to be supported and encouraged to have faith and be patient and in that way take a share of the responsibility for themselves. Supplementation of the breast milk with formula should never be ruled out in principle, but should be well considered. For more information on this topic, see the section on "The Breastfeeding Period". With regard to the loss of weight, it must not be forgotten that the children who are born in an atmosphere of relaxation and patience often don't lose as much weight, because they are frequently not weighed until an hour or two after birth. By that time, they may already have excreted meconium and urine accounting for an ounce or two, as opposed to other babies who are weighed immediately after birth. Babies really are spared stress if they are allowed to arrive in a calm and patient environment.

Nappy Zone/Excretions

When you change the baby's nappies, the need for doing so will now be much more obvious. You'll undoubtedly have to go through the rigmarole after every meal because the amount of urine and stool increases with the increasing intake of food. It is not uncommon for the yellowing breast-milk stool to ooze its way right down to the baby's feet. The colour of the nappy contents ranges from brownish yellow to egg-yolk yellow to spinach green. To your great astonishment, the baby nurse or midwife will inform you that this is all completely normal. The same applies to the consistency of the stool, which can be anywhere from softly formed to mucous to downright runny. In the case of newborns who keep drinking way after their hunger has been satisfied, the nappies will constantly be overflowing and the stool will contain small, firm, linseed-like grains. These are simply undigested protein components of the breast milk. Again, this is no cause for concern. The babies who still receive only sparse amounts of breast milk will have less to show for it in their nappies. These babies often have no bowel movement for days on end. But as long as the nappies are moist or wet six times a day and the child is gaining weight – visibly or "weighably" – this condition is likewise entirely normal. In any case, the midwife will inquire about the contents of the nappies on a daily basis and/or change the baby herself during her house call, and will let you know if everything is alright. Frequently all the midwife has to do during the house call is to allay the parents' concerns and reassure them that everything is as it should be. This is precisely the confirmation parents need during the postnatal period.

Skin Care/The First Bath

In view of the increasing content of the nappies, it is worth your while to wash the baby right in the bathroom sink instead of with a washcloth, soap and a towel. If the baby is changed in the bedroom, where there is usually no washbasin installed, you can have recourse to a small washbowl. In the warm, rather confined space provided by the latter, the baby feels safe and is pleasurably reminded of the womb; this washing procedure is seldom accompanied by crying. Naturally, the baby can also be bathed in the baby bathtub if this proves more practical. Midwives accustomed to providing postpartum care are flexible in every respect and will adapt to the circumstances of your household. It is for the mother to decide whether the baby should be bathed daily or weekly or somewhere in between. It is advisable, though, to wash all of the skin folds and creases behind the ears, in the area of the neck, armpits and groin every two days with water. When you wash the whole baby or give it a bath, the room should be nice and warm or you should have a quartz radiator at your disposal as discussed above. Naturally, the nappy zone has to be cleaned and cared for very regularly to avoid nappy rash.

The baby's first bath at home is nearly always a festive family event. It is ideal to choose a day on which the father and perhaps even the older children can attend. Even mothers who have already had children before enjoy it when the midwife bathes the baby. But in any case, the first-born's first bath is generally carried out solely by the midwife, and the parents are still content just to watch. The second bath is then conducted by the parents themselves. Afterwards the baby is massaged with oil and dressed in its pre-warmed clothing. The parents can decide whether or not to use a bath additive. In any case, they are well advised to use it sparingly and, here as well, to choose only natural products. Essential oils are an excellent choice here, for example *lavender extra, mandarin, rose 10% in jojoba wax, sandalwood 10% in jojoba wax* or *vanilla*. Emulsify (mix) one to three drops of the oil in salt, honey, bran, dairy cream or a neutral soap basis. Among my *Original D® Aroma Blends* are the ready-to-use *Babybad/Baby Bath D®* and *Baby-Kinderduschgel/Shower Gel Babies and Children D®*, which represent a simple alternative to concocting your own additive. The baby products made by natural cosmetics manufacturers – available, for example, in health food stores – are also well tolerated by the delicate skin of a newborn. Bath additives of this kind are preferable to all of the conventional baby brands. Of course I know that the natural skin-care products are more expensive than the conventional ones. If however you're exposing the baby's sensitive skin to ointments, bath additives, oils, etc., they should by all means be natural products, without synthetic aromas, softeners and preservatives. From my own experience I know that you have to spend more money initially on natural products, but you will soon realize that they are more economical for the simple reason that a little bit of them goes a very long way.

Day Five

Need for Warmth

As the child's body temperature stabilizes, the child will gradually find its own sleeping and waking rhythm. It still loves constant warmth in its bed, but a source of heat such as a cherry-stone or herb cushion or a hot-water bottle is no longer necessary. When being held by one of its parents or siblings it should still be wrapped in a cotton or wool blanket, except of course on hot summer days. Naturally, its head still needs protection against the cold as well as the heat, i.e. a cap made of wool, cotton or silk.

Sleeping and Waking Phases/The Protective Instinct

As mentioned above, a certain rhythm now gradually develops; the baby breastfeeds at certain times of day and sleeps for a few hours in between. In very many cases this cycle is about four hours. Some babies already have waking phases of as long as an hour, but they usually want to spend them in physical contact with one of their parents. Sometimes Grandma or a good friend can hold the baby now. You, the parents, will notice that it is difficult for both of you to entrust your baby to the arms of another person. What is at play here is our natural protective instinct, which is still in good working order with us human beings. Even though the Grandma or good friend has raised a couple of children in her day, you'll find yourself trying to explain to these experienced mothers how they should hold or carry your baby. You – the mother – may even break out in a sweat when you see how your newborn is lying in a "stranger's" arms. Things can even get to the point where you react with tears and indignation when the Grandma or aunt says it wouldn't hurt the baby to cry now and then. Your heart will virtually ache when the baby nurse takes your crying baby off to the baby room, saying: "Don't worry, it will calm down…" What you are feeling are entirely normal maternal feelings, which only you can feel. I myself only came to understand them when I had children of my own. From then on I knew what it meant to be a clucking hen that defends her babies by hissing and spitting. I could literally feel the meaning of the expression: "A mother's heart bleeds for her children." Submit to these feelings and defend your child. Your bond with the child will thus become more intense, and the two of you will get to know one another better and better. And don't be disappointed if health-care professionals or your best girlfriends fail to show any understanding for such hen-like behaviour. They have presumably never had children of their own and can't understand such reactions. Try to recall: didn't you and your husband also once come away from a visit to friends who had just had a baby, saying: "That's not how we're going to be when we're parents! Just because they have a child now, there's no more television, no more radio, and they talk in nothing but hushed voices. And they wouldn't let us hold the child for more than about half a minute. We're not going to be like that!" Naturally, some parents really can entrust their children to others quite easily. Maybe you'll be able to cope quite well with this first experience of letting go.

The midwife also proceeds very cautiously when she wants to pick up the child. I would also advise all young colleagues making their first house calls to begin by asking the mother carefully whether it's alright if they take the baby out of its bed. You will find that, at home, the situation is turned around: there the mother has the say. In the hospital it's the nurses who decide whether the baby can be taken from its bed. But whether she is at home or in the hospital, when the postnatal phase is over, the mother will have to make all of the decisions herself – and from the first day on she has to realize that she is responsible and the midwife is merely there to advise her.

The child's waking phases go hand in hand with its first crying bouts. Now it is our job as midwives to enlighten the parents that this screaming is not always indicative of hunger or a stomach ache. We try to explain as gently as possible that the newborn also has the right to use its voice and doesn't always want to be as quiet as a mouse. At the same time, we have to take into consideration that a screaming baby is hard for its parents to endure on the emotional level. On about the fifth or sixth day, the postnatal visit thus often becomes a conversation session. Now the object is no longer to show the parents the "ropes" as regards changing the nappies or giving the baby a bath, but to help them understand why the child behaves the particular way it does. It is advisable to show the parents more about "handling" their baby – to encourage them to carry the newborn in different positions. When the baby is awake, it can be carried around the house lying on its tummy on Dad's forearm, or lie across the lap of one of its parents while he or she is sitting at the table and eating. And then there are various tricks for persuading the baby to burp.

But not only screaming, active children give rise to comforting, enlightening conversations between the midwife and the parents. Consolation is also required in cases of babies who are quiet and almost always sleep. Mothers are often just as concerned when they have a baby who sleeps four or five hours at a stretch during the night without needing to be fed. In these cases it will be necessary to determine whether the baby is healthy and thriving by checking the nappy contents and making sure it is gaining weight. Sometimes it is necessary to encourage parents to wake their child because it requires more frequent meals, for example in the case of infant jaundice or continued weight loss.

Nappy Changing/Excretions

From the fifth day on, the same information applies that was given on this topic for the preceding days. The parents become more and more practiced in handling their newborn, and (unfortunately) the mountain of laundry grows visibly since the baby now not only has to have its nappies changed six or seven times a day, but – often – has to be given a whole set of fresh clothing twice a day because it has spit up or because the nappy wasn't "overflow-proof" after all.

Days Six to Ten

Medical Examination/Weight

There is nothing new to add on the subjects of the baby's weight and need for warmth, particularly with regard to those children who have the opportunity to spend their first days with their mothers at home.

At some point during this phase, the paediatrician or general practitioner will carry out a medical examination of the infant within the framework of a house call. There is often quite a state of suspense surrounding this event, because, for both the parents and the midwife, it is always a relief when the doctor confirms that the newborn is healthy.

On the day of this doctor's visit, the midwife will generally weigh the newborn, since few paediatricians have a mobile, collapsible scale at their disposal. Everyone is always happy when the reading shows that the child has nearly or entirely regained its initial weight. There are even babies who are already above this level, which they don't have to reach, in principle, until ten to (at the latest) fourteen days after birth.

Bathing

It is likewise during this period that the parents will bathe their child themselves for the first time. When the midwife demonstrates the bathing procedure, it is important that she point out to the parents the importance of sliding the newborn into the tub in such a way that it can see the water. In other words, it should be glided in feet first, facing downwards. This way the child sees that it is entering the bathtub and is not surprised by the "enemy" – i.e. the water – from behind, as is unfortunately demonstrated in most infant-care classes. The tummy position is somewhat more difficult to master since the danger of the baby's swallowing some of the bath water is greater. With time and patience, however, the parents will learn the proper way of holding their child. Initially, parents are often amazed when we advise them to let plenty of water into the tub. But when we remind them that we adults also don't take a bath in just ten centimetres/four inches of water, they see our point. And a word of consolation: nearly all babies swallow bathwater at some point during the first few weeks of life. The scare will be greater for you than for the child. Try to calm it down in the water, so that it doesn't leave the tub frightened and crying but calm and blissful. Otherwise the unpleasant experience might be the first thing it thinks of the next time it's put into the tub.

Sometimes, however, the parents have already carried out the bathing procedure before the midwife pays her house call. This is perfectly alright as long as the baby's navel has healed completely. In the latter case, the father is also free to take the baby with him into the big tub. For the new father it is an especially wonderful experience to lie in the bathtub with his child; finally there's a task he can carry out entirely on his own. Most mothers don't like to take a full bath during the first few weeks after birth on account of the bleeding. A father often has to be encouraged to enjoy a bath with his newborn. Maybe you will have an experience similar to that of Mrs. W. …

… the next day she reported happily to me: "With your suggestion that father and daughter take a bath together, you managed to get my husband into the bathtub for the first time in ten years. That's how long he has taken only showers. And now he's even saying the baby has to be bathed at least every two days. After we finished the infant-care class in your practice, he was of the opinion that once a week would surely suffice, and it wasn't necessary to use so much water. So this is how things are when father and daughter …!"

There are countless examples of midwives bringing about changes in the family routine. All of a sudden, a dummy has been introduced or the family's consumption of electricity or water has risen because we advise the fathers to dry the baby with a blow dryer, bathe with it and pacify it with a dummy. Young midwives among my readers should be aware that their words and advice will still be having repercussions years later! Even today, I'm still amazed at the amount of information the parents pick up from the midwife during her house call.

In the case of newborns who spend their first days of life in the atmosphere of the home, it is usually only necessary for the midwife to attend to the child when the navel hasn't healed completely/the stump hasn't fallen off yet. But if everything is alright, there is no reason for the midwife to wake the baby when she comes, unless the mother considers it necessary.

Swelling of the Mammary Glands

In this phase between the sixth and tenth days, the hormonal effect of the breast milk becomes apparent because the babies develop a swelling of the mammary glands. One of the questions which is then posed to the midwife is: "I don't understand it – our child's breasts look so different – somehow swollen. Please have a look, would you?" Sometimes the midwife succeeds in undressing the sleeping baby's top half so carefully that it doesn't wake up. The mother is usually extremely glad if the child is finally asleep and she can lie down herself for an hour.

Parents usually observe this breast growth with mixed feelings, particularly in the case of boys. The midwife is sure to say: "It's a completely normal process." And it's true; the swelling is a sign that the child is being nourished with breast milk. It can even develop to the point where this little bosom produces actual milk. Particularly the fathers are utterly amazed: the things Mother Nature thought up are simply incredible! This lactation is only temporary, but it may nevertheless be important to cushion the little breasts with cotton to which a drop of *lavender 10% in jojoba wax* has been applied, because the child experiences the same pain as the mother during initial engorgement. If the baby's breasts become extremely hard, little curd compresses can also be applied to them. But please don't make any attempt to press the milk out!

A Midwife's Care Following Discharge from the Hospital

It is not until the day of discharge from the hospital – whether six days, fourteen days or, in the case of a premature birth, several weeks after birth – that parenthood starts in earnest for the mother and father. When you pass through your front door, you realize that you are now in charge of the newborn "twenty-four/seven". It is only now that it becomes tangible for many parents that it really is their child for which they now bear the responsibility. The realization that now there is no longer anyone who will appear when you ring a bell and stand by you with advice and assistance is undoubtedly sometimes a bit frightening. I can well remember having rather queasy feelings myself.

On the first morning after you leave the hospital – if not sooner – you will remember hearing about the possibility of having a midwife come to your home. Then of course you can still try to engage a midwife's services, but you may or may not be successful in that endeavour. It is therefore advisable to make contact with a midwife already during pregnancy, and ask her if she can come for a few visits following your stay in the hospital. She will attend to the navel, a task which may turn out to be more difficult for you to carry out on your own than you thought before you left the hospital. Don't be surprised if the midwife doesn't appear immediately, because she is sure to have a number of other women and children to attend to, and frequently a family of her own as well. And don't be taken aback if the midwife's partner asks you some questions on the phone. He is not just being nosy; on the contrary, in most cases the partner of the midwife serves as a kind of "switching centre". Our husbands/partners are usually quite capable of recognizing when it is urgently advisable to notify the midwife by cell phone.

During the house calls which then follow, the midwife will attend to the navel and examine the mother's uterus, answer questions about breastfeeding and discuss with you all of the other topics I went into in the sections on the first six days. Following an in-patient birth, questions concerning the baby's need for warmth, sucking instinct, changing and dressing methods, bathing and handling the newborn, etc. usually come up with a delay of several days.

Essential Oils and the Newborn

Often the question is asked: "What essential oils can I use in the aroma lamp, in the bath water, or in the massage oil?" I am always glad when parents take the time to think about the correct use of essential oils. As I have already mentioned, the newborn child's sense of smell is extremely well developed and should not be exposed to any irritants. Incidentally, childhood memories often go hand in hand with olfactory ones.

If an aroma is to be used at all, then the choice of one the mother associates with her newborn is undoubtedly ideal. In principle, however, it is not advisable to make use of an aroma lamp in the baby's environment. During the first months, the child should be exposed exclusively to the smell of its parents and the immediate surroundings, i.e. the house or flat. When there are unpleasant odours to be dispelled, an aroma lamp with just a delicate trace of a fragrance can be used. In the baby-care products among my *Original D® Aroma Blends*, for example, the proportions of essential oils are very low. I was inspired in the creation of these products by the first words of a new mother, which are frequently something like: "It's a sweet, rosy baby." This description already implies the only aroma oils which are appropriate for the newborn: rose, vanilla and honey. These essential oils are undoubtedly the only ones the baby's nose can tolerate during the first few weeks without the slightest irritation. Mothers frequently notice that their baby's forehead emits a sweet, honey-like smell. One young mother raved about her child: "Mmmh, it smells like a piece of vanilla candy." I have already discussed rose as the most suitable fragrance for mother and child. Many mothers sing this aroma to their babies without even being conscious of the fact: "Lullaby, and good night, with pink roses bedight …" Here it is important to use rose oil diluted in jojoba wax at a ratio of ten percent oil to ninety percent wax; this product allows you to dose the oil as finely as necessary. Later, when the baby is several weeks old, it will enjoy a bath supplemented with *mandarin* or *lavender extra*. The ready-to-use blend *Babybad/Baby Bath D®* is very popular. For the subsequent massage ritual (see p. 319) it is once again rose, as contained in *Babyöl angegriffene Haut/Baby Oil Damaged Skin D®*, which is the most appropriate aroma for the child. In cases of baby acne I also like to recommend *Babyöl pflegend/Baby Oil Skin Care D®*, which also contains Roman chamomile. If the mother gets tired of the scent of roses, honey is a wonderful alternative, as contained, for example in *Babyöl pflegend/Baby Oil Skin Care D®*.

During breastfeeding, it is permissible to expose the baby to low concentrations of the essential oils making up my blend *Stillöl/Nursing Oil D®* – aniseed, fennel, carrot seed, coriander, cumin, lavender and rose – which also serve to stimulate its appetite. The good effects of the essential oils of aniseed, fennel, caraway and coriander in *Fenchel-Kümmel-Öl für Kinder/Fennel-Caraway Oil for Children D®* will be discussed in greater detail later on in connection with flatulence.

Towards the end of the initial phase and during the first months of life, I am frequently asked about suitable aroma blends for restless children. Since many parents have had positive experience with fragrances during pregnancy, childbirth and the postnatal period, they would also like to take advantage of the effectiveness of essential oils to "treat" their lively child in the hopes of maintaining the family peace. They must be aware, however, that a temperamental, active baby will not suddenly turn into a quiet, calm, sleepy baby simply through the effects of essential oils used in the aroma lamp or the bath water. But the essences can, for example, help a wound-up child who has difficulties falling asleep on account of the many new impressions and perceptions. The proper blend may be capable of providing stability to a "fidgeter" who is easily distracted by everything and lacks a sense of inner balance. There are two ready-to-use *Original D*® *Aroma Blends* which are designed to help in these situations. Naturally, you can also allow yourself to be guided by your own sense of smell and try to find an ideal baby-room fragrance yourself. But make sure you avoid all stimulating, refreshing oils, because most children are already little bundles of energy as it is.

For children with difficulties falling asleep, particularly in connection with digestion problems, I consider *Sandmännchen/Sandman D*® with fennel, lavender extra, orange and Swiss pine to be the ideal blend. For those among the little ones who are very bouncy and easily distracted, I like to recommend *Luftikus D*®. It contains honey, Roman chamomile, mandarin and sandalwood.

When using these blends in the aroma lamp, please be aware that two to three drops suffice for very small children. If you want to concoct a bath additive using honey or dairy cream as an emulsifier, three to five drops of the essential oil are enough.

The Care of the Navel

After birth, the umbilical cord stump – measuring about one or two centimetres/half to three-quarters of an inch in length – is usually constricted with a plastic clamp or a catgut thread to keep any blood from oozing out through it. If the child is in the hospital, this umbilical stub is then attended to daily by the baby nurse or the midwife (when the latter has an agreement with the hospital which allows her to tend to her patients on the hospital premises). At home, attending to it is one of the midwife's daily tasks. In either case, the mother – or, when the postnatal period is spent at home, often the father – is instructed to treat the navel according to the method used by the respective hospital or midwife. There is no standard number of days within which the umbilical cord stump has to have fallen off. There are cases in which it already falls off on the second day, and cases in which it hangs on stubbornly until the twelfth day of life. Interestingly, I have observed that the healing process is dependent on what family a child is born into: whereas it takes longer for all the children of one family, the navels of another family's children are all very quick to heal. The time of year also seems to have an effect on this process. Perhaps cosmic forces also have an influence on our bodies, even if we hardly take this aspect into consideration.

In the following sections I will address particularly the other midwives among my readers, but parents are sure to find the topics discussed just as interesting.

The most important rule of thumb concerning the navel is to keep it dry.

To that end I have used a wide range of methods, from the umbilical bandage to the compress – with or without a net – to leaving the wound undressed. As in other contexts as well, it has proven best to decide which the most appropriate method is in each individual case.

The Navel

The mother's opinions and instincts with regard to the care of the navel should always be taken into consideration. For some forty weeks, the umbilical cord was the mother's physical connection to her child. She is very conscious of the fact that it was through this connection that the child was able to nourish itself and grow. The mother will treat the navel with the utmost respect and do everything in her power not to injure the remnant of that connection. It is also worthwhile to think about the fact that the word "navel" also means "a central point; a middle". We midwives should likewise respect this last connection between the mother and child and not treat it thoughtlessly. If the child cries during the process of changing the bandage/compress, the mother will suffer along with it. And she certainly won't be comforted by the careless remark: "That doesn't hurt the baby; there are no nerves in the stump." The older brothers and sisters will then respond with the un"adult"erated perceptiveness so typical of childhood: "But then it wouldn't cry! The midwife is lying, isn't she Mummy?!" We should learn to take a critical view of medical principles such as, for example: "Where there are no nerves, there is no sensation!" Although doctors admit there is such a thing as phantom-limb syndrome following amputation, they don't accept the possibility of pain in connection with the navel stub. I cannot confirm this standpoint, because even the calmest, most relaxed child will scream and kick if we treat the navel too roughly. In many cases there is simply no way to keep the baby from crying during the wound care process – they don't quiet down again until the ordeal is over.

Umbilical Bandage or Net

If the postnatal phases of her older children have accustomed the mother to dressing the umbilical cord stump with an umbilical bandage and she wants to use the same method again, her wish is our command. Many mothers don't like to leave the navel uncovered, because they have an aversion to looking at the navel stump every time they change their baby's nappies. Alternatives preferred by many midwives are compresses or umbilical nets.

Cleaning the Umbilical Cord Stump

In the case of a moist navel stump just in the process of falling off, it is always preferable to use a compress so that the base of the stump dries and the process of mummification takes place rapidly. In these cases it has also proven effective to dry the navel carefully with a blow dryer. Whether the midwife employs *calendula essence,*

Wecesin® Puder, *Rose Hydrolat 𝒟®* or *Rose-Teebaum-Hydrolat/Rose-Tea-Tree Hydrolat 𝒟®* is up to her.

Particularly in cases of foul-smelling navels, I have had excellent experience with *Rose-Teebaum-Hydrolat/Rose-Tea-Tree Hydrolat 𝒟®*. Many midwives still swear by products with an alcohol base; in these cases I recommend mixing equal amounts of *Rose-Teebaum-Hydrolat/Rose-Tea-Tree Hydrolat 𝒟®* and *Calendula Essence (Weleda)*.

If the navel is on the verge of becoming infected, I like to use the essential oil blend *Rose-Teebaum-Essenz/Rose-Tea-Tree Essence 𝒟®* or *lavender extra*, which both have strong disinfectant properties. For the general – i.e. regular – care of the wound, these products do not appear to me to be appropriate, since they are too strong for the sensitive skin surrounding the navel. A word of advice to you, dear fellow midwives: please be very careful with pure essential oils and use them very sparingly! A tiny bit goes a very long way!

Breast Milk in the Care of the Navel

Many midwives and mothers greatly appreciate the qualities of breast milk in the context of caring for the navel. Doctors often still prescribe antibiotic powder or alcohol solutions although the latter don't dry out only the umbilical cord stump but also the sensitive ring of skin surrounding the navel, which can lead to reddening and irritation. I see absolutely no justification for having recourse to antibiotic powders when the healing process is not problematic.

Umbilical Granuloma/Treatment with Silver Nitrate

In my opinion, extreme abstinence should be practiced in the employment of silver nitrate on the base of the navel. With a bit of patience, many umbilical granulomas – commonly referred to as "proud flesh" – heal on their own. Even in stubborn cases, it will suffice to make very sparing use of silver nitrate. All midwives and doctors interested in homoeopathy should acquaint themselves with the pharmacological picture of Argentum nitricum (silver nitrate), a substance associated with restlessness, anxiety and impulsiveness. These behavioural modes can occur in children treated with a silver nitrate stick. With this awareness, perhaps midwives and doctors will think twice before applying a method which merely serves to accelerate the healing process. In my experience, most mothers have plenty of time and patience with regard to the healing of the navel. And it poses not the slightest risk for the newborn if the umbilical stump or wound heals only after fourteen days, or even later. The consequence for us midwives is only that we have to pay additional house calls. Or, if the healing process is extremely slow, the mother will bring her infant to the midwife's practice.

I have often seen a true umbilical granuloma disappear through the administration of the homoeopathic remedy *Silicea*. It is worthwhile first treating the problem homoeopathically and having recourse to the silver nitrate stick only in particularly stubborn cases. If the Argentum nitricum symptoms (described above) occur, precisely these globuli can be used to counteract them. This is just one more example of the principle underlying homoeopathy: "like cures like".

Cloth Nappies during the Navel Healing Process

Following discharge from the hospital, many mothers think they have to wait until the navel has healed before using cloth nappies, because of advice they have received in the hospital to this effect. Even if it is uttered by specially trained personnel, this information is pure nonsense, and an expression of our "throwaway society", where apparently the belief prevails that newborns will only thrive in disposable nappies. For you as parents it is naturally difficult to know what the optimal choice is. Please remember though: simple common sense can tell us that, until the mid 1970s, children were nappied in cloth from Day One until they were toilet trained. Presumably, industry then reacted to our steadily expanding convenience mania by introducing disposable nappies. If you use cloth nappies before the umbilical cord stump has fallen off and the navel wound has healed completely, all you need to know are a few special nappy-folding techniques. Don't allow yourselves to be talked out of the time-honoured cloth nappies, but have your midwife show you how to make proper use of them if your baby still has the umbilical stub. I often have the impression that when babies are put in cloth nappies and woollen panties, the navel heals faster. But this is "only" a midwife's experience and not a result of scientific investigation which can be substantiated by impressive statistics.

Care of the Navel following Detachment of the Umbilical Cord Stump

Even after the umbilical cord stump has fallen off, you may find that the navel generates a bit of ichor, which can even contain traces of blood, for as long as several weeks. Mothers are often disconcerted by this phenomenon and turn to their midwife for advice. We react with understanding, in the knowledge that it really can be quite worrisome for the parents. Your midwife will certainly be able to allay your fears by assuring you that the bloody discharge is entirely normal. Naturally, in these cases she will also have another look at the navel and she may well decide to administer a homoeopathic medication such as *Arnica, Calcium carbonicum* or *Silicea*.

The Care of the Navel after It Has Healed

When cleaning and caring for the navel after the healing process is completed, it is necessary to be very careful. After bathing the baby, do not be afraid to stretch the navel open gently with your fingers and dry the creases and folds of the skin carefully.

Umbilical Adenoma

Some children have a so-called umbilical adenoma. This comes about when the skin of the abdomen grows a little way along the umbilical cord. Once the umbilical cord stump has fallen off, this little piece of skin protrudes a centimetre outward from the abdominal wall. Don't worry; this "navel" will also disappear sooner or later. It may take as long as a year, so be patient. Very few people retain the umbilical adenoma their whole lives long. Incidentally, midwives are not to blame for the appearance of the navel – nor do they deserve any praise when it turns out especially handsome. The form and appearance of the navel are solely a matter of nature and the child's individuality. In the case of an imminent umbilical hernia, we can perhaps advise you to use the trusty navel bandage again for several weeks or show you how to tape the navel, but even we "wise women" cannot work wonders.

Neonatal Jaundice (Icterus)

Infant jaundice is one of the most frequently occurring problems. Despite the frequency of this physiological process, however, people often panic when it occurs.

The following remarks are important for midwives, and as parents you should in any case trust your midwife to decide how to handle the condition and what form of treatment is best. She will also know when the condition has developed to the point where a doctor must be consulted.

Normal Physiological Jaundice

It is entirely normal for bilirubin to be produced in conjunction with the breakdown of red blood cells, and to be stored temporarily in the skin of a newborn due to the immaturity or incapacity of the infant liver. As soon as the liver is capable, it will excrete this substance by way of the normal metabolic process. When this condition develops on the third day of life or later, it is a physiological occurrence which seldom requires treatment.

Jaundice Requiring Treatment

If the skin exhibits too yellowish a hue at too early a date and the bilirubin in the blood exceeds a certain level, the condition can no longer be considered normal. The danger of a rising bilirubin level leading to permanent brain damage is only present during the first forty-eight hours of life. Moreover, even within this period, such high levels are extremely seldom in infants which have been carried to term. After that time, the blood-brain barrier closes, and the bilirubin can circulate only in the body, but not in the head. Constant monitoring is still necessary, but from Day Three you can relax and rest assured that there will be no dramatic consequences. Once again, I am reminded of the old Allgaeu midwife who once remarked: "Listening to you young midwives, one would think we were all idiots, because here in the valley almost everyone was born at home. The children I attended to were all as yellow as Chinamen but they all turned into healthy, intelligent people." I can only confirm these words; my three children were also as yellow as quinces and all three of them are intelligent and healthy. But I can also remember the worrisome postnatal days only too well, and the growing concern for each child. And my state of mind was not improved by such careless statements as: "Oh, that's completely normal, you'll see." Or, worse still, the cheerful comments of some visitors about this healthy-looking newborn, followed by the question: "What did you do, eat carrots all the way through pregnancy to give your child such a beautiful complexion?" Remarks like these often leave the new mum lying in bed with tears running down her cheeks, feeling grievously misunderstood. After all, she is experiencing true concern and fear for her child for the very first time and has the distinct impression that no-one understands what she is going through.

The In-Patient Situation

In the hospital, either the free-lance midwife from the outside or the maternity ward nursing staff will keep an eye on the infant jaundice in consultation with a paediatrician. At the first signs, blood is taken from the child's heel, and as soon as the bilirubin exceeds a certain level the baby is put under a "blue lamp". The ultraviolet radiation is relatively harmless for the baby and very effective. Often the baby's condition improves distinctly within twenty-four hours. There are newborns, however, which have to lie beneath the lamp in the incubator, their eyes bound, for several days. This is very hard for the mother, because she is separated from her baby, and the sight of the blindfolded eyes and the child lying in the artificial environment of the incubator makes her heart ache. Hospitals are rarely equipped with mobile units allowing the phototherapy treatment to be carried out right next to the mother's bed.

Infant Jaundice at Home

When the mother and child are at home, the midwife will assess the degree of the jaundice, checking and documenting it regularly by comparing the tip of the baby's nose with a colour scale known as an icterometer. She will see to it that the necessary measures are carried out at the right time.

As in many other situations, preventive action is extremely important in this context. The midwife regularly reminds the parents to adhere to the method which has been agreed upon. As she has already explained to them during the preliminary discussions conducted during pregnancy, the measures are undertaken to avoid having to have the baby admitted to the hospital. Unfortunately it is not yet possible to treat babies at home with mobile phototherapy units. This is a circumstance which, in my opinion, merits action. Midwives, doctors and health plans should join forces to ensure the availability of such units. Already the cost savings alone would justify such a system, aside from the fact that keeping the baby at home is much nicer for the whole family.

Preventive and Naturopathic Measures

Constant Body Temperature

The absolute top priority in the effort to keep the degree of jaundice as low as possible is to ensure a constant body temperature, i.e. to avoid undressing the baby unnecessarily. The nappies should therefore be changed as seldom as possible, a quartz radiator should be installed above the changing table and the baby should have a hot-water bottle in its cot/bassinette or lie in its mother's arms.

Abstinence from Medication

A further aspect is the abstinence from medication during labour as well as the postnatal period. This is generally not an issue when the mother and baby spend the postnatal phase at home; as a matter of fact, the desire to avoid unnecessary medication is often one factor in the decision to leave the hospital after the birth or to give birth at home. The infant liver is thus not exposed to any additional stress.

The Mother's Diet

It is very important that the mother adhere to a "liver diet", i.e. eat foods that stimulate the liver function and avoid foods that represent stress for the liver. In particular, you should avoid animal protein (meat and sausage) during these first few days. Reduce your intake of hydrogenated (solid) fats and legumes to the greatest extent possible. I especially recommend that you go without tomatoes, since they contain a large amount of Vitamin A, which puts a burden on the liver. Drink a lot of fluid and remember that mothers used to be fed soup, rice or oat gruel and potato dishes during the postnatal period. If the mother consumes a lot of fibres and takes a teaspoon of cold-pressed vegetable oil (e.g. olive oil) twice a day, her digestive system will soon be functioning smoothly, a further means of keeping the jaundice at bay.

Intake of Fluid

At the slightest sign of icterus, the baby's intake of fluid should be increased, for example by feeding it corn silk or fennel tea. Fluids serve to stimulate the excretion processes; an activation of the kidneys in turn activates the liver.

Herbal Medicine

In cases where the yellowish hue appears early on, i.e. on the second day of life, or in stubborn cases of icterus or slightly raised bilirubin levels, mother and child alike are given the special, liver-stimulating *"Boldo" Midwives' Tea* containing: celandine, milk thistle, dandelion leaf and root as well as boldo leaf. The proportions are as follows: three parts each of milk thistle, dandelion leaf and dandelion root, and two parts each of celandine and boldo leaves. It is important to know that celandine is one of those tricky herbs which should only be administered by a health-care professional. It contains alkaloids which, if consumed in excess, are harmful – even toxic – for human beings. If you adhere to the doses cited, however, there is no cause for concern. Once again, we have to hand it to Paracelsus, who was right when he said that it is the quantity alone that makes something poisonous! So don't allow yourself to be fazed by "experts" who don't know everything. I frequently receive phone calls from parents telling me that the pharmacist was appalled about the employment of celandine in the context of neonatal jaundice. In such cases, the entirely physiological infant jaundice is often confused with infectious jaundice (viral hepatitis type A). I would therefore like to advise my fellow midwives to keep a package of *Boldo Tea* in their bags so they don't have to send the father to the chemist's where his request is most likely to be turned down: in any case, in Germany celandine is clearly contraindicated for use by women who are pregnant or breastfeeding.

The mother should take care not to drink more than two or – at the very most – three cups of the tea a day, and no more than a teaspoon of warm tea should be fed to the newborn before every feed. If you follow these instructions, you will not exceed the permissible daily dose of celandine. Where necessary, the child can be given more fluid following its meal of breast milk; here corn silk tea suffices. Very many children are content to drink this tea without sugar. If, however, the newborn stubbornly refuses every offer of tea but exhibits a distinct rise in its bilirubin level, the parents should sweeten the tea with dextrose or, better still, maltose (also known as barley or malt sugar). But please do not exceed the usual dose of one teaspoon of dextrose to 100 ml/3.5 fl. oz. of tea. Moreover, please be advised that you should not use honey as a sweetener during the first year of life, since it not only has a laxative effect but can also lead to botulism, a form of food poisoning which can be fatal. Honey can contain bacterial spores which can multiply unchecked in the immature infant intestinal flora and form botulism toxin, a neurotoxin. The latter can lead, in turn, to respiratory paralysis and the death of the child. If the tea really does have to be sweetened for the baby to accept it at all, you should begin reducing the amount of sweetener you use as soon as possible!

◎ Homoeopathic Treatment

I would no longer want to do without homoeopathic remedies in the treatment of infant jaundice. But no matter how often I have pointed it out elsewhere in this book, I must remind you once again that these medications must not be administered indiscriminately by laypersons. Only midwives and doctors with the appropriate knowledge will be able to make the right choice. The globuli I use most frequently in the therapy of infant jaundice are: *Aconitum, Chelidonium, China, Lycpodium, Sodium sulfuricum, Sepia, Sulfur.*

◎ Aroma Therapy

Essential oils have also proven effective in the treatment of neonatal icterus. During the acute phase, two to three drops of the aroma blend *Karotten-Limetten-Öl/Carrot-Lime Oil 10% in jojoba wax 𝒟*® can be massaged into the baby's upper right-hand abdominal zone every time its nappies are changed. The essential oils contained in the blend – Angelica root, carrot seed, lime, litsea, rosemary and juniper – stimulate the metabolic processes.

Checking the Excretions

It is important to keep an eye on the quantity and consistency of the infant's stool. If the baby has only excreted small quantities of meconium and transitional stool, the administration of sweetened tea after jaundice has set in should be ceased immediately, since sugar has a constipating effect! In these cases, the mother should be supported in producing enough milk. One means of doing so is to put the baby to the breast more often. During the postnatal period at home, it has proven best not to feed the baby glucose solutions as is unfortunately still common practice in many hospitals. I am firmly convinced that the natural fasting during the first few days following birth is one of the best forms of prophylaxis against infant jaundice.

Treatment with Sunlight

As soon as the skin starts to take on a yellowish hue, the midwives accompanying the postnatal period in the home will request that the parents expose the child to direct sunlight frequently for brief periods, or at least to take sufficient advantage of daylight. In these cases, the baby has to go without the canopy over its cradle or bassinette for a few days. The simplest method is to clear off a windowsill, cover it with a warm sheepskin and lay the baby down on it with a hot-water bottle to enjoy natural phototherapy. At home we don't have to blindfold the baby since it will close its eyes of its own accord when the sun shines directly on its face. The parents take a seat next to the windowsill and watch to make sure that their baby doesn't get too warm. Almost immediately, the yellowish shade begins to disappear on the side facing the sun and the baby will have to be turned around to expose its other side to the daylight. In other words, depending on the bilirubin level, it will be necessary to expose only the baby's face to the sunlight or its naked back or tummy. Naturally, this therapy is also dependent on the time of year, the possibilities offered by the interior of your home and the family situation.

Midwives' Knowledge

During my years as a postnatal midwife, with the aid of the *Boldo Midwives' Tea* and the right globuli I always succeeded in averting the dangers that can be associated with jaundice. Interestingly, in cases where these risks cropped up, I was able to convince many parents of the effectiveness of homoeopathy, even those who had previously regarded it more or less as a form of witchcraft. In some cases it took a lot of effort on my part to cite Samuel Hahnemann's fundamental ideas and teachings to counter biases and clear up misunderstandings about this school of thought. Otherwise I refuse to proselytize for homoeopathy, because I regard it my obligation to accept every outlook on and approach to life, but in the case of infant jaundice there is simply no alternative. Therefore I would like to urge all of my colleagues to become thoroughly acquainted with the subject matter in order to be able to conduct discussions with concerned parents and answer their questions.

In general, the care of a child afflicted with jaundice will depend very much on the midwife's previous experience. She will ask herself again and again whether she really came to the right conclusions on the basis of the icterometer (a colour scale used to determine the bilirubin level), because waiting too long could have negative consequences for the child's health. But drawing blood causes the child pain, loss of energy and thus represents a further burden on the metabolism and should not be undertaken at the drop of a hat. What is more, over-reactions on the part of the midwife will cause the parents unnecessary worry and fear. The child will sense these feelings and thus likewise be negatively affected. In these situations the midwife must exhibit powers of intuition and good judgement as well as recognize her own limits. A newborn which has been admitted to the hospital is rarely discharged right away again, even if the midwife or paediatrician merely wanted to "check". Children with jaundice are always a reason to pay one house call too many or stay too long, or make one phone call too many rather than one too few. I am all too well aware that a case of infant jaundice can be associated with sleepless nights.

Initial Minor Illnesses

Conjunctivitis

Unfortunately, newborns and infants often contract eye infections. In many cases it already happens during the first few days after birth, and the mother therefore asks for advice when she comes home from the hospital, because she doesn't want to use the antibiotic eye drops prescribed by the doctor there.

Preventive Measures

To prevent the baby from contracting conjunctivitis, it should always be handled and cared for with clean, freshly washed hands. Its older brothers and sisters should be taught this rule as well. The mucous membranes of the baby's eyes are very sensitive and must be protected from impurities of all kinds. The nappy or cloth you have on hand for when the baby spits up should also be changed regularly.

When you wash the baby's face, it is advisable to use only water and clean the eyes solely from the outer corner towards the bridge of the nose, and never in the opposite direction.

When airing the room, always make sure the child's face and eyes are not exposed to a draught. Move the bassinette away from the open window or close the canopy around it.

Natural Treatment Methods

If the eyes of the newborn are already slightly infected and pussy, the above-mentioned preventive measures are also the first steps in the treatment of the infection.

To wipe and clean the sticky pus away from the eyes, I recommend using *water sterilized by boiling and allowed to cool to room temperature*. Add a pinch of salt to it and, naturally, use a fresh gauze pad for each eye each time you carry out the cleaning process.

In the case of an eye infection during the breastfeeding period, the mother can naturally also treat the child's eyes with *breast milk*, which essentially can be used to treat any infection. This simple and natural method is always successful.

No matter what method of natural treatment she chooses, the mother of the newborn should know that there are no miracle cures which make the problem vanish into thin air from one day to the next. "Gut Ding will Weile haben": Good things take time. But with very few exceptions, naturopathy actually always leads to success within a week.

ꙮ Homoeopathic Treatment

If the eyelids are already reddened, I recommend *Calendula D4 eye drops* and *Euphrasia D3 eye drops,* administered by the mother alternately every time she changes the child's nappies or breastfeeds it. This treatment almost always clears up the conjunctivitis.

Naturally, the two substances mentioned can also be administered in the form of homoeopathically potentiated globuli. In addition to Euphrasia and Calendula, the midwife can also choose from among: *Argentum nitricum, Pulsatilla, Sulfur* or *Thuja.*

ꙮ Herbal Medicine

In the initial stage, when the eyes are tearing, I recommend Wala-brand *Euphrasia* (common name: euphrasy or eyebright) eye drops in one-way disposable pipettes. The mother should administer the drops to the afflicted eye regularly every time she changes the baby's nappies. She can of course make the solution herself by steeping euphrasy leaves in water, but this home-made solution should be applied to the affected eye on compresses in order to prevent any microparticles from making their way into the eye, where they might irritate the mucous membranes. For this reason, it is also advisable to use a very fine tea filter when making the solution.

ꙮ Aroma Therapy

The use of *Rose Hydrolat 𝒟®* to rinse out the eyes supports the healing process and suffices as a treatment when the eyes begin to discharge pus. Obviously, it is absolutely essential that the rose hydrolat not contain alcohol. It was precisely the desire to have an effective remedy against conjunctivitis that originally led the Bahnhof-Apotheke in Kempten to bottle rose hydrolat without alcohol under sterile conditions.

I frequently advise the mother to use a 0.2 percent solution of the *Original 𝒟® Aroma Blend Sitzbad/Sitz Bath 𝒟®* both for cleaning the eyes and for an eye compress applied while the child is feeding at the breast. To prepare this solution, add a pinch of the bath salt to sterilized water. Make a batch of it once a day and use a fresh cotton pad for each application. Often this method alone is already successful.

An alternative remedy for conjunctivitis is an *isotonic saline solution* supplemented with *lavender extra*. This solution can be purchased from any chemist; the proportions are three drops of lavender extra essential oil to 30 ml/1 fl oz. of saline solution.

Nappy Rash

Nappy rash is a topic which will demand the parents' and midwife's attention again and again, during the postnatal period and later on.

Preventive Measures

You can guard against this problem by carrying out the simple measures I mentioned previously in the discussion of the newborn's Day One, as well as by washing its behind with somewhat cool water and olive oil or curd soap. For washing, a natural sponge or raw silk washcloth is suitable, because they gently stimulate the circulation in the affected area. A pleasant form of inurement carried out early will protect your baby from nappy rash better than any baby wipes promoted by the advertisements. For the daily massage of the skin in the nappy zone – a means of stimulating both the circulation and the natural resistance to rashes and irritation – use cold-pressed organic plant oil. Before putting the fresh nappy on, apply a cream with a natural basis which is free of preservatives, additives and zinc oxide. I moreover recommend using cloth nappies and changing them regularly; in my experience these are the most effective ways of preventing nappy rash.

General Measures

If the baby has developed nappy rash despite your efforts, the following measures will facilitate the healing process:

- *Nappy-changing:* Change the nappies often, making sure to use an extremely absorbent type of nappy. If you are using disposable nappies for a child who passes a lot of water, it is advisable to buy a somewhat larger size and supplement it with a nappy insert. Disposable nappies should not be too tight-fitting, but should leave a bit of space for the circulation of air in the nappy zone.
- *Air and sunlight:* As often and as long as possible, the child should be allowed to lie with a naked behind in a warm place where it is well protected from the danger of taking a chill. Air and, if possible, sunlight, are time-tested natural means of supporting the healing process of the skin.
- *Drying, warmth:* Following a sitz bath (see the section on Aroma Therapy below) it is a good idea to dry the newborn with a blow dryer, because skin afflicted with nappy rash hurts when it is touched. The use of the blow dryer not only spares the child pain, but also administers air and warmth and keeps the skin dry. **Please be sure to cover the male baby's penis with a washcloth or nappy during the blow-drying process to protect it from a fatal shock if it passes water.** After the cleaning procedure, the baby's behind can be exposed to infrared radiation for a few minutes. The fact that the child should not be left unattended during this treatment is surely obvious.
- *Silk nappy inserts:* Another good method of healing nappy rash is the use of nappy inserts made of raw silk. These inserts are helpful regardless of whether you use cloth or disposable nappies for your baby. Start using them as soon as you notice a slight reddening of the skin. Silk draws the moisture away from the skin and supports the healing process of the skin. In my opinion, every mother should have some of these silk nappy inserts. After use, it is best to wash them out immediately with curd soap under hot water. The inserts dry very quickly and can be used right

away again. If washed frequently in the washing machine with water near the boiling point, however, pure silk wears out quickly.

- *Breast-milk treatments:* Here as well, breast milk can be very helpful. At the first signs of nappy rash, it is advisable to apply the extremely valuable breast milk to the baby's behind and the rash will never actually develop. I would like to relate one of my first experiences with the use of breast milk for this purpose:

… Brigitte, a friend of mine, was just in the process of changing her newborn's nappies when I arrived for a visit. I was astonished to see her dip her hand into a light yellowish liquid in a glass on the changing table. With the affection of which only a mother is capable, she massaged her baby's buttocks and the creases of skin. "Stop ogling at me! If it helps me keep my nipples from getting sore it won't hurt my son, will it? Yes, you guessed right, it's breast milk!" This was an event I experienced very early on in my career as a self-employed midwife and it taught me that there's a lot to be said for alternative methods. Since that time, the advice to use breast milk for healing purposes has been indispensable for me. How wonderful that there are women who show us midwives how children can be treated, simply and naturally, with means that go beyond what we learned during our vocational training!

- *The breastfeeding mother's diet:* The question as to the mother's diet (if she is breastfeeding) should not go unasked. Not always, but relatively often, the nappy rash is caused by hot spices or an excess of vitamin C consumed by the mother. With a bit of intuition and recollection work, it will soon become clear whether it was the pepperoni on the pizza, the kiwi in the breakfast cereal or the freshly pressed apple juice which caused skin irritations in the baby's nappy zone by way of the breast milk.

Aroma Therapy

The *Sitzbad/Sitz Bath $\mathcal{D}^®$*, containing the essential oils yarrow, lavender, chamomile blue, rose and rose geranium on a Dead Sea Salt basis, has been proving its excellence in the treatment of nappy rash for nearly two decades now. You can bathe your child's bottom in a bowl of *Sitz Bath $\mathcal{D}^®$* water, or clean it with a washcloth dipped in such water, once to several times a day. Add half a teaspoon of the bath salt blend to a litre/quart of lukewarm water.

Herbal Medicine

In minor cases of nappy rash evidenced by a superficial reddening of the skin, *Ringelblumensalbe/Calendula Ointment $\mathcal{D}^®$* will provide relief; if the condition has already reached a more advanced stage with bleeding or even oozing patches, *Beinwellsalbe/Comfrey Ointment $\mathcal{D}^®$* – likewise time-tested for twenty years – is an optimal choice. Like all of the *Original $\mathcal{D}^®$* Aroma Blends, these two ointments are produced by my pharmacist from high-quality natural substances. Please be advised that the products of other companies frequently contain preservatives such as zinc oxides.

◎ Homoeopathic Treatment

Homoeopathy is always an extremely effective means of treating nappy rash. In addition to the more well-known substances *Arnica, Calendula, Hypericum, Sulfur* and *Symphytum*, the so-called *miasmatic remedies* can also be administered here; they are capable of clearing up very severe cases even when the child has a natural genetic predisposition for this condition. This therapy is time-consuming and should be carried out only by trained homoeopathists. If none of the other treatments described on these pages is effective, the time has come to enlist the help of such a person to investigate the possible causes and look for the suitable remedy.

Zinc Ointments

Grandmas often ask whether the problem could not be dealt with very simply by the use of good old Penaten® Cream (or its equivalent in their country). It is true that with a thick dab of such a cream, nappy rash really can be avoided, because it quite effectively protects the skin from the stool and urine which may well contain irritants and acids. But I would like to point out here that all of these extremely thick and pasty ointments which, according to the advertisements, protect the baby from nappy rash contain zinc oxide to a greater or lesser degree. Zinc oxide in salves and ointments really does heal raw wounds quickly. But that is no reason to use creams containing zinc on a regular basis as a preventive measure, thus constantly exposing the child to zinc, not to mention the fact that disposable nappies also contain zinc and are therefore not biodegradable: the soil would be heavily polluted with metal. After nappy rash develops, zinc cream heals the raw skin quickly, but does not eliminate the cause. Toxins which are otherwise excreted by way of the skin in the nappy zone now have to find another route. They are forced back into the baby's organism, where they may well put a strain on an organ or other part of the body. Repression is rarely a good solution. On the contrary, in homoeopathy there is a rule of thumb – the "Hering Rule" – according to which: "Healing takes the proper path when it proceeds from top to bottom and from inside to outside." I therefore urge you to try to tolerate raw, wounded skin for a little bit longer and support the baby's body in its self-healing mechanisms by using natural remedies.

Wind

In the newborn phase and throughout the first three months of life, the question most frequently posed by mothers during house calls, on the phone, or during consultation in the midwife's practice is: "What can I do? My baby has such a bad case of wind."

Waking Phases

The first step is to determine whether the baby really is suffering from flatulence, or whether it just can't find anything better to do during its waking phases than cry. I would like to take this opportunity to point out that a baby should be allowed to use its voice now and then. Every mother should be capable of determining that the child doesn't have its nappies full, isn't hungry and doesn't have wind, cold feet or hot feet. If all of these possibilities have been ruled out, perhaps the child is purely and simply bored. It wants to be carried around and occupied, but its mother would like to take a shower, has to cook dinner or take care of the older children. In these situations the mother has no choice but to put the baby in its bassinette. It will whimper and whine, may even yell at the top of its voice. What I mean to say is: the baby should be allowed to complain, i.e. have a proper scream. And you don't have to have a guilty conscience if you think to yourself: "I'm granting my baby the right to protest, but in this case I cannot comply with its demands." I am quite sure that the baby will either stop crying after five minutes without having incurred any damage, or the mother will have taken care of her needs and obligations and will rescue the baby from its predicament. Incidentally, a very suitable aid for children who want to be carried all the time is a baby sling. If used properly, it will take a load off your back; what is more, it leaves your hands and arms free for your household work, the baby takes part in the action and is content. But please don't allow yourself to be swayed to the contrary by opponents to the baby sling; it is advocated not only by millions of mothers, but by many doctors as well. All sceptics and critics should be asked to take over your baby – and all of your housework – for several days and then see what they think.

Crying Phases/Genuine Flatulence/Infantile Colic

It is almost impossible to distinguish between genuine flatulence or infantile colic on the one hand and the typical evening crying phase on the other. The latter typically begins between five and eight o'clock p.m. and lasts two to three hours. In many cases, you can almost set your clock by these crying or wind phases.

One sign of a crying phase is that nothing you do calms the baby down. Breast-feeding only helps for a little while, as does carrying the baby around. A bath followed by a massage may also provide temporary relief. Whenever I talk about this topic I am reminded of what my sons told me when my youngest child, a girl, was so restless in the evenings: "Mama, that's just the way it is: babies cry in the evening." This remark was very comforting for my husband and me, because children often have an instinctive understanding of their little siblings' needs. They often succeed in getting the baby quiet, or even making it laugh, much faster than the parents.

True flatulence, on the other hand, really does cause the child pain. Its face may be bright red – or very pale – as a result, and you may even see beads of sweat on its forehead or between its eyes. The newborn usually has quite a bit of wind, a phenomenon reflected in the term "drum belly". Some babies remain still when they scream, but others pull their legs up and then stretch them out again with a jerk, often passing quite a bit of wind in the process. When it is being carried, the baby will prefer to lie face downwards with its tummy on its mum's or dad's lower arm. When you are carrying your child, try to see to it that its abdominal muscles are relaxed, i.e. its back rounded, its head and arms hanging downward loosely, on your arm, over your shoulder or – when you are sitting – on one of your thighs. A good way of calming down a newborn, particular during the restless hours of the day, is a Pezzi or Togu ball. These are gymnastic balls with a diameter of about 60 cm/24 in. and provide parents with a very comfortable seat. Sit on the ball with your baby lying on its tummy across your thighs, and bounce on the ball or describe small circles with it. These movements are sure to provide the child relief. And you take a load off your spine as well as your neck and shoulder area into the bargain.

If what the baby has is colic, its screaming and pain attacks – accompanied by jerky doubling-up movements – will alternate with quiet phases. The pains of colic are similar to contractions; they come and go. Nothing seems to give the baby relief.

Underlying (Emotional) Causes

These belly aches are usually caused by digestion problems. During the first twelve weeks, the newborn's digestive tract has a lot of trouble performing its function. Maybe it really is hard for the newborn to "digest" life outside the womb. When these screaming attacks occur, we have to try and take a holistic approach: Why does a newborn inflate to such an extent? Does it want to attract attention? Does this reaction perhaps mean that it can't accept the way it is being handled? Does it have to scream and rebel against the overprotective care or the loud television, the constant visits or the glaring colours that keep it from falling asleep? A child who started out quiet and cheerful but then starts screaming when it is being held may not always be expressing pain but the desire to be left lying in its bed. It often takes several children for parents to learn to respond to their child's screaming by putting it to bed and being rewarded by a baby who drops off to sleep. For my husband and me it was the same: It wasn't until our third child that we began to point out to each other that maybe the newborn would rather be in its bed. I would like to encourage you to risk putting your child down in its cradle/cot/bassinette when it is screaming. It's certainly worth a try; maybe the child really does simply want to be left alone. Many children turn off their screams like a light switch, turn their head to one side and fall asleep. If I hadn't experienced this happening with my second child, I would never have believed it.

Children of Smokers

Maybe some children really have to kick up a fuss by whatever means they can to draw attention to adverse circumstances. They want to get the parents to stop smoking, because studies show that the children of smokers suffer from abdominal pains much more frequently than those who grow up in non-smoking families. Incidentally, it is above all the children of smokers who die from SIDS.

So be strict with yourself, the other members of the family and your visitors and put a ban on smoking in your home in general, if only to spare your baby its stomach pains. It doesn't suffice to prohibit smoking in every room but one, because the smoke drifts through every opening and the clothing smells of it; the child is exposed to nicotine by way of its sense of smell. Protect your baby from this threat like a mother hen!

Breastfeeding Times/The Breastfeeding Mother's Diet

Breastfeeding mothers whose children are prone to suffer from wind should make an effort to breastfeed at regular times of the day. If possible, they should avoid putting the baby to the breast at intervals of less than three hours. The reason for this is that it takes three hours to digest breast milk, and every gulp of fresh milk that is introduced to the stomach before the fermentation process has been completed will further aggravate the digestion problems. Try to stick to strict times for a day or two; the problem with flatulence will often be allayed. And if no improvement comes about, at least you will know for sure that the wind has not been caused by irregular meals. I am well aware that breastfeeding mothers are bombarded with advice and instructions as to what they should and should not eat. And I'm sorry to have to join the ranks of the advice-givers, but one cause of flatulence in an infant really is often to be found in the mother's diet. I stress the word *one*, because diet is never the sole root of the evil. Very many babies who are fed with infant formula likewise suffer from severe digestion problems and wind, and in those cases the tummy ache certainly isn't caused by red cabbage, sauerkraut or Allgaeu cheese spaetzle. But in cases of breast-fed children, the mother often feels as if the problem is all her fault.

All you really have to do as a mother is avoid everything that causes you and your partner digestion problems. After all, the child inherited its disposition from the two of you. Also, be careful with foods that didn't agree with you during pregnancy, because it is your child, and perhaps it already signalled to you that it doesn't like this or that before it was even out of the womb. In this context, I also consider it necessary to address the topic of milk. It wasn't until my own experience with breastfeeding that I was able to believe that cow milk just doesn't agree with many children. This was just one more situation in which I had to admit that my dear older colleague knew more than I did: "But don't you realize that our babies aren't calves? The milk you get from the farmer down the road is too fatty for both of you", she said when she saw me with my screaming baby. I happily stopped drinking cow milk, because actually I had only been drinking it by the litre during the breastfeeding period because I thought it was sensible, but not because it tasted good to me. Two days later, my newborn was only crying half as often. I don't want to imply that this is the be-all-and-end-all solution to the problem of flatulence, but it has helped in a great number of cases – particularly those in which the mother thinks she has to drink milk during the breastfeeding period for the baby's sake, but actually senses an aversion to it.

Moreover, it is certainly advisable to avoid hot and foreign spices. And I have ascertained time and time again that Italian pizza, with its yeast crust, does not agree with newborns. The same goes for tropical fruits rich in vitamin C. Babies often not only contract nappy rash but also wind when the mother eats non-native foods.

I highly recommend that the mother start experimenting by consciously eating one particular kind of fruit or vegetable on a particular day and then closely observing the baby's reaction. The conclusions will be different from one child to the next. One thing is sure: during the first several weeks you should avoid eating fresh plums. After three months, however, you may well discover that the baby no longer gets wind from foods which initially caused it terrible tummy aches. Foods which are quickly digested cause wind more quickly than those which are more difficult to digest; in the latter case it can be half a day before the wind develops.

Bottle-Fed Children

As mentioned above, flatulence can just as easily occur in bottle-fed children. One simple explanation can be that the wrong kind of nipple is being used – a nipple with too large a hole, causing the newborn to swallow too much air while it is drinking. Make sure that only a drop or two of the lukewarm infant formula comes out of the nipple hole when you hold the bottle upside down. Another important pointer is to let the bottle stand for a little while after preparing the formula and before feeding the baby. The reason is that shaking the formula to mix it leads to the formation of foam, which should settle first. When you boil the water to sterilize it for the formula, see to it that the lime contained in the water stays behind in the pot and doesn't make its way into the baby bottle. In many areas, the tap water contains a lot of lime. Signs of this are greyish water and the lime residue found in the pot you use to boil the water. In many cases it helps to prepare the formula with suitable mineral water (indicated on the label) or with weak fennel tea (see p. ■).

Means of Treating Flatulence

The following measures can be used to treat flatulence and colic. Naturally, they often serve initially just to relieve the symptoms, but they can also influence the causes.

⌒ Aroma Therapy

One sensible method of treatment is massage with *Fenchel-Kümmel-Öl für Kinder/ Fennel-Caraway Oil for Children 𝒟®*, also known as the "four-winds oil". With this *Original 𝒟® Aroma Blend* consisting of aniseed, fennel, coriander and caraway in cold-pressed plant oil, the baby's abdomen is massaged circularly in a clockwise direction (!), preferably during a nappy-changing session before the time of day when the flatulence usually sets in. Later, when the flatulence has developed, this massage can be repeated. If the baby shows signs of not wanting such a massage, however, apply a moist, warm oil compress to its abdomen. To this end, soak a gauze swab (or Kleenex) with *Fenchel-Kümmel-Öl für Kinder/ Fennel-Caraway Oil for Children ℑ®* and then place it on the infant's abdomen. Leave the compress on as long as possible; it doesn't matter if the baby falls asleep; the compress won't cause it any discomfort. Incidentally, the oil will be absorbed entirely by the skin. Another means of bringing about the desired relaxation is to give the baby an aroma bath. In this case the oil has to be emulsified in honey, Dead Sea Salt, dairy cream or breast milk. After such a relaxing bath, you should take the baby out of the tub quietly, speak to it very calmly and soothingly while you dress it, breastfeed it if necessary and then put it down in its bed.

This oil is equally effective for adults, as I would like to demonstrate by telling you the following story…

… with this fennel-caraway oil blend I had a very strange experience at a further-training course at which we were served lentil stew. Soon after eating, everyone asked for a break. We all stood by the windows, passing wind and rubbing our inflated bellies. Not one of the midwives felt like getting back to work. We didn't know what to do until I suddenly thought of concocting an oil blend for us. In no time flat, our problem was literally gone with the wind and we were able to concentrate on our work again.

With *Stillöl/Nursing Oil ℑ®* you can also obtain the same results, but it should be mixed with olive or sunflower oil at a ratio of 1:1. Mothers have told me that their newborns had less wind when they, the mothers, had applied this oil to their breasts.

Herbal Medicine
It is often helpful to offer the baby a teaspoon of *Fennel-Caraway Tea* before it is fed. You can also add a bay leaf to the seeds before steeping them. A spoonful of this weak tea (a bare ½ teaspoon to 100 ml/3.5 fl. oz.) will suffice to have a positive effect on the baby's digestion. I advise mothers who are breastfeeding to drink one to two cups of this tea themselves every day, or have a few swallows of *Fennel-Caraway Tea* with bay leaf ten minutes before putting the baby to the breast.

Homoeopathic Treatment
Homoeopathic remedies are among the most effective methods of relieving severe flatulence in newborns. I would like to provide detailed descriptions of several substances, because there are always parents who have a collection of homoeopathic remedies in the house. If the first one you try doesn't bring about any improvement, don't start experimenting, but get in touch with a homoeopath or a midwife experienced in homoeopathy.

Belladonna –
When the baby has a screaming fit, its head turns bright red
Its forehead sweats

It prefers to lie in its bed, wants to have its peace and quiet
A warm hot-water bottle helps

Chamomilla –
The baby's main restless period is around nine o'clock in the evening
The basic mood is tense and irritated
It wants something and the next moment it's not happy with that thing
During screaming fits, often one cheek is pale, one red

Cuprum metallicum –
The baby is badly cramped, has colic-like cramps
Holds its thumb firmly in its fist
Its skin is pale-bluish
The abdominal wall is tense and sensitive to the touch

Colocynthis –
The child has severe flatulence colics which occur in waves
It rears up and then doubles up
Its favourite position is over the mother's shoulder
The pressure (shoulder) relieves the pain somewhat

Lycopodium –
The child has difficulties burping and frequent hiccoughs
It drinks greedily, but not very much at a time, and tires easily
It has a swollen belly and loves to be undressed
The worst time of day is from four to eight o'clock pm but at night it sleeps calmly

Magnesium carbonicum –
The child has colic-like flatulence pains which often already begin while it is being breastfed or shortly thereafter
It frequently spits up sour milk
The stool smells sour and looks foamy green
It loves pressure on its tummy and the pain causes it to double up

Magnesium phosphoricum –
The child has colic-like pains which crop up abruptly
The stool is greenish and comes out in a spray
Every movement and the slightest bit of cold make everything worse
Warmth and abdominal massages help the baby

Oral/Systemic Candidiasis (Yeast Infection)

One of the unpleasant and often tedious and stubborn problems newborns and infants have as long as they wear nappies is a yeast infection. These fungi are a symptom of our modern affluent society. The newborn unfortunately doesn't receive any protection from its mother against this fungal infection the way it does against other pathogens; on the contrary, it is helplessly exposed to them from the first day on. It takes about a year until the immune system is relatively capable of reacting. The preventive measures should therefore be carried out very conscientiously, since the struggle against yeast can be very wearisome and an infection of the mouth is almost always accompanied by an infection of the entire intestinal tract and ultimately appears in the nappy zone in the form of a rash. Candidal dermatitis in the nappy zone frequently comes and goes throughout the period in which the child wears nappies – developing whenever its immune system is weakened, e.g. on account of sniffles, a cold or a vaccination.

Preventive Measures

As important as it is to keep the baby warm on the first days of life, as early as the second week it is just as essential to protect its skin from a fungal infection by washing it with cold water and exposing it to the sun and air. Remember, a moist, dark, warm milieu provides the yeast fungi with ideal conditions for growth. And if you add sugar, the fungi fairly thrive. This is just one more reason to replace the sweetened ready-made baby tea with unsweetened home-made tea as soon as possible. Incidentally, fruit juice also contains sugar! When your child gets to the point where it starts drinking juice, always dilute the latter with water. A mother who is breastfeeding should avoid sweets, because the sugar she consumes increases the chances of her baby's contracting oral candidiasis, commonly known as oral thrush. Another important preventive measure is to see to it that neither you yourself nor your other children put the dummy or the bottle nipples in your/their mouth/s. This bad habit is the Number One means by which yeast spores are passed on.

The old adage about keeping a cool head (not referring to the baby's head-covering but to fresh air) and warm feet represents the best prophylaxis against oral thrush in an infant. See to it that the warmly dressed baby sleeps in the fresh air or a cold room as often as possible, and you will rob the fungal infection of the conditions it needs to spread and worsen. Over and over again, I witness that the incidence of oral thrush infections increases when the heating is turned on in the autumn.

In the nappy zone, the same preventive measures apply as described above in connection with nappy rash (see p. 354 f.).

Oral Candidiasis – Methods of Treatment

One sign of oral thrush is a white coating on the tongue which cannot be wiped off – very difficult to distinguish, incidentally, from the normal milk coating on the baby's tongue. However, if it is accompanied by white or grey furring with stipples on the insides of the cheeks and lips and/or on the gums, you can be sure your baby really does have oral thrush. It is well worth your while to take a look in the baby's mouth regularly – whether you are its mother or the attending midwife – since the sooner an oral yeast infection is recognized, the better and more quickly it can be treated with naturopathic means. In severe cases, however, usually the only thing that will do the trick is an antimycotic agent prescribed by a doctor.

Aroma Therapy

Oral thrush which is detected right at the start can be treated very effectively with *Rose-Teebaum-Hydrolat/Rose-Tea-Tree Hydrolat 𝒟®*. The infected areas are dabbed with a cotton bud/Q-tip soaked in hydrolat, or the entire oral cavity is wiped out with a small cloth soaked in that solution. Naturally, a freshly laundered cloth must be used each time you repeat the procedure.

Homoeopathic Treatment

See the section on "Systemic Candidiasis".

Systemic Candidiasis – Methods of Treatment

In the initial stage, systemic candidiasis can easily be mistaken for normal nappy rash. Ask an experienced homoeopath, your midwife or paediatrician to take a look, because only a practiced eye recognizes the infection immediately. The yeast infection in the area of the genitals is characterized by small, perfectly round spots with a red centre, surrounded by a fine white ring. These spots usually spread rapidly through-out the entire nappy zone. The first method of treatment to be undertaken is the same as described in the section on "Nappy Rash" (see p. ■f.).

No matter what treatment is used to cure the yeast infection, success will only be attained if the therapy is carried out long enough, preferably several days after the infection has healed completely. It is also important to observe all preventive meas-ures such as cold water for washing, exposure to air and the use of silk nappies. In many cases the yeast fungi merely lie dormant and break out again the next time the immune system is weakened, for example when the first tooth comes in or the baby has the sniffles. Let me console you by reminding you that, sooner or later, the child will be out of nappies and then the problem will be a thing of the past.

Aroma Therapy

Systemic candidiasis can be treated with *Rose-Teebaum-Essenz/Rose-Tea-Tree Essence 𝒟®*, a blend of the essential oils lavender extra, manuka, rose and tea tree. To this end, a drop of the essence is dabbed onto each of the affected areas of the skin. This procedure, however, should only be carried out a maximum of five times a day for a period of two or three days, every time the nappies are changed. When the fungal infection has already spread to a large area of skin, it is better to spray the afflicted zones with *Rose-Teebaum-Hydrolat/Rose-Tea-Tree Hydrolat $\mathcal{D}^\circledast$* , followed by the administration of *Rose-Teebaum-Balsam/Rose-Tea-Tree Balsam $\mathcal{D}^\circledast$* . It suffices to apply this balsam to the affected areas of skin twice a day. When the infection has been subdued and the skin is dry, *Beinwellsalbe/Comfrey Ointment $\mathcal{D}^\circledast$* *(PA free)* should be employed to conclude the healing process.

⊙ Homoeopathic Treatment

Homoeopathy represents a good supplemental therapy in cases of oral and systemic candidiasis alike. Remedies commonly used in this context are: *Borax, Graphites, Kalium muriaticum, Lycopodium, Medorrhinum, Mercurius, Sodium carbonicum, Sulfur.* As has been mentioned repeatedly, these substances should only be administered by an experienced practitioner with precise knowledge of the corresponding pharmacological pictures.

Coryza: The Sniffles

I am always pleased when a mother has developed so much trust in her midwife that she also asks the latter for advice even after the period paid for by the health plan is over (in Germany eight weeks). In many cases, the baby's first case of the sniffles is cause for enough concern to prompt the mother to call or come to the midwife's practice.

Natural Methods of Treatment

• *Breast milk:* The simplest form of nose drops I can recommend to you is breast milk (if you are still breastfeeding). You can carefully allow a drop of it to run into each of the baby's nostrils – that will help better than anything else. The healing powers of breast milk have been discussed frequently in this book. An alternative is to obtain a *physiological saline solution* from your chemist, a much better choice than any of the commonly used medicinal nose drops, which are not entirely free of side effects.

• *Mucus suction devices*: Since the infant is not yet capable of blowing its nose and thus emptying it, the mother must take over this task. A simple Mucex mucus suction device for newborns, likewise obtainable from the chemist's shop, is a helpful method. Rubber clysters are often offered, but they are too large for the baby's tiny nose during the first half year of life.

⊙ Aroma Therapy

Naturally, I can also recommend an ointment containing essential oils: *Engelwurzbalsam/Angelica Balsam $\mathcal{D}^\circledast$* . It helps congested noses start to run and soothes irritated mucous membranes in the nostrils. Rub it very sparingly into the forehead and bridge of the nose. In the case of newborns, it suffices to apply a dab of the ointment to a gauze swab and attach it to the inside of the bassinette/cradle near the baby's head. I created *Erkältungsöl wärmend/Common-Cold Warmth Oil $\mathcal{D}$°* especially for our littlest ones, as well as for older folks receiving homoeopathic treatment, since I was unable to find any product on the market which is not too strong for baby noses and is free of mint, menthol and camphor. This common-cold oil has become extremely popular; it can either be used in the aroma lamp or a drop of it can be applied to a Kleenex and fixed to the canopy over the baby's bed. But please do not apply it directly to the baby's clothing!

⊙ Homoeopathic Treatment

Cases of the sniffles afflicting newborns and infants should be taken seriously since it is very difficult for the baby to breathe when it is being breastfed if its nose is congested. It also struggles to breathe properly when it is put in its bed, and can't fall asleep. These are the very symptoms corresponding to the "guiding symptoms of the time-tested homoeopathic remedy *Sambucus*. But there are also other substances – *Allium cepa, Arsenicum album, Euphrasia, Luffa, Pulsatilla* and *Nux vomica* which can be taken under consideration.

This topic is discussed in more detail in my book *The Homoeopathic Home and Travel Medicine Chest*, where the use of the remedies for small children is also described.

The First Tooth

No sooner has the family gotten through the days and weeks of wind and screaming phases when they are confronted with the next problem: "Our baby is whiny and starts screaming at the slightest provocation – it can't already be teething, can it?" the mother asks when she sees the midwife at the postpartum gymnastics class or runs into her on the street. At my seminars as well, this is one of the questions most frequently asked by worried mothers. Strictly speaking, we midwives are not the person to go to about teething problems, but the latter often spark questions relating to breastfeeding since the mothers are unsure whether the baby's desire to be breastfed quite frequently is really normal. My simple answer to this question is yes, but it usually doesn't suffice, since the mothers would like to know what else they can do to cope with the situation and help the child. I would therefore like to introduce you to the various methods of treatment provided by naturopathy.

The teething period generally lasts from the sixth to the twelfth month, followed by a second phase – when the molars come in – in the second year of life. When the nighttimes start to become strenuous again, you will be grateful that you can accompany your baby through such healthy and important stages and comfort it when it suffers pain, and you can look forward to the day when you can proudly present your child's first tooth to your friends. Incidentally, the first tooth is no reason to stop breastfeeding.

When applying the various methods described below, try to remember: Wonders take time and occur only rarely, while teeth – in the literal as well as the figurative sense – are something every human being needs to survive in this world.

⟨⊙⟩ Herbal Medicine

One traditional means of relieving the pain of teething is orris root. Already our grandmothers knew of the relaxing and analgesic properties of this root. The dried root is offered to the infant to bite on.

Amber necklaces are a method whose popularity has spread far beyond the anthroposophic circles where its use originated. In the context of healing with minerals, amber is referred to as the "teething stone"; it is recommended that it be worn for a lengthy period in order to give it a chance to take effect. Many of these necklaces contain one particularly large clump of amber which can be used by the baby as a biting stone.

⟨⊙⟩ Aroma Therapy

At the first sign of teething problems, you can use *Zahn-Öl/Tooth Oil 𝒟*®, a blend of Roman chamomile, lavender and cloves on a St.-John's wort oil basis. Cloves and Roman chamomile are oils with analgesic properties, which – although they cannot work wonders – at least help the baby get some sleep. Massage a small amount of the oil onto the baby's cheeks.

⟨⊙⟩ Homoeopathic Treatment

As always, homoeopathy has an appropriate remedy for all of the symptoms that arise in connection with teething, as long as the simile rule is observed. Unlike allopathy, however, the aim of homoeopathy is not freedom from pain but normality, which in this case means: The child is teething but is nevertheless relatively easy to cope with; the parents don't have to get up hourly, but probably only once or twice during the night. The following substances can be considered in this context: *Belladonna, Chamomilla, Coffea, Nux vomica* and *Phytolacca*. Please be advised that high homoeopathic potencies can only be administered once!

More information on this topic can be found in my book *The Homoeopathic Home and Travel Medicine Chest*.

Concluding Remarks

Officially, the midwife's responsibilities towards the child end with the healing of the navel and the certainty that the child is gaining weight and thriving. As mentioned previously, however, the midwife's advice often goes beyond that point. The list of topics on which a midwife is also consulted include not only sniffles and teething but also vaccinations, vitamin K and vitamin D prophylaxis and many other questions mothers ask themselves and each other.

One of my chief aims is to try to understand all of the parents' worries myself, but also to provide help in the form of references to literature. Perhaps even more importantly, I want to impress upon the parents that it really is worth the effort for them be there for their children on a full-time basis during the first years of life. In view of the various events and stages in the baby's development – some of which I have just described – you can see that there is never a dull moment when you are parenting. Soon you'll be confirming from your own experience that, no sooner have you coped with the first case of the sniffles and the arrival of the baby teeth, the next issues come knocking at your door. Don't allow yourself to be overwhelmed by the constantly growing task of parenthood, however, but be proud of your child and enjoy it to the fullest every day. Soon it will be giving you a kiss (with however runny a nose) and calling you "Mama" and "Dada". The carefree shine of its eyes and the cheerfulness with which it approaches life will be a constant source of joy for you. Feel yourself swell with parental pride and enjoy every moment with your baby while it is small, because it will grow, and the worries will grow with it. The last teething pain will be replaced by attacks of rage, followed by all kinds of kindergarten and school stories; you'll hardly notice the transition to the pre-adolescent phase and finally your big children, equipped with their newly earned driving licences, will be headed for adulthood.

But of one thing you can always be sure: Parenthood not only means a lot of responsibility but also, to an even greater degree, pride, joy and the unconditional love your child feels for you. There is absolutely no doubt in my mind: parents grow and mature through the challenges presented them by their children on a daily basis.

Among these challenges are the illnesses the children suffer. In addition to the wonderful possibilities of aroma therapy and the healing powers of herbs, homoeopathy is an outstanding holistic method of treatment which can also be employed by parents independently once they have learned enough about how it works. That, however, is the aim not of this book, but of my *The Homoeopathic Home and Travel Medicine Chest*. I moreover offer regular seminars in Kempten, not only on aroma therapy and herbal medicine, but also on homoeopathy. But perhaps my homoeopathy booklet and the manual *Aroma Therapy from Pregnancy to Breastfeeding* will provide you with enough orientation on their own. The publication of further practical manuals on aroma therapy is planned to help you employ this excellent treatment method successfully when your child becomes ill.

Another highly recommendable book on all methods of homoeopathic treatment and the questions that come up in that context is *Homöopathie und die Gesunderhaltung unserer Kinder und Jugendlichen* by Dr. med. Friedrich Graf. There you can also read more on the topics of vitamin K and vitamin D prophylaxis as well as on the ins and outs of vaccinations. In this connection, it is important for me to point out that the fluoride prophylaxis was discontinued in the U.S. in the late 1990s. On the subject of vitamin D, you should know that there is no such prophylaxis in the Scandinavian countries. There people are still taking cod liver oil in the winter as they have done for ages. If you decide against administering vitamin D, you should inform your paediatrician of this fact. I know that many women shy away from doing so, but otherwise the medical profession will never find out that, even though the pills have been prescribed and duly fetched from the chemist, they are often not actually given to the children – whether because the mother simply forgets to administer them or because she has an aversion to the idea of giving a baby pills on a daily basis. I can well understand their point of view, because today it's vitamin D, tomorrow painkillers and maybe sooner or later Ecstasy. Scientists agree that, due to the sufficient administration of vitamin D, rachitis, or rickets, has become a thing of the past, but I nevertheless wanted to tell you my views on the subject. Incidentally, vitamin D is a substance which makes its way into the breast milk. Take it yourself as long as you breastfeed, because it is much easier for you to recognize the possible side effects in your own body than in that of your child.

I don't want to discuss the topic of prophylaxes in any greater depth here, however, because that would exceed the scope of this book. Obviously, we midwives are obliged to be well informed on these issues, because we are often asked to give advice on them during our house calls. In my responses to the parents, I discuss the matters from the point of view of conventional medicine as well as naturopathy. Ultimately the parents must decide what route they will take. Please remember one thing: Saying no to the vaccination means saying yes to the illness! Consider very carefully whether you feel prepared to cope with the illness and what doctor will support you in the process. Also take into account that vaccinations are not only a form of protection but can also be harmful. You can find out more about this subject through the media, particularly the Internet. Leave yourself plenty of time for all of these decisions; there really is no rush because these are decisions for an entire lifetime and cannot be reversed once they are made. With a sufficient amount of knowledge and information under your belt you can calmly and confidently embark on the first two years of your child's life.

THE BREASTFEEDING PERIOD

It was a long-deliberated decision on my part to discuss this topic on its own rather than in the sections on "The Postnatal Period" and the "Newborn". Breastfeeding is a subject the mother should already devote her attention to during pregnancy so as to be able to prepare well for the demands it will make on her. In my opinion, the mother should think of breastfeeding as her "profession" for the next several months. What that means, of course, is that she should be well informed and better "trained" than any nursery nurse or midwife. The topic of breastfeeding will not only preoccupy her during pregnancy and following childbirth. New questions and uncertainties will continue to come up throughout the breastfeeding period. Perhaps her child will be born too early and she will only realize several weeks following discharge from the hospital that she still has questions, for example concerning what is normal and what is out of the ordinary. The section below is intended to serve you as an initial reference work and also as a reminder that it can be very helpful to make contact with a midwife or the breastfeeding coordinator at the hospital.

For us midwives, breastfeeding represents an important informational obligation during our clients' pregnancies. Expectant mothers frequently come to the midwife's practice to obtain information and advice to ensure that, "this time around", everything will go more smoothly. During the postnatal period, during the daily house calls, whether the child was born at home or in the hospital: advice on breastfeeding is often the top priority. Women who have had children before can discover the same uncertainties as those who have just had their first baby. Even months after childbirth, many mothers still come to the midwife's practice or breastfeeding group to get answers to various questions. I frequently advise women to attend breastfeeding groups for a while – an ideal setting in which to learn from one another's experience. But if group talks and like-minded women don't help, or if a pathological problem arises, it is not at all unusual for a mother with a seven-month-old baby to request that the midwife pay her a house call. Fortunately, doctors have begun to send women with breastfeeding problems to midwives more and more often – after all, midwives are the experts when it comes to treating a blocked milk duct and getting the milk to flow again. In Germany, this service is covered by the public health plans – and I hope that will continue to be the case in the future.

As in the other sections in this book, I will try to provide useful pointers and pass on my midwife's experience to my readers. My views may not always conform to those held by the women responsible for breastfeeding issues in the hospitals: I have occasionally found that their statements are quite theoretical and do not always jibe with reality. A lot of the advice they give, for example, is difficult to put into practice in a family with several children. Not only that, but there are also mothers who already have gathered quite a bit of experience themselves, which naturally must be respected. Individuality shouldn't be the price for all those new findings and breastfeeding guidelines. Guidelines are necessary, of course, but deviations from them in all directions should be allowed. Life is not a straight line but proceeds with ups and downs, quite in keeping with the basic law of polarity. Every woman who has more than one child, for example, can confirm that the experience she gained with one child can be thrown overboard lock, stock and barrel when the next baby comes along. In the following section I would like to relay to fellow midwives and mothers in all directions the fruits of my many years of professional practice as a way of helping them through the unique breastfeeding period with joy and success.

I acquired most of my knowledge while caring for mothers and during my own breastfeeding periods. I would like to take this opportunity to express my gratitude to the breastfeeding group leaders who helped me so much while I was going through these phases myself. Just as they did, I would now like to share my experience with other women so that they are truly well informed – and accordingly independent as mothers.

The Prerequisites for Successful Breastfeeding

Conviction is Everything

A mother should be convinced of the rationale and benefits of breastfeeding. On the basis of my experience as a midwife, I can report that 99% of all women are capable of breastfeeding. Only comprehensive information, however, will enable them to breastfeed for a long period and not give up after the first rueful attempt. The mother should not go about it with the attitude: "OK, I'll give it a try if you (girlfriend, husband, midwife, doctor) think it's so great", or just because breastfeeding is 'in' these days. Every woman should know that breast milk provides her child with the best possible nutrition. There is not a single brand of industrially manufactured infant formula which really corresponds to the composition of breast milk. Infant formula is never more than a substitute based on cow, mare or soy milk. Our newborns, however, require human milk. This is the only milk that contains the antibodies they need to protect them from illness during the first months of life.

In my view, a mother can be confident in her ability to breastfeed her child for at least eight weeks and, naturally, much longer, if she is adequately informed. The first thing she should know is that, as I just explained, during the first weeks the mother's milk is the sole source of the immunoglobulins (IGMs) which are so important for the baby's immune system. In the antenatal classes the parents – i.e. the fathers as well as the mothers – have to be enlightened comprehensively about these fundamental aspects of breastfeeding during the first weeks of the child's life. The aim is not to talk the expectant mother into something – that would only cause breastfeeding problems anyway, because her body would not cooperate for very long if it was being forced to do something the woman didn't want to do: on the contrary, it would react with physical symptoms of one kind or another. Whether or not you are ultimately satisfied with several weeks or, like countless women, nurse your child for months, is initially neither here nor there. Emancipate yourself from time pressure and the pressure to perform; you know only too well: first of all things don't always happen, second of all the way you expect, but, third of all, the way the baby wants them to! The first thing you have to do is begin breastfeeding, and then life will decide how long you can and want to breastfeed – and how long the baby wants to be nursed. In many publications on this subject, the mother's resolutions are discussed, but in reality the infant also has something to say about the matter.

I have known families in which the children were breastfed for months, even as much as a year or longer, and child "no. 8" suddenly refused to follow suit. It categorically rejected the breast! The mother, herself a breastfeeding counsellor, was accordingly at her wit's end, but ultimately had to accept the fact that knowledge is one thing, the child another! Never try to force it! Set your sights on getting through the first eight to twelve weeks successfully and accept all of the ups and downs you experience. After that, things will go like clockwork. It really is true that the breastfeeding crises occur primarily during these initial weeks. The child grows, gains weight, and simply wants more to eat, which means more frequent breastfeeding until the balance between supply and demand has once again been found. It is during this very period that the mother's hormone cycle readjusts. I call this phase the battle of the hormones: which will prevail, the oestrogen, which is trying to usher in a regular menstrual cycle and renewed fertility, or the breastfeeding hormone prolactin, which is responsible for lactation and, during the breastfeeding period, almost has a right to victory on the hormone battlefield. The influence of oestrogen is detectable in the increased desire for sexuality, pangs in the lower abdomen when the ovaries become active again, perhaps even the first menstruation. According to scientific theory, the latter is actually to be regarded a pathological occurrence because when a woman breastfeeds regularly every four hours an increase of oestrogen is impossible. But textbooks and reality are often two different things! I have attended to women who menstruated throughout the entire breastfeeding period, and women who did not have their periods for as long as two years after the birth of their child. Please be advised that breastfeeding is not a reliable form of birth control. Moreover, there are babies who actually start sleeping five to seven hours at a stretch during the night, and an interval of that length suffices for the hormone system to bring about a regular menstrual cycle once again. It is important to breastfeed regularly during this phase so as to support the prolactin, i.e. to activate the breasts as often as possible. When the child wants to drink frequently, it's wonderful! Even if the relatives are worried the baby is being spoiled, hang in there – during menstruation, put the child to the breast as often as possible and you will see that the breastfeeding hormone will prevail.

Do not regard breastfeeding as a must, even if the World Health Organization justifiably recommends a nursing period of six months. See it instead as a gift and a pleasurable, unique experience with this particular child. Enjoy breastfeeding for as long as possible, because there are babies who start wanting to try something from your dinner plate at the tender age of three to four months, while others are still adamantly refusing solid food in the ninth month. Children do not always conform to the descriptions found in books!

Allergies and Breastfeeding

Many people are of the opinion that there is a connection between the enormous increase in allergies and the decrease in the number of mothers who breastfed their children in the 1960s and 1970s. The mothers of many children afflicted with eczema are of a generation in which babies were fed exclusively infant formula from birth. Back then, these products corresponded even less to human breast milk than they do today. Unfortunately however, these insights now cause mothers who suffer from allergies to put themselves under massive pressure to breastfeed their children for six months, whatever the cost. Already this pressure alone often seems to me to be the cause of problems that arise in connection with breastfeeding. It simply must not be forgotten that mental attitude has a substantial influence on the human hormone system; worry and anxiety eat away at the soul! And a mother who is anxious or under pressure to perform will have a high adrenalin level which will interfere drastically with the interplay of hormones and neurotransmitters such as serotonin, oxytocin and endorphin so important for breastfeeding, leading in turn a low level of prolactin or delaying its secretion. Moreover, I would also like to point out that the absence of breast milk is not the sole cause of allergies; environmental toxins and, even more importantly, vaccinations also play a role. The pharmaceutical industry has a huge interest in vaccinations, and can perhaps even be considered the "chief producer" of allergies. People who speak out against vaccination are nevertheless ignored and branded as irresponsible. What is important for me in the context of this book is that not all of the blame be dumped on the mothers, but that the fathers and men in our society also learn something on the subject of allergies. For as many as four generations now, our genes have been burdened with wide range of preservatives and environmental toxins. This is to say nothing of the fact that many mothers these days were not breastfed themselves and at the same time were given the complete range of vaccinations – with the consequence that their children can no longer receive full protection from their mothers' milk! Ask your midwife to recommend you good literature on the pros and cons of vaccinations.

I would like to advise all mothers who suffer from allergies not to put themselves under any pressure whatsoever. This advice is particularly difficult to follow during the postnatal period. Try to protect yourself from the feeling that everyone around you is worrying about whether the "poor child" of a mother with allergies is getting enough breast milk. Don't subject yourself to too much of these well-meaning but entirely unhelpful concerns; enjoy motherhood to the fullest, enjoy parenthood with your partner and avoid every form of stress, because adrenalin and cortisol inhibit both prolactin and the immune system.

False Information/The Partner/The Family Situation

As a mother you should always critically question discouraging accounts of negative breastfeeding experiences and people who advise you against nursing your child. Remember that these stories and opinions are often rooted in a negative experience the respective person has had herself. In the context of my advisory activities, I frequently discover that a serious problem lies at the root of a woman's supposed inability to breastfeed. Usually she has received false information, or has false conceptions about breastfeeding, about the limitations it places on the mother's body and the supposed irreversible changes breastfeeding subjects the body to. Problems between the woman and her partner and difficulties a mother has in accepting herself as a woman are the most frequent causes of this inability to breastfeed. There are still men and women who have sexual motives for rejecting breastfeeding. Even if it is often not done consciously, the male partners exert a lot of influence on their partners when they say things like: "Now her breasts belong completely to the child. My wife is no longer anything but two milk-producing breasts; she's totally forgotten everything else!" Many mothers are strongly – and negatively – influenced by jealous husbands in their attitude towards breastfeeding. In the past few years, the general opinion has finally changed somewhat in favour of breastfeeding, and a woman who nurses her child doesn't have to withdraw from society anymore. But many women are negatively influenced in their own homes, above all by their partners, whether in connection with their sexual relationship or their cooperation as parents. In this context it is important to know that, as soon as the postnatal phase is over and the hormone system has become readjusted, women take pleasure in sexuality and experience sexual desire regardless of whether or not they breastfeed (also see the section on "Sexuality after Childbirth" on pages 427 f.).

The breasts of a woman who is breastfeeding her child must not be treated as a taboo zone by her partner during lovemaking. Both partners will notice a new emotional sensitivity in their relationship.

Girlfriends and grandmothers cause women quite a bit of uncertainty with remarks like: "What, you really want to nurse? It didn't work with me. I can hardly imagine you breastfeeding either. Of course it's your decision, but I think you should save yourself the trouble and forget about the whole messy business."

I advise all expectant or new mothers to ignore comments of this sort, or react the way Marion did …

… "I'm going to show my mother and my sister that I certainly am capable of breastfeeding a child, even if both of them claim that the women in our family aren't 'milk mothers'." She really did have quite a struggle, and it took a lot of effort, staying power and encouragement from me for her to be

able to breastfeed her child fully. One day the grandmother – who was now proud of her daughter for nursing her baby – remarked to me admiringly: "It's all thanks to you that a woman from our clan is able to breastfeed; my midwife and the one who took care of my daughter weren't that persistent." I was grateful for this recognition, especially since the hours and hours of advice and aid for the young mother with her inverted nipples could never have been paid for, least of all by the health plan. But recognition is one of the mainstays of our profession, and praise of that kind does us no end of good.

The Nursing Bra

Many a woman shies away from the thought that she won't be able to go without a nursing bra for months to come, although she perhaps never wore a bra before. The widespread opinion that a nursing bra is absolutely essential could hardly be further from the truth. Every woman can and should decide for herself whether she wants to wear a nursing bra or not. Not even a doctor has any business telling a woman it's high time she started wearing a bra.

Many women feel they need the support a bra offers; others feel confined and handicapped by it. In the case of breasts from which the milk tends to flow out between and/or before breastfeeding sessions, the young mother will look for a means of keeping the absorbent breast pads from slipping, but a camisole will serve this purpose equally well. Many women wear a bra during the first four to eight weeks; after that, habits change again. The breastfeeding mother will decide on her own whether she can do without her "armour" at least at night. She takes it in stride that she is likely to wake up somewhat milk-soaked, or, contrary to expectations, nice and dry. The woman's partner might also try to encourage his wife to try sleeping without the bra. But be careful: she may interpret this remark as an expression of sexual expectations and she herself may not be ready yet!

Changes in the Breasts

Every woman should know that her breasts will change on account of the hormonal adjustment, but not merely because of breastfeeding.

During the first few days after childbirth, the breasts will become fuller and fuller and a feeling of tautness will soon develop. This initial swelling and sensitivity is quite similar to what women experience at the beginning of pregnancy or in conjunction with ovulation.

But already on about Day Three, when the milk "comes in", the breasts can become firm, lumpy, even hard, and in many cases painful. The term "initial engorgement" means that the breasts are beginning to fill up with milk. By around the sixth day after birth, the woman will experience an unpleasant tension only shortly before she puts her child to the breast. And those who do not breastfeed according to a fixed schedule but simply according to need won't become acquainted with this tension at all.

For the first several weeks, until about the end of the postnatal period, breasts which produce milk are uncommonly beautiful, and most women – certainly along with their partners – are proud of them. One morning in the hospital room, a woman remarked: "They're gorgeous! I wish my breasts could stay this way!" Her roommate, on the other hand, said: "I don't know; I can't really get used to my humongous bust. When I was pregnant, I couldn't see past my belly to my pubic hair, and now, thanks to my "balcony", I can't even see my belly anymore." Wait and see how your breasts change and gather your own experience. You are likely to determine soon that your breasts fill up and become a bit tight shortly before the baby wants to be fed. It can also happen that you don't feel the tingling sensation of the "engorgement" until the baby begins drinking. In many cases, a woman need only think about her baby and her nipples will begin dripping, and especially when the baby cries her breasts will fill with milk and milk spots will appear on her blouse. You will quickly become accustomed to this "leaking", however. You can cope with the situation best by wearing easy-to-launder clothing and absorbent breast pads.

By the end of the late postnatal period at the latest, and frequently as early as the end of the second week, the breasts will soften again and return to their normal size. Like all women, you will think to yourself: "If I didn't hear my baby swallowing and see the milk in the corners of its mouth and feel the steadily increasing weight on my arm while it is drinking, I would think the poor child was starving: that's how small my breasts have gotten again." It's high time we stopped judging a nursing woman by the size of her breasts. All that really matters is that the milk production is activated the moment she puts the baby to the breast. It is not the form and size of the breasts but the lactation glands which are of decisive importance for the production of milk.

I can furthermore reassure you that, after you have weaned your child, there will be more left to your breasts than limp pouches of skin, a rumour still unfortunately making the rounds. Naturally, the mother of a child who has been breastfed exclusively for eight months can't be expected to have breasts as bouncy and firm as those of a young woman. But it is simply not true that a woman breastfeeds at the cost of her feminine beauty. The breasts will be softer and perhaps hang down a bit more than they used to, perhaps even be a bit smaller than before, but with exercises of the upper torso and breast muscles – part of the postnatal gymnastic programme, incidentally – the breasts will firm up again. After the breastfeeding period is over, a lot can be achieved by massaging the breasts with the *Original 𝔇® Aroma Blend Brustmassageöl/Breast Massage Oil 𝔇®*, containing the essential oils of Angelica root and rose geranium, among others. For the partner, a massage can be a wonderful way of rediscovering his wife's breasts. So don't hang your head and your breasts when the breastfeeding period is over, but straighten up your breastbone while you're still breastfeeding and, later on, care for your breasts and "work" them. As one reader informed me, *Brustmassageöl/Breast Massage Oil D®* can even make stretch marks on the tummy and thighs disappear again.

One thing is certain in any case, and applies not only during pregnancy and childbirth: Other people, your partner included, will only like you as much as you like yourself. If a person doesn't love him/herself, he/she is not loved by others! After the birth of a child, learn to look at yourself in the mirror and to accept yourself as a mother in all your roundness and softness. Children don't like sharp-boned mothers! A mum is for cuddling up to and leaning on, and a soft tummy and breast are the most important prerequisites for that function.

Being a Breastfeeding Mother

It takes a considerable amount of self-confidence and healthy trust in Mother Nature to be convinced that you are a good breastfeeding mother. Nature knows women are strong enough to bear children and children are strong enough to endure natural childbirth, and she also saw to it that the children can be fed by their mothers. You can rest assured that the composition of the breast milk will always correspond to your child's individual needs. It will always have the right temperature and be available in plenty night and day. As a mother, learn to defend yourself and your child and don't allow well-meaning questions from relatives or friends – for example: "You really think the baby is getting enough from that thin, watery milk?" – to unsettle you. And don't let yourself be talked out of breastfeeding by a paediatrician who advises you to stop because the baby has gained fifty grams/two ounces to little. Stick up for the optimal form of nutrition for your child; show your teeth and growl like a lion mother, because you will soon ascertain that your instinct is leading you in the right direction. The principle of allowing yourself to be guided by your feelings applies not only during pregnancy and childbirth, but, more than ever, also once you have become a mother. And in many respects, motherhood starts during the breastfeeding period.

Be convinced of yourself and your actions and remain true to the thought that breastfeeding is the best and only right thing for your child. At the same time, however, inform yourself about the most natural thing in the world by asking your midwife or a breastfeeding counsellor. Remember that many women have lost precisely this normal, natural aspect of life because it is no longer passed down from generation to generation within the family.

Outer Peace and Quiet

Along with the will to breastfeed, the second of the three main prerequisites for success in this endeavour is: peace and quiet! What I mean by this, first of all, is a peaceful and quiet environment. It should be completely accepted by everyone around that, in the presence of a breastfeeding woman, no loud discussions are conducted, no radios or televisions are blaring and no cell phones are constantly ringing. As I have been happy to note, I am not the only midwife who refuses to conduct a postnatal house call or give advice on the breastfeeding position when there's a television on in the room. Particularly during the entire postnatal period, it is essential that the mother's surroundings are quiet. She should be able to devote herself entirely to the job of breastfeeding. In my experience, the older children never really have to be told to hush, because they generally gaze at a breastfeeding mother with widened eyes and a tangible sense of awe. I often have the impression that adults, on the other hand, have no idea how to behave in this situation. Either they ignore the breastfeeding procedure entirely and cheerfully start a conversation or, worse still, they make jokes about it as a way of covering up their inhibitions. As incredible as it seems, the following is a true story …

… the newborn had to stay in the hospital under constant observation. It had cost the mother a great amount of effort to persuade the hospital staff to allow her to breastfeed her child, or at least to try. After a tense fifteen minutes, she had finally succeeded in getting the baby to suckle at her breast. Right at that very moment, she was told: "Please go and sit over there on the other chair; we need this chair immediately!" A workman needed a chair in order to change a light bulb. I have nothing against doing work that has to be done, but was it really necessary to bother this mother, of all people? By the way, after that interruption, the baby refused to be put to the breast again; the meal was over.

Inner Peace and Quiet

For successful nursing, a factor even more decisive than quiet surroundings is a calm and relaxed mother. If all she has besides conviction is a lot of textbook knowledge, it won't suffice, and the midwives and baby nurses will groan: "another one of those mothers who thinks she can breastfeed just because she's read a lot about it". But with the addition of a further ingredient – a sense of inner calm – the mother can peacefully watch her baby suckling. She has organized and delegated the necessary household tasks and left the responsibility for the business phone to the answering machine. The older children are in the capable hands of a babysitter, and the mother can patiently wait for the baby to find the nipple, latch onto it properly with its mouth and begin to suckle. The mother can relax when she puts her baby to her breast and doesn't have to worry about whether her newborn should be drinking 90 ml/3.2 fl. oz. or 110 ml/3.9 fl. oz. of breast milk. She is well informed and knows that what really matters is not the actual amount but whether or not the baby drinks its fill. When all of these conditions have been met, the mother will be able to relax. And if she then also allows her breath to flow freely, the breast milk will likewise flow freely and abundantly. In other words, a mother should not be constantly subjected to nonsensical or unnecessary demands for which the postnatal bed is not the place. She should be in a position to remain calm on the firm foundation she has built for herself with her preparations, which include her conviction that Mother Nature will not allow her child to go hungry.

I have no doubt that if you have prepared for the postnatal period as recommended in this book, you will have the necessary inner and outer peace and quiet and will have no major breastfeeding problems.

All too often, however, I find that parents don't really understand the necessity of following well-meant words of advice concerning preparations for the postnatal period in general and breastfeeding in particular. This can lead to a situation like the one Andrea experienced …

… she had given birth to her second child at home and everything had gone well; the parents felt as if hey were in seventh heaven. Already on the second day, things were almost back to normal; the mother was lying in bed, but she felt responsible for her older daughter, who was two at the time. The mother was surrounded by toys and picture books, and, armed with a bottle; the little girl also took her nap in mum's bed. This state of affairs is actually not unusual during the postnatal period. But somehow it seemed to me that the mother paid more attention to the older child with every day that passed. Andrea got up to look for her daughter's slippers, gave the help complete instructions as to what needed to be done in the household and complained that her partner was already devoting himself entirely to his work again. She put the older girl to bed at night and in her (overly?) maternal manner she saw to everything having to do with the household and the children. She "merely" gave directions, but nevertheless, all in all it was too much. It wasn't long before I arrived to find her with tears running down her cheeks because the newborn refused to suckle. It took the baby at least ten minutes before it would latch onto the well-filled breast, and then it would take its time, drinking pleasurably for at least half an hour. She was at her wit's end: "This time I'm producing plenty of milk and I'm entirely confident that the baby is getting enough; what is more, it's putting on weight. But it makes such a fuss; my daughter also keeps asking why the little tyke always cries so much and takes so long to find my nipple and start drinking. What am I going to do, how will things be when my help stops coming and more people stop in to visit?" We had a long talk in which it became clear that, with its behaviour, the baby was asking for more attention, because if it merely latched onto the nipple and got the job done quickly, its presence would presumably not even be noticed and the mother would have long since left her postnatal bed. The mother realized that she was expecting too much of herself and, more than anything, longed to have her husband at her side and be alone with him. We decided that now she would devote herself entirely to her newborn. We arranged that the older child would go and stay with an aunt and the grandmother would turn all importunate visitors away. I explained to the father that a lot of the work he was doing could probably wait for the time being and he would be well-advised to experience the postnatal period with his wife because, while there is always more work, but you can never make up for missing the postnatal phase.

When I arrived the next day I found the mother in her nightgown, her husband at her bedside, both of them beaming and happy. The "big" girl had cheerfully gone to her aunt's house, Grandma was presiding over the kitchen and the visitors, and it was impossible for anyone to cross the threshold without being informed that there was a postnatal mother in the house. And to top it off, the mother laughed and remarked: "My little one still takes its time finding the nipple, but now we both enjoy the procedure. It's true; otherwise I really would have a baby that did nothing but sleep. Thanks for getting us on the right track."

Staying Power

Another factor needed for successful breastfeeding in addition to conviction and calmness is persistence. Often this quality is required right at the beginning because now and then there really are babies who can virtually only be "tricked" into suckling at the breast, no matter how many nursing books say that all you have to do is stroke the baby's cheek and it will turn its head to the mother's breast, latch on to her nipple and drink. In reality, there are children who don't seem to be aware of this procedure because it simply refuses to suckle just because the mother or the baby nurse or the midwife wants it to. With patience, however, the day will come when the mother is able to breastfeed her child without assistance.

Many a new mother has to wait ages for lactation to begin in earnest. Instead of the frequently cited two to three days after the birth, it can sometimes take five days until the tension in the breasts is finally felt.

You will have to exhibit another form of patience when the baby suckles for half an hour instead of the five to ten minutes per breast promised by the books. Many babies simply cannot drink their fill that quickly! As if that were not enough, it might then take the child another half an hour until it finally burps. And finally, it may turn out to be the kind of baby who wants to be carried around for a while before dropping off to sleep.

Patience will be required to get through the period of hormonal readjustment which is frequently accompanied by a shortage of milk requiring the mother to put the baby to her breast often. Staying power will be needed to nurse a sick baby every hour because swallowing causes it pain. And it can also demand a lot of effort on the part of the mother to explain to those around her why she is feeding her child exclusively with breast milk, and that it will not go hungry as a result.

Persistence, staying power and the patience to sit and wait – these are qualities demanded of women in connection with becoming and being a mother. It starts with a girl's longing for her first period, followed later on, when she is a woman, by the desire to have a child and the longing not to have her period. The beginning of pregnancy demands the patience it takes to endure the nausea, and the hopeful waiting to feel the child moving inside her. A certain amount of persistence is required to live through the forty weeks of pregnancy and wait patiently for labour to begin. And in many cases, quite a bit more of the same is needed to get through the hours of labour. As described in the present section of my book, there is no end to the tests of a mother's patience presented her by the breastfeeding period. But that's not the end of it. As the child grows, patience and staying power will be required of the parents again and again. If all goes well, the day will come when they can say: "Our persistence paid off;

now our child is big and on the way to becoming independent. What are a few years of waiting in comparison to a whole life?"

I would like to encourage you and help you to develop these qualities right from the start of your life with your child. It will be worth all the effort you put into it, because this intimate connection is absolutely unique and can never be made up for later. And when the child is older and goes through illnesses and difficult adolescent phases, you will remember that persistence and patience already proved their worth once before. Nothing you experience in your life with your child will be for nought, even if it takes time. Many people these days are unfortunately of the opinion that they don't have time. With your child, you will learn to have time and be patient all over again. In later years, the memory of the breastfeeding phase will be a happy one. Don't allow yourself to be robbed of this experience. A wonderful task is waiting for you, a task that will give you great satisfaction and confirmation.

The Wonderful "Business" of Breastfeeding

Perhaps the last few pages have left you with the impression that breastfeeding is extremely difficult – and less confident than ever of your ability to box your way through all of these difficulties. I would therefore now like to tell you a lot of very positive things about breastfeeding.

It is a phase which belongs entirely to you. In later years, you will think back to these moments of togetherness again and again. You will perhaps never again gaze so deeply and lovingly into your child's eyes. Look into your baby's eyes and you will realize that the two of you have built up a little world around you in which no-one can disturb you.

There are so many practical aspects about nourishing your child with breast milk that you won't fully appreciate them until the weaning process is over. Already for this reason alone, many women have much regretted not having been better informed about the advantages of breast milk: the mother's milk always has the right temperature, will never be too cold in winter, will never be able to spoil. You don't have to rush out shopping before the stores close because you discover you are out of infant formula. You won't have to curse another rise in the price of the formula. You can go to parties and take long hikes with your breastfed baby. Holidays are wonderful, because your baby doesn't have to adjust to different water and different food. The only thing you'll have to think of is the nappies, and since they will be made of cloth (at least if I have managed to convince you not to use disposables!), there will likewise be no problem, since water, laundry soap, air and sunshine are available all over the world.

You will be aware that, as long as you breastfeed, your baby will be well protected against illness, and as soon as you start supplementing its diet with infant formula it will come down with its first case of the sniffles.

In my mind there are lots of pros to breastfeeding, and not one of the cons is strong enough to convince a woman not to breastfeed. I wouldn't want to miss a single day of my own breastfeeding periods; on the contrary, today I would nurse my children with all the more conviction and confidence in light of all the experience I have gained in the meantime. It is my great wish that, with my knowledge and my experience, I will enable you to have a positive and wonderful breastfeeding experience yourself.

Following the preparatory talks in the group, a dear colleague of mine who was expecting a baby remarked to me: "It won't really be such a problem, will it?" I responded to her by saying: "At the beginning it will be something of a 'G'schäft' [literally: 'business', Allgaeu dialect for hard work], but once the initial difficulties are overcome it's fun." The very next day, this same colleague was a mother, and we both laughed when she put her baby to her breast. "You're right, it is something of a 'G'schäft', breastfeeding." And several weeks later, the beaming, breastfeeding midwife confirmed to me: "Inge, this is the most wonderful 'G'schäft' I've ever experienced."

Practical Information on Breastfeeding

The First Time

If at all possible, the baby should be put to the mother's breast immediately after its birth, while the two of them are still in the birthing bed. Most newborns exhibit an extremely well-developed sucking reflex during the first hour of life outside the womb. In nearly all hospitals, midwives will see to it that women can put their babies to their breasts and assist them in doing so. Incidentally, this is also possible after a caesarean.

Putting the Child to the Breast/The Breastfeeding Position

Another prerequisite for successful breastfeeding is a relaxed position. Initially, the mother should lie in bed, on her side, so as not to put a strain on the pelvic floor and the wounds that may have come about during childbirth. She should brace both her back and her head with cushions so as to be able to relax in this position, because the milk will not flow properly otherwise. If the baby is put to the breast when it cries, and if it moreover exhibits a clear sucking urge by sucking on its fingers or making sucking motions with its mouth, it will find the breast of its own accord. If the mother attempts to nurse her baby at a previously established point in time, on the other hand, she may well run into problems. I have rarely encountered any major obstacles to breastfeeding or difficulties in getting started when the baby is at home where it can determine its own sucking and sleeping phases. I nevertheless advise mothers to be well informed about the various positions for breastfeeding. But please, don't treat yourself and your baby like a machine! Remain calm, remember your conviction and don't give up! It will work.

Try to have your baby lying next to you in such a way that you can hold it firmly to your body and your breast with your lower arm. See to it that the child's tummy is facing yours; i.e. it should not be lying next to you on its back and merely turning its head towards you. That would be like sitting sideways at the dinner table and merely turning your head towards your plate. If you try that out sometime, you will immediately notice the twisted position of your body and you will furthermore be able to imagine that it is not good for the nipples to be made use of so one-sidedly. This "latching-on" error is one of the mistakes most frequently made in the breastfeeding context. On the other hand, be careful not to press the child to your body or even hold it too firmly, because it may well feel confined and try to defend itself by crying. Before you offer the child your breast, stimulate the nipple to make it hard and erect; the baby will be able to latch onto it much more easily as a result, and will automatically take a sufficient amount of the areola into its mouth. Now use the hand opposite the child to offer it your breast. Hold your breast in such a way that it is nestled between your thumb on one side and your fingers on the other, and stretch the surface of the skin slightly by pulling your hand gently towards your ribcage, i.e. away from the child. Doing so is certain to get the nipple sufficiently erect. By applying slight pressure to the breast – as though you wanted to feel your fingers with your thumb – you will aid the baby in bringing about the "let-down" or milk ejection reflex. In the further course of the section on breastfeeding, I will refer to this way of holding the breast as the "pressure grip". This milking motion – often erroneously described as a stroking motion – gets the milk flowing more easily and more quickly. And the "pressure grip" is particularly advantageous in cases of children who have trouble with suckling or breasts quite swollen with milk, because in both cases the baby can't get a proper grasp on the nipple or enough of the areola between its jaws to stimulate lactation. Often it simply doesn't put enough energy into sucking. Once the milk is flowing and the baby is drinking properly, however, you must release the pressure immediately, because otherwise your child will have the feeling of drowning in milk. Towards the end of the feeding session at one breast it can be helpful to apply the pressure grip once again to squirt a bit of milk into the baby's mouth as a way of showing it that it would be worth its while to take another good pull since the breast is not completely empty yet. In this way you can help to ensure that at least the first breast offered is really emptied completely.

This "technique" may appear a bit complicated in the written description of it, but don't worry, you'll soon master it. And besides, you are sure to find an experienced mother who can give you a pointer or two. It doesn't always have to be the nurse or midwife, both of whom may shy away from touching your breast. A close girlfriend – a "bosom buddy" in the truest sense of the word – who has breastfed children herself, often has more time and more experience and is more relaxed to boot.

Many a woman is afraid her baby could smother if its nose is pressed too firmly against her breast – another piece of information which is still circulating even though it is complete nonsense. Before a child suffocates at its mother's breast it will be intelligent enough to let go of the nipple and pull its head away. Or it will kick and writhe as a way of demanding that its mother change position.

After several days, you will prefer to breastfeed in a sitting position. Again, what matters most is that you are relaxed. Remember: inner and outer peace and quiet. Pay attention to your position, relax your shoulders, have something to rest your lower arms on, and a stool for your feet. One of the first tasks during the midwife's initial house calls is to remind the breastfeeding mother to relax. If she doesn't have a stool, we just improvise, using the nearest armchair, the edge of the table, a pile of old books or a beer crate as a footrest. However you manage it, make sure you can put both feet on the floor or on some type of footrest. This applies not only to the tips of your toes but to the whole foot. Sit in such a way that, by adding the necessary number of cushions, the child can lie on your thighs. As soon as you have the feeling of having to hold your child's weight with your arm, tensing up your shoulder muscles in the process, or of having to bend forward to take the burden off your arms, it means you haven't bolstered yourself properly. All partners are hereby called upon to check the mother's "working position" and correct it, if necessary, by adding more cushions. Physical tension during breastfeeding can lead to sore muscles. But if you sit in an upright but relaxed position, you can breastfeed for months without any physical discomfort.

The Duration of the Breastfeeding Session/Changing Sides

During the first forty-eight hours, newborns are rarely interested in suckling for any great length of time, and their tendency to tire easily can last for several days. Five to ten minutes at each breast accordingly suffice. You will hear a lot of conflicting information about this aspect but, as mentioned previously, your child will let you know what it needs. When it stops actually drinking and just sucks at your nipple playfully – the way it may well have done in the womb with its fingers for hours at a time – you should remove it from your breast after five minutes, as hard as it might be for you. Many problems with sore nipples already start on the birthing bed.

If it's your first child …

… it is advisable to begin by always offering both breasts at every meal. Change breasts after the above-mentioned five to ten-minute period and lengthen the duration every day until, beginning with the initial engorgement, the child can decide for itself how long it drinks at each breast.

You will find that the amount of time spent at each breast averages off to about twenty to thirty minutes. A robust newborn who drinks quickly may even empty one breast within about ten minutes. Here I would like to quote a colleague of mine who drew a nice comparison: "A lactating breast is not a bottle! So there's never really 'bottle empty!' Milk is produced continually; it's just that it doesn't always flow in abundance."

If the child is one of the type who drink slowly and pleasurably, the procedure will take longer. Be aware of the fact that, for the time being, a newborn's purpose in life is to suckle at the breast. It is seeking to satisfy not only its hunger there, but also its sucking urge, and the two tasks together take at least thirty to forty-five minutes per meal. Moreover, after a short break and a breather, it will tend to empty the second breast more thoroughly than it did the first.

During the first few days it is advisable to change to the second breast after about ten minutes, so that the latter is also "emptied". The baby can stay at the second breast until its needs are satisfied.

At the next meal, you should begin with the breast you ended with last time around. That way, the mammary glands in both breasts will be stimulated – and both breasts will be emptied – alternately. If you have trouble remembering which breast to start with, tie a little ribbon to the strap of your nursing bra or pin a pretty brooch to your nightgown. If you forget to give yourself that reminder, nothing much will happen. One look in the mirror, or even just the tension you feel in one breast and not the other, will tell you which side's "turn" it is.

Beginning on the day of initial engorgement, one breast per meal may well suffice. I highly recommend that you offer the first breast until it has become tangibly softer and empty. After changing the baby's nappies you can put it back to the same breast and then, if it is clearly still hungry, offer it the other breast. From now on, the length of time spent drinking will be determined by the baby itself, but you can still employ the above-described pressure grip to get it to empty the first breast. The reason for doing this is that changing sides too quickly may stimulate lactation unnecessarily.

Experienced Mothers

Mothers who have breastfed before will take the circumstances accompanying initial engorgement with her previous children, as well as the amount of milk she had then, as her orientation. If lactation didn't cause her any problems, and if she always had to let the child drink at both breasts, it will be advisable for her to proceed as described above.

However, if initial engorgement was very unpleasant and accompanied by an excess of milk, it is probably better to begin offering only one breast per meal beginning on Day Two at the latest. Perhaps you belong to the category of women who almost suffer from their overly abundant production of milk, i.e. whose babies didn't even drink half of the milk in one breast at every meal. In these cases I urgently recommend that, from the beginning, you offer the child only one breast per meal. You should also avoid breastfeeding too frequently during the first couple of days in the hope that this time your initial engorgement will be normal. On the fourth or fifth day, you will be able to determine whether one breast really is enough, or whether it is necessary to offer both after all. Your midwife will undoubtedly be able to give you the right advice. These are things I learned from mothers who had experience with excessive milk production and I am very grateful for this knowledge. Even if it is contrary to the guidelines generally given, in the care of mothers afflicted with this problem it has proven its value many times over! It just goes to show that practical experience is sometimes better than some scientific finding which says, for example, that in the first twenty-four hours after birth it is essential to breastfeed for altogether 110 to 120 minutes in order to stimulate all of the prolactin receptors and bring about lactation. This requirement is also met if the newborn is nursed altogether six times, for twenty minutes – but only at one breast – each time. But I have also witnessed situations in which the baby only wanted to be breastfed three times during the first twenty-four hours and then went on to be breastfed exclusively for a full year. Thanks to the children, there is simply no breastfeeding rule without an exception.

Taking the Child from the Breast

Babies almost always let go of the breast on their own when they have had their fill. But there are some who like to doze off with the nipple in their mouth. If a woman has irritated or sore nipples, however, it may be necessary for her to gently remove the child from her breast. Try sticking your little finger into one corner of the baby's mouth. This will interrupt the sucking process, and you can pull your nipple out of your child's mouth easily.

Burping

During the first few days – and from the time of the initial engorgement at the latest – it will already be necessary to get the baby to burp. The best method is to put your baby over your shoulder. You can help the child in what is sometimes a strenuous process by patting its back rhythmically between its shoulder blades with the hollow palm of your hand. Naturally, your baby may already burp while it is still at your breast, in between two gulps of milk, or when you turn it into an upright position immediately after breastfeeding. But there are also cases where patting the baby's back and stroking its head from back to front don't suffice, and it has to be carried around and gently bounced for ten minutes during a breastfeeding break before it finally burps and it can resume its meal. Children are just different. Incidentally, the fathers almost always take over on the "burping ritual" when they're home.

In many cases, the parents decide that it's ridiculous to wait around for ages for the baby to get rid of gas which it might not have in its tummy to begin with, and the mother puts it back to her breast. And, lo and behold, the baby falls asleep quite peacefully. Not all babies have to burp; it depends entirely on how they suckle. Children who drink greedily and hastily swallow a lot of air have to be "burped" to avoid wind and tummy ache. A child who drinks slowly, almost as if it was bored, calmly swallowing each individual gulp, may never have to burp at all.

The Composition of Breast Milk

100 ml/ 3.5 fl. oz. contain	Breast milk (BM)			Cow milk, fresh
	Colostrum	Transitional BM	Mature BM	
Protein (g)	2.7	1.6	1.2	3.3
Fat (g)	1.9	2.8	3.5	3.5
Carbohydrates (g) (Lactose)	6.5	7.0	4.8	
Mineral salts (g)	0.33	0.24	0.21	0.72
Calories (kcal)	65	70	70	66

(From: Das Hebammenbuch; Lehrbuch der praktischen Geburtshilfe; Mändle et al., Schattauer-Verlag)

Colostrum

From the first day until initial lactation, the breasts produce colostrum. Often no more than a few sticky yellow drops, this fluid contains twice as much protein as the mature milk produced later on. The proportion of fat is lower at first, and ultimately almost doubles, as can be seen in the table. In relation to the amount of fluid, the proportion of lactose is already high, but gets even higher in the course of the weeks that follow. Thus even if only a few drops are produced at a time, the baby will certainly be able to drink its fill and its little stomach can gradually become accustomed to the increasing amount of milk

Transitional Milk

This is the milk produced from the time of initial engorgement onward. Now it takes on the shade of an egg yolk, a clear sign that the proportion of fat is increasing rapidly so that the child can quickly compensate for its loss of weight. The percentage of protein sinks by about one third as the amount of fluid increases, and the lactose content rises. The milk newborns receive is decidedly sweet. Even in this transition phase, the milk now flows abundantly and provides for the baby's satiation and weight-gaining needs; it will normally keep this composition for about two weeks. Not infrequently, however, this transitory milk is produced for several weeks. Since the amount of milk does not increase, the proportion of protein likewise remains constant, and therefore even those newborns who – according to the table – should be drinking a lot more manage to gain weight.

Mature Breast Milk

From about the third to (at the latest) eighth week of life, the mother's mammary glands produce mature breast milk. This milk has a watery, bluish appearance. The protein content will decrease to about half of what it was in the colostrum, while the fat content is nearly double and the lactose has increased again. It is important to be careful with such generalizations, however, because the composition of breast milk will be determined to an extent by how much the baby drinks. The breasts of a woman whose baby drinks less frequently will produce more satiating milk than breasts at which a child wants to suckle constantly. The fat content of breast milk alone can fluctuate between 0.8% and 4.5%, as numerous studies have shown. The way the mother's body adjusts to the needs of the infant always has been and always will be a remarkable phenomenon.

Once these adaptation processes are clear to you, you will understand why industrially manufactured infant formula can never do justice to the individual needs of the child in the first weeks of life.

Initial Engorgement

The so-called initial engorgement of the breasts with milk takes place approximately between the third and fifth day of the postnatal period. This is the point at which milk production begins in earnest. In many cases, particularly when the mother is spending the postnatal phase in her own home, this much-feared day comes and goes without the slightest discomfort. There is no doubt in my mind that this is due to the holistic postnatal situation created in the home. Whether in the hospital or at home, the woman usually notices that her breasts swell, fill up and become taut. She has the urge to lie in bed with her arms crossed in front of her breasts to keep anything or anyone from touching them. Contact with the breast can be unpleasant or cause the milk to flow. Most mothers are happy if they are not greeted and embraced all too stormily by family members and visiting friends on this day.

The unpleasant side effects are usually over after a day or two. On the one hand the mother's body quickly adapts to the needs of the baby and produces only as much milk as necessary; on the other hand the mother has learned to handle her full breasts.

It does happen, however, that a woman will complain of difficulties putting her child to her breast and of pain during initial engorgement. This pain is caused by hard lumps and overheated breasts stretched to the very limits of their capacity. As mentioned above, this state of affairs usually comes about when the baby is fed by the clock and not according to its needs.

Reread the sections on "The Postnatal Period" and "The First Hours, Days and Weeks of Life", and maybe you will be able to avoid these discomforts for the most part.

Preventive Measures

The prerequisite for avoiding problems in conjunction with initial engorgement is undoubtedly breastfeeding according to demand. Moreover, the aspects described in the section on "The Duration of the Breastfeeding Session/Changing Sides" should also be taken into consideration. Think carefully about whether you really should always offer the child both breasts. Remember that every time the baby is put to the breast and suckles at it, lactation is stimulated all the more.

As soon as you notice a feeling of swelling and tension in your breasts, you should avoid drinking constantly yourself. Two litres/quarts of fluid per day is the norm! Be aware that the air in the hospital tends to be too dry, leading you to drink too much. Furthermore, you should now reduce your consumption of *Stilltee/Nursing Tea* partially or completely, because this blend promotes lactation. Be careful not to toast the birth with too many glasses of champagne, even if many hospitals recommend its enjoyment in moderation because it likewise stimulates lactation.

Before breastfeeding, it is advisable to massage the swollen breast (on the side to be offered to the child) gently with *Stillöl/Nursing Oil 𝒟®*, which will make the milk flow better.

⑤ Natural Measures to Take in Cases of Discomfort

Painful, swollen breasts and problems with an already **overabundant** flow of breast milk can be relieved by taking the following measures.

- Reduce your daily intake of fluid to a normal amount.
- Only offer the child one breast per meal.
- Before you breastfeed, get the flow of milk started in the breast you intend to offer by applying a warm compress to it and massaging it gently with *Stillöl/Nursing Oil 𝒟®*. It is also important to stimulate the nipple to make it erect so that the child can latch onto it well despite the bulging areola. It may be helpful to hand express a bit of milk at the start, a measure which will aid the child in drinking.
- While you breastfeed, cool the other breast with a cold pack or ice cubes wrapped up in a washcloth, to prevent it from producing even more milk. This instruction applies only if you offer the child one breast per meal. You can hold the ice pack to your breast by clamping it into your armpit.
- Cool both breasts after breastfeeding, preferably with a compress of cold quark to which two to three drops of *lavender extra* per breast have been added. To support the reduction of the milk with essential oils, it is advisable to mix the quark with *Salbei-Zypressen-Öl/Sage-Cypress Oil 𝒟®*, an *Original 𝒟® Aroma Blend* which contains mint and lemon in addition to sage and cypress. This oil should really only be used in cases of overly abundant lactation, because otherwise it may cause you to stop producing milk altogether! Also take into account that mint works as an antidote to homoeopathic medications, so if you are taking the latter you should not use the oil. My essential oil blend *Rosengeranie-Lavendel-Massageöl/Rose-Geranium-*

Lavender Massage Oil $\mathcal{D}$®, developed specifically for this purpose, has proven effective. After breastfeeding, and even when the baby is taking a short breastfeeding break before drinking again, carefully apply the oil to your breasts, or mix three to five drops of *Rosengeranie-Lavendel-Öl/Rose-Geranium-Lavender Oil $\mathcal{D}$®* into about three spoonfuls of quark and spread the mixture onto a gauze pad. Then repeat the process with a second pad and apply one to each congested breast.

- If it is really necessary, the homoeopathic medication *Phytolacca* can be administered here. The choice of potencies requires a sure instinct. A low, medium or high potency is selected, depending on whether the milk is to be reduced in quantity, made to start flowing or increased in quantity. I can look back on any number of successful treatments with this remedy. Here I allow myself to make diagnoses over the phone or by E-Mail when women turn to me using those means of communication. But please never use this medication without expert advice, and never, ever, for a long period of time! Remember: where there is an effect there is also a side effect, even in homoeopathy.

There are many means of treating swollen, painful, lumpy breasts which nevertheless produce too little milk:
- A talk about what obstacles to maternal happiness there might be on the emotional level.
- Regular loosening-up exercises for the shoulders and gentle massaging of the breasts in radial and circular motions with *Stillöl/Nursing Oil $\mathcal{D}$®* before every breastfeeding session.
- The application of warmth before breastfeeding in the form of infrared radiation or hot-water compresses, administered to breasts which have been massaged with *Stillöl/Nursing Oil $\mathcal{D}$®* or, in a pinch, with the leftover *Dammmassageöl/Perineum Massage Oil $\mathcal{D}$®*.
- Possibly with the aid of a midwife or baby nurse and the application of the "pressure grip", help the newborn to empty one breast completely. It will be necessary to massage the breast firmly, stopping now and then to apply hot compresses. This is painstaking but very worthwhile "handiwork". Naturally, the child is then also offered the second breast.
- In these situations, the most helpful homoeopathic remedies are *Pulsatilla* and *Bryonia*. The former is the right choice when everything is clogged: the woman's emotional state, her milk, her lochia and, where applicable, her painful varicose veins. Under the effect of the Pulsatilla, a cheerful mood will set in and the milk will begin to flow. Bryonia is taken when the entire breast feels taut and hurts no matter how gently it is touched. Expressing the milk by hand is out of the question. Often the tension and pain in the breasts can be reduced or even "conjured away" (as one woman put it) within ten minutes of the administration of Bryonia.

Further Engorgement

Ten days after initial engorgement and a further three weeks later, a condition much like initial engorgement can come about. These phases of increased milk production nearly always go hand in hand with growth spurts on the part of the baby, who then naturally requires more nutrition. As a result, the mother usually does not experience any discomfort and in many cases she hardly even notices the engorgement because her breasts do not swell up painfully with milk.

The final engorgement between the eighth and twelfth week after birth is usually accompanied by an abrupt change in the mother's hormone balance. This phase is often followed by another period of inadequate milk production. The mother's body is essentially trying to decide whether oestrogen will play the leading role, bringing about ovulation, or whether the prolactin – the lactation hormone – will continue to dominate. By breastfeeding frequently during this period, the mother can influence the outcome of the debate and ensure that she will continue to have a sufficient amount of milk for her child's needs. Within a few days, her patience will be rewarded by another gentle engorgement. The baby's needs will continue to be met, even if the intervals between breastfeeding sessions now become longer.

What all of this means is that the "breastfeeding train" will wait at the station for you for at least eight weeks and you will have several opportunities to climb aboard. If for some undoubtedly justified reason or another you have only partially nursed your baby and supplemented your milk with infant formula, you can still manage the transition to full breastfeeding. Particularly if you yourself have been ill, or have given birth to a premature or ill child, these eight weeks of "deliberation time" can be a glimmer of hope for you. In situations like these, the aid of a midwife and the accompaniment of the other members of a breastfeeding group can provide you with loads of support and encouragement. In this context, I am always reminded of Mrs. H …

… her baby had been born abroad, prematurely and by caesarean section. In that country it was common practice for women who had undergone caesareans to be given a shot to stop milk production. Saddened and disappointed, she turned up in our practice fourteen days after the birth without her baby, and told me how very much she would have liked to breastfeed her baby. I encouraged her to go out and get an electric pump immediately, drink plenty of fluids and pump her breasts diligently. The baby came to Germany in its third week of life; at the sight of her child the mother immediately produced more milk, and seven weeks following its discharge from the hospital, the baby's diet consisted exclusively of breast milk. Naturally, this was only possible by way of the mother's iron will, firm conviction, inner calm and exemplary staying power.

Milk Quantity/Weight Gain in Breastfed Children

As already mentioned previously in various contexts, the amount the baby drinks will depend on the baby itself and the mother's milk production. There is no rigid rule for breastfed children! I strongly advise mothers against checking the amount consumed by weighing the baby before and after every meal; it only causes a lot of unnecessary worry and tension. All that really matters is that the baby gains weight. The midwife will monitor the baby's weight and provide you with the necessary advice.

If you yourself have a set of scales at home or have borrowed one from the chemist's shop, lay the baby on it either naked or dressed only in an undershirt, having first spread a thin cloth on the surface of the scale. Make a note of the weight along with an indication of whether the baby's tummy is empty or full. Wait several days before repeating the procedure, making sure the baby is in the same state as the first time. The difference will tell you whether the baby has gained weight and, if so, how much.

Here it is extremely important to be aware that a newborn can initially lose as much as ten percent of its birth weight. This weight loss is an entirely normal and natural physiological process caused by the excretion of meconium and loss of fluid after birth. The child will not begin to gain weight until the quantity of breast milk increases, i.e. until the fourth or fifth day of life. Recent studies show that that this ten percent weight loss is a reference value that was calculated in the years in which breastfeeding was very uncommon, in other words applies above all to bottle-fed babies. The newborn should reach its birth weight again by ten to fourteen days after birth. For the eight weeks that follow, the simple old rule of thumb still applies: 100 g/3.5 oz. per week are necessary; 200 g/7 oz. per week is an excellent average. Don't allow yourself to be disconcerted by the paediatrician or well-meaning relatives. While the mother is breastfeeding, the father can do the arithmetic!

When the child is examined by the paediatrician (in Germany a routine examination is carried out between the fourth and sixth weeks of life), its weight will also be checked. If its weight really is worrisomely far below the average, the mother can talk to her midwife or the paediatrician about how it should be monitored in the following weeks. Don't panic; simply ring up your midwife like so many others who have been doing that for years. Of course I am well aware that you can't just overlook the situation if there are signs that the baby is underweight, and that you urgently need the advice of an experienced mother or midwife, because otherwise the doctor's worrying diagnosis will already cause your milk production to decrease rapidly. You should never have to be alone with these typical maternal fears. The consolation of a friend who has no children of her own won't help much: "Stop worrying; the child won't starve to death that quickly." Clearly, only well-founded encouragement and like-minded mothers are really helpful in situations such as these.

But also think about the fact that children are not statistics and refuse to conform to norms any more than you do. There are weeks in which your baby drinks a lot and gains weight. And then there are phases in which it is content with a minimum of milk. The same is frequently true of adolescents. First they seem to be living on air and then they'll have a phase of several weeks in which they eat like a horse. These growth spurts and development phases already begin during the first weeks of life. The weight curve will be accordingly jagged. So please spare yourself the stress of regular weighing! The only parents who derive pleasure from such log-keeping are statistics analysts. Rather than constantly entering the baby's weight and height onto a list, use the time to play and cuddle with it.

In rare cases, the midwife or paediatrician will request that you monitor the quantity consumed per day. This involves weighing your child before and after every breastfeeding meal over a span of twenty-four hours, without changing its nappies in between the two weight checks. In other words, the baby shouldn't be given a fresh nappy until after its post-nursing weight check. This is the only means of keeping track of the overall quantity consumed as a basis for deciding how to proceed with regard to the child's nutrition.

However, I would also like to point out to you that you can determine very well whether the baby is getting its fill just by observation. A normally growing baby will demand between five and eight meals a day, wet its nappies five to six times a day and have bowel movements numbering from as little as once a week to as many as several times a day. Its little belly will visibly become fuller and wider. One sure sign that it is gaining weight is that its newborn clothing no longer fits and it has to graduate to the next larger size. If you are unsure whether your child is thriving, ask a competent woman for advice. Do not allow yourself to be upset or disconcerted by tables and units of measurement. If you as parents are of small, lightweight build, neither you nor the paediatrician can expect your baby to gain as much weight as the baby of your neighbour who is 1.80 m/5 ft. 11 in. tall and whose husband weights 100 kg/220 lbs. I would nevertheless hereby like to urge my colleagues to carry out weight checks whenever they are uncertain. After all, we shouldn't err in the opposite direction, going from checking the weight five times a day to never weighing the baby at all! Even today, there are children who don't grow properly, and however committed we are to breastfeeding, we should not lose sight of reality. I highly recommend that you as a breastfeeding mother really turn to "your" midwife for advice, and not just any midwife. Your midwife already knows you and your baby and can provide better help as a result. If for some reason you do consult with a different midwife, it is helpful to show her pictures of the baby taken in the course of the preceding weeks.

I could write reams about supposedly undernourished infants who are allegedly in urgent need of nutritional supplementation with infant formula, merely because they don't conform to the German norm. With words of consolation for the mother and a bit of advice, these children thrive anyway, even without the formula. Isn't it really much more important that the child is healthy and exhibits constant developmental progress? How would we adults react if we were forced to conform to some norm or other?

Influencing the Milk Quantity

The two most important **rules of thumb** throughout the breastfeeding period are:
- *Offering both breasts at every meal increases the quantity of milk!*
- *Offering one breast per meal reduces the quantity of milk!*

Increasing the Milk Quantity

Frequent Nursing

Breastfeeding the baby frequently serves to increase milk production and, conversely, a reduction in the number of breastfeeding sessions decreases the production. By breastfeeding according to demand, the relationship between demand and supply of milk is regulated automatically. It generally takes four to eight weeks until the baby's hunger and the supply of milk correspond. I often cite an example from economics to explain this rule: If a woman asks for a fresh bread roll once a day, the baker won't change his production quantity. But if she starts turning up in his shop ten times a day, he will try to meet her wishes, even if it takes a few days. Here as well, persistence pays off. The same applies to the production of breast milk: Following several days of breastfeeding at two-hour intervals, the milk quantity will increase and the child will lengthen the intervals entirely of its own accord. Breastfeeding according to demand is practically guaranteed to be successful. For this reason, the mother should neither supplement her own milk with infant formula nor try to force a four-hour rhythm onto the baby, but should put it to her breast when it cries and visibly searches for the breast. Once again, I could recount hundreds of stories of stress situations following discharge from the hospital. In Germany there is a seal of approval called "stillfreundliches Krankenhaus" – "baby-friendly hospital" – but surprisingly few hospitals have been awarded it or even made any effort to fulfil the respective requirements. Maybe this is because there's no financial advantage in doing so. In any case, to this very day, upon discharge from the hospital, mothers are still often advised to supplement the baby's diet on grounds that they do not produce enough milk. But by following this advice, the supply-and-demand cycle is disturbed and the breast really does offer the child an insufficient quantity. If the above-mentioned customer started going to the bakery across the street, the first baker would have no further incentive to bake additional rolls. Simply by reducing the amount of infant formula or omitting it entirely, most children receive an adequate supply of breast milk within a few days. It is true that this frequent breastfeeding takes a lot of time, and the parents are in urgent need of a midwife's support and encouragement. The conditions for successful breastfeeding described at the beginning of this section – e.g. patience, staying power, peace and quiet – should once again be called to mind.

Nursing Bra or No Nursing Bra

One simple but very effective method of increasing the quantity of milk to the sufficient level is to stop wearing a nursing bra. Merely due to the feeling of "liberation" and "room to breathe", the breast will automatically produce more milk. Mothers are often happy to hear this advice, take off their bras immediately and usually report that they think they feel a tingling in their breasts even before the house call is over for the day. In many cases, taking off the bra is what triggers initial engorgement.

⊗ Herbal Medicine

The mother's intake of fluid influences the milk quantity within three days. This aspect should not be underestimated! The main thing is to increase the amount of fluid in general. But you will soon notice that the most helpful fluids for increasing milk production are non-carbonated water and suitable herbal teas (no sage or peppermint tea!). Since its invention in 1979, *Stilltee/Nursing Tea* has proven by far the best when it comes to increasing the quantity of milk.

This blend consists of equal parts of aniseed, fennel, black cumin, dill, marjoram, milkwort and lemon balm. I know how difficult it can be to obtain genuine bitter milkwort – Polygala amara – and that it is unfortunately often confused with Polygala vulgaris (common milkwort) or Senecionis herba, also referred to as Senecio ovatus (wood ragwort), which contains harmful pyrrolizidine alkaloids. So be very careful! My many years of good experience with *Stilltee/Nursing Tea* are confirmed again and again. Many mothers report that their milk production increased the very first day they started drinking this tea. An important aspect to take into account is that the seeds have to be freshly crushed. The essential oils maintain their effectiveness for as long as three weeks if the tea is stored in an opaque container or dark-coloured package. After that, the lactation-inducing properties decrease to about half their original strength. Moreover, the maximum daily dose of one litre/35 fl. oz. should only be consumed on the first few days; after that, three cups (0.75 litres/26 fl. oz.) a day will suffice. Of course, you can "spread out" the three teaspoons of *Stilltee/Nursing Tea* (1 per cup) over a litre or even more water. In other words, the amount of fluid can be increased, just not the amount of herbs, because otherwise the tea can easily have a laxative effect on you and your child. Fathers have reported to me that they got their emotional balance a bit out of whack by joining their wives in the enjoyment of this tea for a week or so. This is just one more proof of the effect of the herbs and seeds on the hormone system. Of course, some men would say that those fathers were just going through paternal postnatal downs.

If the baby suffers from wind, it can be given this tea in strongly diluted form.

Many years ago, my friend Gina, a midwife in Berlin, asked me if I had ever heard of *"barley water"*. She said it was a popular and very effective beverage particularly appreciated by mothers who didn't like tea or simply wanted a change from *Stilltee/Nursing Tea*. This lactation-inducing drink is extremely cheap and easy to make. Fifty grams/1.75 oz. of barleycorn are boiled in two litres/70 fl. oz. of water for an hour and a half; then the liquid is poured through a sieve to remove the barleycorn, and left to cool. It can then be flavoured with a tablespoon of apple juice and the juice of a fresh, organic lemon and sweetened with one tablespoon of honey. This beverage is then taken in sips over the course of one to two days.

Homoeopathic Treatment

Homoeopathy is another effective natural means of supporting lactation. Here again, it is essential to make contact with a midwife or other health-care provider well-versed in this method. Only on the basis of thorough knowledge of the individual pharmacological pictures is it possible to determine the right remedy on the first try. I do not by any means want to convey the impression that I myself am always able to help women quickly and easily by homoeopathic means. Success is much more likely if the midwife already knew the mother during pregnancy and is accordingly familiar with her basic constitution and personal life situation.

As already mentioned, Pulsatilla is often a suitable remedy. All women who have had positive experience with this substance during pregnancy don't have to think twice about using it again – for themselves and for their children – during the postnatal period. Pulsatilla is perhaps the very best example of the holistic approach of homoeopathy; it runs through this book like a red thread. Go back to the previous chapters and reread the descriptions in order to determine whether you are the "Pulsatilla type". As always, of course, the correct potency must be chosen; in this particular context a higher potency will be required.

The following remedies can likewise be considered: *Agnus castus, Bryonia, Calcium carbonicum, Lac caninum, Lac defloratum, Secale* and *Sepia*.

Aroma Therapy

Like everywhere else in the area of midwifery, essential oils can also be helpful in cases of insufficient lactation. Actually, they are my favourite aids, because applying massage oil automatically means giving the mother attention on the physical and emotional level. An aroma which supports you in your motherhood will boost your mood. Moreover, you can treat yourself with essential oils and do not have to rely on medication and other healing methods and their practitioners. Essential oils thus lead to a certain amount of autonomy which strengthens your self confidence, something no mother can ever have too much of.

Here I would above all like to recommend *Stillöl/Nursing Oil $\mathcal{D}^{®}$* which has already been mentioned in various contexts. This is an *Original $\mathcal{D}^{®}$ Aroma Blend* containing aniseed, fennel, carrot seed, coriander, cumin, lavender and rose on a fatty plant oil basis, and is a very trusty aid when it comes to stimulating milk production.

Beginning on the first day of the postnatal period, you can massage your breasts with this oil several times a day to help ensure that lactation will set in quickly and smoothly. If the quantity is still not adequate, massage your breasts with this product, using circular and radial motions, before every breastfeeding session, following the same procedure discussed in conjunction with preparing the breasts for nursing during pregnancy. Throughout the entire breastfeeding period, whenever a problem arises – be it insufficient milk production, congested or painful breasts – this oil will be a wonderful aid.

Reducing the Milk Quantity

Breasts which produce too much milk are undoubtedly just as much of a burden as the reverse. With the following pointers I have helped many a woman solve this problem. If you want to take preventive measures, you will find advice in the first pages of this section.

- *Breastfeeding:* As described in the previous section on this topic, the first step will be to offer only one breast per meal. As you feed, you will also have to cool the other breast with a cold pack or bag of ice cubes. By applying strong pressure to the nipple with your thumb for one to two minutes you can also keep the breast from producing additional milk
- *Bra:* Between breastfeeding sessions it is helpful to wear a firm, tight bra and/or, if possible, to lie on your front for a while.
- *Quark:* Cold compresses, containing quark (milk curds) for example, should also be applied in between breast-milk meals.

☉ Homoeopathic Treatment

Homoeopathy has a useful plant for overproduction of this kind: *Phytolacca* (pokeweed). Administered only temporarily and at a low potency (D3–D8) it is sure to reduce lactation. The choice of potency and dose requires a certain amount of skill, but an experienced midwife will surely determine the right treatment quickly.

☉ Aroma Therapy

In this situation, the essential oil of *sage* is an effective aid in reducing the milk quantity. One option is to apply a few drops of sage oil to the nipples after breastfeeding – a method recommended in many hospitals and by many midwives. Please be advised, however, that sage should really only be used in cases of overabundant lactation! Sage oil can also be mixed with quark and applied in the form of a quark compress. An even better choice is *Salbei-Zypressen-Öl/Sage-Cypress Oil 𝒟®*, which is used for weaning, because pure sage oil can have too high a ketone content, which can lead to respiratory depression in the newborn. I am grateful that, for the protection of infants, the production of the *Original 𝒟® Aroma Blends* is accompanied by very detailed laboratory controls, and that a harmful degree of ketone can therefore be ruled out.

A lot of sensitivity is required in applying all methods of breast milk reduction, so as not to make the mistake of stopping milk production entirely.

The Care of the Breasts

Women frequently ask me how they should care for their breasts. There really isn't much to consider in this context. Mother Nature did not develop any special measures for breast care, and women in the postnatal period accordingly don't have to do anything different from usual. All that remains to be said is that postnatal mothers tend to break out in a sweat with some frequency and therefore have a heightened craving to wash or shower. Normal bodily hygiene is entirely sufficient.

Preventive Measures in the Care of the Breasts

In order to avoid sore nipples, you should see to it that you keep your nipples soft and supple. In practical terms, you should protect them from excessive warmth, moisture and extreme cold. The correct breastfeeding position is another important aspect. If the child does not latch onto the nipple correctly, one area of the nipple will be subjected to more "stress" than another, a circumstance which can also lead to soreness. It's like wearing shoes that don't fit properly; they pinch in certain places – with painful consequences.

Moisture and warmth represent favourable conditions for the development of a fungal infection, which is extremely unpleasant, itches and can lead to sore, cracked nipples. It is therefore highly advisable to allow your breasts to "air dry" after every breastfeeding session. Remaining drops of breast milk do not have to be removed, but should in any case be allowed to dry!

Extreme cold can likewise lead to cracks or rhagades of the nipples. Just as our hands and lips get cracked and dry in the winter, this can happen to the nipples of a mother who breastfeeds her child. No matter what you do, don't go out without warm, protective breast pads throughout the winter months or when a cold wind is blowing. Also consider carefully before swimming in a cold lake or unheated swimming pool. Even going out to the balcony to hang up laundry can lead to problems in this respect. In extreme cases, you can even suffer from a so-called "vasospasm" if you put your child to your breast immediately after it has been exposed to the cold. This is a condition in which the breast does not release the milk at all, or only in conjunction with a lot of pain. The result is often a congested breast, which can be accompanied by a fever (see p. ■f.).

In the case of exposure to extreme cold, you should warm your breast immediately. In the summer, you should dry yourself off immediately after your swim in a cold lake, dress warmly and soak in the warm sunshine. In the autumn and winter you can administer infrared radiation or hot compresses. These measures are sure to help you avoid the cracks, congestion or reduced lactation that can be caused by cold.

In some children, the frenulum linguae – the cord of skin connecting the tongue to the floor of the mouth – is too short, a condition called tongue-tie which can cause breastfeeding problems to a degree that should not be underestimated. In these cases the child cannot get enough of the nipple into its mouth, leading to stress for the outer tip of the nipple, and the attendant soreness. This problem can really only be solved by cutting the frenulum linguae, an operation which naturally can only be conducted by an experienced surgeon.

Nursing Pads Made of Natural Fibres

The best means of preventing any of the various problems that can arise is to wear breast pads made of natural wool and wild silk. These textiles will help you to avoid moisture, heat and cold. Since women started using these nursing pads, sore nipples and the accompanying problems have decreased to a minimum. When I started out in my profession, cracked, bleeding nipples were the most frequent reason for making house calls. The use of natural breast pads relieved me of that work almost overnight. It is simple to explain how they work:

Wool and silk are animal protein fibres, which repel bacteria. They accordingly do not provide favourable conditions for the spread of germs; on the contrary, they have anti-inflammatory and healing properties. They are breathable and thus guarantee good air circulation around the nipples and breasts.

Wool warms the breast and absorbs as much as forty percent of its own weight in moisture. The breast remains dry because the moisture is conducted to the outside. In comparison, cotton only absorbs six percent, and the moisture it does absorb stays in the fibres longer. A little experiment with a shot glass full of water which is poured onto a piece of cotton and another one onto a piece of pure natural wool will illustrate these properties. Or imagine a wool sweater in comparison to a cotton shirt in the washbasin: which article of clothing sinks into the water immediately and which goes down slowly but then soaks up all of the water?

Silk feels smooth, fine and soft, does not cause any skin irritations and can be worn by women who react sensitively or are allergic to wool. This natural fibre is particularly suitable for breastfeeding women because it has cooling properties when the environment is warm and vice versa. I have already discussed the healing qualities of silk in conjunction with sore baby bottoms. And to top it off, silk is also absorbent without feeling moist.

If you use natural-fibre nursing pads made of wool or silk, you won't need the nipple ointment often recommended in hospitals. What is more, wool and silk pads are economical, because one or two pairs are entirely sufficient. They don't need to be sterilized, they don't cause any refuse, you don't have to keep going out and buying disposable breast pads, and when you're done breastfeeding you can use them to treat wounds and sores in the family. Milk spots can be removed by washing them by hand with curd soap.

Cotton nursing pads are certainly better than using disposable ones, but they do not possess all the wonderful properties of wool and silk. Cotton pads should be changed on a daily basis and regularly sterilized in boiling water.

The Breastfeeding Mother's Diet

In the sections on "The Postnatal Period" and "The Newborn" I made repeated reference to the diet of the breastfeeding mother. Please reread those passages.

In the context of diet, you should be aware that the baby feels "newborn" until the eighth week of life, and you are in a phase of hormonal, emotional and physical readjustment for about the same length of time. In the previous chapters I have frequently discussed the signals of a healthy body; and this is a principle that applies during the breastfeeding period as well. A healthy, balanced diet of food your body is accustomed to will not harm your baby. Eat and drink the food and beverages of the region you live in and avoid changing your dietary habits during the breastfeeding period, particularly where exotic cuisine is concerned. Don't use any hot spices. If you like cabbage in all its different forms, start out by carefully testing cauliflower and broccoli. These are the two types which are least likely to cause the newborn wind. Potatoes and carrots, which can be prepared in any number of delicious variations, represent a balanced, healthful diet. Particularly if you flavour them with caraway and fennel seed you – and your baby – won't have the slightest difficulties. Vera, to whom I attended during her postnatal phase, told me, however, that she could only eat storage potatoes since freshly harvested ones had caused her baby a tummy ache. The same undoubtedly applies to a number of other types of vegetables and, especially, fruit. If it is harvested before it is ripe, it can lead to severe digestion problems. Choose fruit and vegetables according to what grows in your garden or surroundings. In other words, do not eat fresh pineapple, kiwi, mango and other exotic fruits on a daily basis, since they are extremely acid.

Alcohol and Coca Cola are presumably not your standard drinks. A glass of red wine or low-alcohol beer will have a relaxing and enjoyable effect and accordingly will not harm your child. The same applies to coffee. If this beverage has been contributing to your happiness for years, now is not the time to subject yourself to withdrawal, because the baby will be subjected to it right along with you. Do, however, reduce your intake of coffee and try switching to a coffee substitute such as grain coffee. As everyone knows, coffee has a stimulating effect. Particularly after four o'clock in the afternoon, I urgently recommend that you not drink stimulating beverages. Adherence to this last piece of advice, incidentally, has reduced the length of many a baby's daily (or nightly) "screaming phase" or made it vanish entirely. It is likewise important not to eat foods which are difficult to digest or any big meals past this time of day. Easily digestible foods such as vegetables and chicken soup are suitable for the evening. Since this is something I learned from my mother, I was astonished to read in a specialized journal about a colleague of mine who did not learn this wisdom until she attended a course on traditional Chinese medicine.

I have often witnessed that it is not the composition of the diet that causes a mother problems, but finding the time to sit down for a meal. Not only does the baby demand a lot of attention, but the mother herself is in the midst of her transition from a well-structured professional life to the irregularities of life as a housewife and mother. She forgets herself and she feels that it's too much trouble to cook for herself alone. It is absolutely essential, however, that a woman who is breastfeeding eat adequately, because breastfeeding takes a lot of energy. She should moreover avoid going below her initial weight on account of the excretion of toxins that goes hand in hand with weight loss. These toxins are stored in the fat tissue and they stay there if the mother keeps her weight. As a means of getting a balanced diet without constantly having to cook – and to keep mothers from trying to live on coffee and chocolate – I recommend that they make themselves so-called milk balls or milk pralines. The latter keep well in the refrigerator, can therefore be made in large batches, are easy to make and yummy. The recipe is as follows:

Brown in a pan 1 kg/2 lbs. of a blend of coarsely ground wheat, barley and oat
Stir in 300 g/10.5 oz. of cooked brown rice and
350 g/12.3 oz. cold butter along with 1 glass of water.
Then add 300 g/10.5 fl. oz. of honey.

Form balls from this mixture, measuring about 2 cm/¾ in. each in diameter, and roll some in sesame seeds, some in sunflower seeds and some in dried, grated coconut. Warning: Midwives and men love these calorie bombs, too!

You may want to start out by making half the recipe to see if you like these milk balls.

Special Circumstances in Connection with the Mother

Flat or Inverted Nipples

One problem which can cause some temporary discomfort is flat or inverted nipples. Neither type will prevent you from being able to breastfeed. You are likely to have a consulted a midwife about this problem during pregnancy. Now the phase begins in which you have to get the baby to latch on to your breast with lots of patience and a few tricks. Don't hesitate to ask the nursery nurse of midwife for help. It is advisable to put the breast shells on your breasts about half an hour before nursing (see p. ∎f.). The warmth of the body creates a vacuum and the nipples become erect. Take your baby into your arms and only remove the breast shell immediately before latching it to your breast. If you follow this instruction, the baby will have no problem grasping the nipple. In many cases it will also be advantageous to use a nipple shield when breastfeeding, at least for a while. But do keep trying to manage without it.

During many a postnatal house call, my first deed was to have the mother try putting the baby to her breast without a shield. In many cases, the child latches onto the breast without objection and the mother is surprised that her baby does so well with-out this aid. Sometimes I ask myself who in the world is advising young mothers to use this spacer consistently, without trying out any other possibilities. In my opinion, true breastfeeding advice has everything to do with interpersonal closeness, but of course there are always people who require a bit of a safety margin. Try to accept that not all nurses and midwives can deal so directly with your breasts, but you yourself don't have to keep this distance from your own body and from your child.

Cracked/Sore Nipples

However conscientious you are about taking various precautions, sore, cracked or bleeding nipples can develop. This is unfortunately a very painful condition, particu-larly when the baby latches on. Following its first few gulps, however, the pain dwin-dles and your baby can drink its fill without causing you any further discomfort.

The first thing to do if you are suffering from this affliction is ask your midwife for help. With all of her experience, she will be able to provide you with advice and natu-ral methods of support to achieve rapid healing and crack-free nipples. Sore nipples are no reason to advise a woman to wean or pump, but an occasion to see to it that she receives plenty of good advice on breastfeeding while she still has the problem and to treat it until it's gone.

Treatment can begin by checking the breastfeeding position. The baby should be able to grasp as much of the areola in its mouth as possible, and should not put un-necessary strain on the breast by suckling for longer than it needs to. Furthermore, when it has finished drinking, don't just pull it away from the nipple, but release the vacuum by sticking one of your fingers into a corner of the baby's mouth.

Adhere to all of the preventive measures discussed repeatedly in the previous sec-tions of this book, e.g. the healing effects of air, light and sunshine, the use of nursing pads, the correct latch-on technique, etc.

Irritated Nipples

Irritated nipples can usually be dealt with effectively by the general breast-care meas-ures discussed and adhering to a three-hour rhythm. Interestingly, women with sore nipples almost always correspond to the pharmacological picture of the homoeo-pathic substance *Silicea*. One of the main criteria here is: she feels better in a context of regularity and structure. The holistic approach allows a woman to be advised to honour her own individuality, even if its means violating all kinds of breastfeeding guidelines. The child will certainly fare best when the mother is feeling well and happy. And if this structure is what she needs, then the baby will be fed at three or four-hour intervals without further ado.

Natural Treatment

Rule Number One in cases of sore nipples is: wear silk breast pads to achieve optimal healing and ventilation of the affected zones.

⟨◎⟩ Herbal Medicine

Cracks of the nipples can be treated with undiluted *calendula essence* or *rathania tincture*. Wet a cotton bud/Q-tip with a bit of one of these remedies and carefully clean the wounds with it before and after breastfeeding..

⟨◎⟩ Aroma Therapy

Bathing the nipples in *Sitzbad/Sitz Bath $\mathcal{D}^®$*, which has excellent wound-healing properties, can be helpful. To this end, dissolve a pinch of these bath salts in a shot glass full of sterilized, lukewarm water, as often as you want to. Bathe each of your nipples in the glass for a few minutes. Afterwards rinse them off with clear water and dry your breasts with a blow dryer or infrared light. Twice a day, apply a thin coating of *Beinwellsalbe/Comfrey Ointment $\mathcal{D}^®$* or *Ringelblumensalbe/Calendula Ointment $\mathcal{D}^®$* (both likewise excellent aids in the treatment of wounds) to the nipples after the bath or, alternatively *Rosenbalsam/Rose Balsam $\mathcal{D}^®$* or *Melissenbalsam/Lemon Balm $\mathcal{D}^®$*. It is not at all a good idea to apply compresses thickly spread with ointment, because this will make the nipples too soft, prevent proper air circulation and provide fertile ground for bacteria and fungal spores.

A good, fast, first-aid measure in this situation is the application of *Rose-Teebaum-Essenz/Rose-Tea-Tree Essence $\mathcal{D}^®$*. Apply a single drop of this oil, undiluted, to the wound after breastfeeding. As soon as the wound has closed, spray *Rose-Teebaum-Hydrolat/Rose-Tea-Tree Hydrolat $\mathcal{D}^®$* (instead of the essence) on the affected area after every breastfeeding session for several days.

⟨◎⟩ Homoeopathic Treatment

The homoeopathic remedies *Arnica, Castor equi, Causticum, Phytolacca, Sepia, Silicea* and *Sulfur* often prove helpful in the effort to heal sore nipples quickly.

Midwives' Knowledge

With the appropriate homoeopathic medication, a suitable essential oil blend and natural fibre nursing pads, the problem is nearly always soon overcome and forgotten. The midwife should always do everything in her power to ensure a fast healing process. From my own experience, I unfortunately know what it means to breastfeed the baby for weeks with tears of acute pain in my eyes. I warmly recommend to all midwives that they stand by any woman with sore nipples and provide her with loads of encouragement to help her continue breastfeeding. In these situations, it is often quite worthwhile to think about whether there is any discord in the family: perhaps the mother's nipples are indirectly calling attention to some grievance with which she is afraid to ask for help.

Breastfeeding Aids

Nipple Shield

In many situations it is advisable to offer a woman a nipple shield to wear during breastfeeding to avoid putting further strain on the nipple. In this case it must be determined, however, whether the nipple shield is really providing protection or only aggravating the condition. Sometimes it's not so much the nipple as the woman herself who needs relief from stress. Then the nipple shield is not the solution. If it is used for a lengthy period, however, the newborn's weight should be checked once a week. The reason for this is that, when the mother uses a nipple shield, the baby's tongue can't "milk" the breast properly, but sucks primarily with its lips instead of the velum palatinum (soft palate) – a phenomenon the midwife will be able to recognize immediately. It tires from suckling at length but may not really have managed to drink its fill. If at all possible, the nipple shield should be taken off after the first few minutes so that the baby can properly satisfy its hunger.

In cases of emergency I have often used a bottle nipple in place of a nipple shield. I first puncture one or two extra holes in the nipple with a hot needle so that the baby can accustom itself to the fact that several milk ducts secrete milk in the breast, and that it can and should regulate the quantity of milk and the speed at which it drinks. With this aid, babies who have been bottle-fed for one reason or another will usually drink at the breast immediately and without any trouble. This trick is also helpful when the mother's breasts produce too much milk and the baby constantly chokes during the initial vigorous pulls and then, as is often the case, refuses to keep drinking or merely licks the milk which flows out of the breast of its own accord, but never really gets enough. Many women report that their milk is constantly "leaking", the baby constantly wants to be fed, but never really makes a satiated impression. Here it suffices to breastfeed the baby with a bottle nipple during the first few minutes in which the breast is virtually overflowing, but without adding extra holes. In the course of a few weeks, this aid can usually be omitted again. The bottle-nipple method can also be used when the milk flows abundantly and the child drinks hastily, swallowing a lot of air in the process and suffering from wind as a result. With a converted bottle-nipple breast shield, this problem will be overcome because the baby will drink more slowly.

Always keep your sights on getting to the point where you don't need the breastfeeding aid any longer; direct contact is always the best.

There is another somewhat more expensive but time-tested method of healing sore nipples: tin breast caps (sometimes called cappellinos) worn in between breastfeeding sessions. Consistent alternation between air and tin caps, which can also sometimes fill up with breast milk, will help the sore or irritated nipples to heal quickly. Colleagues of mine on the North and Baltic Sea coasts have also shown me seashells which look like little caps and can likewise be used to protect the breast between nursing sessions. According to these midwives, they likewise facilitate the healing process immensely. Again and again, it proves worthwhile to talk to midwives and mothers about the customs practiced in their regions.

Breast Pump

In my view, the use of an electric pump is only rarely justified. It nearly always leads, in effect, to a triple burden on the mother, because now she has to pump her breasts, then feed the baby this milk from a bottle, and then clean and sterilize all of the equipment. It is really no wonder, therefore, if the nipples become all the more irritated, lactation decreases and you are just short of weaning before finally turning to a midwife for help. I would like to advise all mothers to contact a midwife as soon as the breastfeeding problems come up, because in gridlocked situations even we can't work wonders overnight. Before starting to use an electric pump, try to find a midwife who will help you to avoid taking this drastic measure. When I embarked on my career as a self-employed midwife I swore to myself that I would never leave a woman pumping who had a healthy baby. In my eyes, a pump is only necessary in true – and temporally limited – emergencies. Machines are simply no substitute for breastfeeding. Often it takes several time-consuming house calls and a lot of enlightenment effort, but in the end, all women and midwives will agree that, once the postnatal phase is reached, the in-depth lactation counselling received during pregnancy really pays off. A midwife will nevertheless never shy away from helping a mother during the postnatal period and showing her how to get the baby accustomed to the breast. The young mother will be grateful when she has been liberated from this machine.

No pump can empty the breast as thoroughly as a healthy baby. This is something I experienced personally – it taught me a lot, but it was both painful and disappointing. The machine can really be no more than a brief substitute or a means of relieving a mother whose baby is sick and cannot drink properly for a time. If pumping cannot be avoided – e.g. if the child is ill or premature – it is important to recommend the modern interval and double breast pumps. In Germany, the costs are covered by the public health scheme; find out if this is likewise the case in your country. Incidentally, with enough patience and persistence, it is possible to accustom a baby to the breast even if it has been fed with pumped breast milk for months! An additional aid in cases of prematurely born children is a "supplementary nursing system". It is highly advisable to obtain the help of a professional in learning to use this method.

Pumping and Freezing Breast Milk

In order to store excess milk in the freezer, manual breast pumps, used on a temporary basis, can be a help. Be advised that the transitional milk can be used in this way only for a few days, until the fourth week of life at the latest. A three-month-old baby will refuse this early milk for the simple reason that it tastes different. Mature milk can be kept in the refrigerator – at a temperature of 4 to 8 °C/39 – 46 °F – for a maximum of 72 hours, i.e. not in the door but in the back of the refrigerator. It can also be kept for quite a while in deep-frozen condition. For this purpose, store the milk in glass or lightproof plastic containers (for example those made by Medela or Ameda and available at the chemist's) or the plastic bags which are manufactured specifically for this purpose. The information regarding the storage life of deep-frozen breast milk varies between three and six months. If you have no separate freezer but only a refrigerator with a deep-freeze compartment, please be advised that the latter is not cold enough to keep the milk for more than a few weeks. The portions of milk collected in the refrigerator in the course of the day should be put in the freezer after no more than twelve hours from they time the milk is pumped. The milk is thawed by placing the container into warm water. Any leftovers must be thrown away and should not by any means be reheated! Also, never warm up breast milk in a microwave!

It is a great relief for a mother stuck in a traffic jam, for example, to know that the baby can be fed by her husband with warmed-up breast milk if necessary. Such feedings should not be carried out on a regular basis, however. Even if freezing is an extremely gentle method of preservation, it does have a negative effect on a few of the nutrients.

It is also possible to hand express. Initially it is a bit awkward to squirt the milk into a sterilized container, but with a bit of patience and practice, you will soon be an expert. This, by the way, is the least painful method of emptying a breast, and is a particularly good alternative in cases of sore nipples. Learning the hand expressing technique with the "pressure grip" described previously (see p. ■) confirmed me in my conviction that we midwives really do practice a handicraft. This is how it's done: The woman takes hold of the breast with her thumb and index or middle finger about 3–4 cm/1 ¼ – 1 ½ in. behind the nipple, i.e. around the edge of the areola, pulls the fingers backwards towards her ribcage and then presses them together. Now milk will appear on the tip of the nipple or come squirting out of the milk ducts, and is collected in a sterilized container of some kind. This process is continued until any excessive pressure (caused by excess milk) on the breast is relieved and the breast feels softer again, or until the amount required for a single meal has been collected. I myself made a habit of expressing milk by hand and thus relieving the pressure on my breasts whenever my baby had a relatively long sleeping phase. I could then relax and let the baby sleep and I always had some milk in stock in the freezer, so my husband was never faced with any breast-milk emergencies when I was out. In the phase when

I started supplementing the breast milk with solids, the leftover milk was a perfect basis for baby cereal.

Blocked Milk Ducts/Inflamed Breasts (Mastitis)

One of the crises most feared by women during the breastfeeding period is congestion or inflammation of the breast(s). This situation is as threatening for the midwife as it is for the mother. An inflammation of the breast afflicts the woman in her femininity and intimate sphere. Thanks to naturopathic methods, however, I can reassure all women and relieve them of their fears. I regard it as highly important to refute the widely circulated rumour that a woman with a febrile blocked duct or an inflammation of the breast has to stop breastfeeding immediately because otherwise an abscess can form, treatable only by surgical means. In all my years of self-employment as a midwife, there was only one single case in which I attended to a woman whose breast infection ended in an abscess and who accordingly had to undergo surgery. After the ordeal, however, she continued breastfeeding and was free of all discomfort a few days later. Sometimes I think that if I had known then all I know now, this surgical intervention might not have become necessary. Only a handful of women I have cared for have had to take an antibiotic or have stopped nursing on account of a febrile breast incident. These were cases in which the mothers were essentially happy to have an excuse to wean their babies. Again and again, I witness situations in which the body of a woman "lays down the law" when she herself doesn't manage it. Naturally, this is a principle which applies to all kinds of situations in life, and to men and children as well. Physical discomfort nearly always has an emotional cause. It is no surprise that the percentage of psychosomatically ill persons is increasing. Sooner or later, nature rebels when the person's symptoms are repressed, but he/she is not truly healed.

Emotional Causes

A blocked milk duct is one of the best examples I know of the physical consequences of emotional problems. The true cause is often not immediately obvious, but it is usually worthwhile for the midwife to join the mother in the search for problems in the family, in her relationship to her partner or in connection with her new motherhood. Most breast congestions occur at the beginning of the week. When the midwife asks whether the husband still has leave from work, the answer is almost always: "That's just it; he has to go back to work and there's just no way I can manage everything without him." When the midwife digs a little deeper, some mothers tell her about all the things that have "dammed up" in her life in the meantime, as in the case of Mrs. A. M. ...

... "To tell you the truth, I don't know what to do. My husband and mother-in-law keep telling me I should bottle-feed the baby, now that I've breastfed for four months. But now, with my full, congested

breast, what choice do I have but to feed the baby with it?!" We talked, and in the course of the conver-
sation it became clear that the mother was very grateful for this problem and it didn't really bother her
that much. She was a mother who took great pleasure in breastfeeding her child. We agreed that she
should stand up for her opinion and her wishes, and I assured her that a child really could be breastfed
for half a year or longer without any cause for concern, no matter what anyone said. She subsequently
explained this to her husband and told her mother-in-law that the baby would not be given a bottle as
long as she enjoyed nursing it. Mrs. A. M. was happy when we said goodbye and remarked: "It's good
I got this blocked milk duct; it gave me a chance to talk to you about things — I never would have been
so bold as to call you just to talk."

I would like to take this opportunity to encourage all mothers to contact their midwives or a breast-
feeding group leader whenever they are unclear or uncertain about something, even if they are not
experiencing any physical discomfort. Try to overcome your inhibitions and don't be embarrassed
about your problems and questions — other mothers go through exactly the same thing.

Distinguishing between a Blocked Duct and an Infected Breast

In many cases it is difficult to determine whether the problem is congestion caused by increased milk production similar to initial engorgement, or whether it is a true blocked duct threatening to become febrile or perhaps already at the point of infection. In my opinion, the midwife's first task is not to make a correct diagnosis but to provide first aid to the mother.

Blocked milk ducts are painful; the breast is swollen and taut, initially similar to the way it was during initial engorgement. Breastfeeding and contact of any kind can often be extremely unpleasant in this situation. A breast can also be congested just in one area, producing a lump which is likewise sensitive to the touch and perhaps slightly reddened. A congested breast is initially not accompanied by a fever.

A *breast infection* exhibits all the same symptoms as a blocked milk duct, but the afflicted woman feels physically unwell and has pains of the limbs and joints of the kind accompanying flu. In most cases the body temperature rises rapidly, often to as high as 40 °C/104 °F. The afflicted breast is reddened in the area of the congestion and almost always painful to the touch. The reddening can affect one limited area or the whole breast. Stripes of redness can also appear.

Causes of Breast Congestion

A variety of causes can lead to this condition. As mentioned above, emotional problems are among the foremost causes of physical stagnation or congestion. In any case, it is important to consult a midwife as soon as at all possible, since she is the health-care provider who has the most experience with breastfeeding mothers. Don't wait too long, and don't shy away from calling the midwife on the weekend, because a congested breast which is treated improperly or not at all can become infected in the twinkling of an eye.

- Another possible cause is increased milk production brought about by a renewed *engorgement* which can take place anywhere between the fourth and ninth weeks of life.

- The breast can become congested when the *child is ill* and suddenly stops emptying the breast, leading to an imbalance between supply and demand.

- *Positive experiences* can also sometimes have unpleasant consequences: perhaps you have recuperated well in the holiday sunshine, maybe gone to a party on top of it, and enjoyed some sparkling wine or wheat beer, both of which promote lactation. All of these factors can lead to an abrupt increase in milk production. Your baby is full after just one side, and you have to go several hours before it drinks from the other one. It can also be the long-hoped-for first time a baby sleeps through the night that causes the congestion. The baby sleeps for an eternity of seven hours while the mother sits in bed with painful, swollen breasts.

- The *nursing bra* can lead to congestion if it is too tight or slips up at night.

- Another – particularly painful – possibility is that the mammary gland has become clogged with a *bubble* formed when the baby was suckling. A congestion of this kind is initially not accompanied by any symptoms. The mother merely feels pain and reports that her child lets go of the breast right away again and refuses to go on suckling even though she is certain that the breast has not been emptied yet. After the breastfeeding session you merely see a tiny yellow spot on the nipple; on closer inspection you discover that a transparent membrane is blocking the "entrance" to one of the tiny passages. In these cases, you have no choice but to puncture the bubble with a sterilized needle and press the milk out manually. Often it suffices to have the baby suckle from that breast afterwards and hand express in addition. I will never forget my first experience of a bubble leading to a congested breast …

… Mrs. M. called me early one morning and asked me for help, a distinct note of concern in her voice: "Could you possibly come by sometime in the course of the day? Something is wrong with my right breast. It hurts so, and it's hard and taut. And the baby refuses to drink from it properly; it lets go again right away and screams, even though there is still milk in the breast. I have no idea what's going on!" I promised to look in on her right away. In the intervening time, she should make quark compresses. She didn't have a fever, or even reddening of the breast, but it is nevertheless important to give a woman a means of finding relief for her taut, swollen breast and accordingly for her state of mind. When I arrived, I was astonished myself: there was no reddening, no temperature and the cause of the pain was not visible, but the upper outer quarter was clearly full of milk. Mr. M. was carrying his son around to calm him down, because the child was restless and whiney. I used the "pressure grip" to see whether the milk would flow out properly. Milk dripped from two ducts, but suddenly a small golden yellow spot appeared, tinier than a pinhead. "What in the world is that?" I asked, amazed. After repeated at-

tempts to press milk out of the upper outer zone of the breast, the little spot got a bit bigger and I could now see that a tiny, delicate membrane was covering the end of the milk duct. I asked the father to bring me a pin. I suddenly remembered that the father was a doctor, a thought that sent shivers down my spine. 'I wonder what he'll say when he sees me fiddling around with an ordinary pin?' I thought to myself. But I quickly came to the conclusion that the most important thing was to help the mother and I told the father what I was planning to do. "Do what you think is right, as long as this little guy can drink his fill again and my wife is relieved of her pain. I already resigned myself to the fact that I can't do anything to help her with this sometime in the middle of last night." I dipped the needle in Calendula Essence, dabbed a bit of the latter onto the breast as well and, gathering my courage, punctured the bubble. A "mini milk plug" landed in my eye, the milk began flowing out and as we were all laughing about this course of events the "little guy" was already back at his mother's breast, which he noisily emptied. The mother beamed happily about the relief she was feeling as the breast emptied, and the father clapped both hands to his head and declared with equal relief: "You midwives always have another trick up your sleeves! I already had visions of my wife on the operating table and coming back with a big ugly scar. Thank you!" I replied proudly: "And you doctors are always so pessimistic. Your wife didn't even have the slightest signs of an infection. But now I understand why you were so restlessly pacing the floor with your baby in your arms. I didn't even think about such dire consequences." I was happy that I had been able to provide the breastfeeding mother with such quick help, just by being perceptive and a bit creative. During my years as an independent midwife I used the pin successfully any number of times.

Methods of Treating a Congested Breast

If you are afflicted with congestion of the breast, begin by reading the information provided in the section on "Initial Engorgement" (see p. ■ ff.). All of the pointers given there are also helpful and quickly effective here.

- The most important thing is to let the baby suckle *as frequently as possible* and, if in doubt, wake it to ensure that the breast is emptied as soon as possible. Interestingly, most mothers report: "It's amazing; my baby seems to sense that it's supposed to drink a lot. Since I've had this congested breast, it drinks often and then goes back to sleep again for an hour or two." I am quite certain that the natural connection between the mother and child functions wonderfully in these situations. Often the only thing we lack is faith.
- Please be advised that a suitable breastfeeding position provides relief quickly. The baby's lower jaw should be on the side where the blocked duct is. This can be achieved by leaning over the baby in the all-fours position and letting it suckle on the hanging breast. It may look a bit comical, but it does you good and helps right away, thanks to the law of gravity, i.e. the fact that fluid flows downward.
- Other helpful means of treatment are *Stillöl/Nursing Oil $\mathcal{D}^{®}$*, quark compresses and white cabbage leaf compresses with *Rosengeranie-Lavendel-Massageöl/Rose-Geranium-Lavender Massage Oil $\mathcal{D}^{®}$*.
- The homoeopathic aids to be considered here are *Bryonia* and *Phytolacca* as

well as *Arnica, Aconitum, Belladonna, Pulsatilla, Silicea, Borax* and a number of others.

If you should happen to be in possession of the Homoeopathic Home and Travel Medicine Chest offered for sale by the Kempten Bahnhof-Apotheke, the first thing you can take when you become aware of the problem is *Aconitum*, followed by consulting the accompanying booklet (of the same name) to determine whether one of the time-tested substances *Bryonia, Phytolacca* or *Pulsatilla* is suitable for you. If not, make contact to a midwife or other health-care provider versed in homoeopathy. This person will ask you about your symptoms in detail and, with the aid of a reportory (an index of symptoms and pharmacological pictures) find the appropriate remedy for you. Don't be surprised, therefore, if your midwife pulls a book out of her bag and calmly begins looking for the substance exhibiting the greatest similarity with your symptoms. All midwives with training in homoeopathy are certain to have a copy of the repertory by Dr. Friedrich Graf, which is extremely helpful and will undoubtedly allow her to find the right remedy. It is the sign of a good homoeopathic therapist if she frequently refers to books, because otherwise she would have to be a computer on legs. Nobody could possibly remember all of the myriad remedies and all of their holistic effects. Scientific medicine has no medication for a febrile breast infection aside from alcohol compresses, which sink the fever, but cause dry skin, and antibiotics. Naturopathy, for its part, has a whole spectrum of treatments to choose from, as illustrated by this example.

Methods of Treating Mastitis

A true febrile breast infection (mastitis) is an extremely painful illness which can only be cured with bed rest. If a breastfeeding mother initially has only a slightly above-normal temperature, she should nevertheless stay in bed. She will get over the infection all the more quickly. From experience, I believe there is a correlation between lack of rest and mastitis: precisely those women who do not observe the recommendations pertaining to the postnatal period are the ones who develop febrile congestions of the breast. Once again, we observe that the body sees to it that it gets what it needs. Sometimes it has to expend a lot of energy (in this case fever) to call attention to its needs.

Midwives' Help

These situations are a double challenge for us midwives. On the one hand, we have to instruct the woman on how to proceed, aid her in putting the child to her breast properly and press the remaining congested milk out of her breast afterward. On the other hand, however, we also have to allay the entire family's fears of a breast infection, while at the same time making it very clear that the mother belongs in bed and the father belongs at home. If this is absolutely not possible, the services of a housekeeper have to be engaged. In Germany it is possible to apply to the health plan for financial aid to pay the house help in such cases. If this is likewise the case where you live, and you need your doctor to approve the application, the midwife should make sure that the doctor understands the following: The mother is not to be put back on her feet by giving her an antibiotic, and weaning is not the solution either! The doctor must only fill out the necessary form. This is one of those situations in which good cooperation between a midwife and a gynaecologist or general practitioner pays off. In moments like these I long for the return of the postnatal nurse's profession, which unfortunately no longer exists. How useful these women must once have been! But who knows, maybe along with our old remedies we'll also dig up an old occupation. In any case it would be desirable and extremely sensible.

Fortunately, most physicians have once again accustomed themselves to the fact that a midwife's help can and should be enlisted to treat a breast infection. Gynaecologists frequently ring up the midwife's practice and request support for one of their patients. In other words, word has spread that, with our methods, we can get a case of mastitis under control well without reverting to an antibiotic – which doesn't mean that the latter is not sometimes necessary after all.

Initial treatment is based on the principles of breastfeeding explained under the sections on putting the child to the breast, initial engorgement and congestion of the breast.

It is also important to get an idea of the woman's emotional situation and physical condition right at the start, and to assess whether the family is prepared to take responsibility for naturopathic treatment. During the first consultation, the midwife usually examines the breasts manually to determine where the congestion or centre of inflammation is, and how large it is. Here it is extremely important to pay attention to the size and intensity of the redness so as to have a basis for comparison as treatment proceeds. As she examines and observes, the midwife explains to the afflicted woman how serious she considers the situation to be. Then she will attempt to press some milk out so as to judge its colour and consistency. Next, it is absolutely essential that the breast be emptied. To this end, the midwife and the mother will attempt to put the hungry child to the breast. In the process, they should see to it that the baby's lower jaw is on the side where the congestion is located. This will enable it to draw out the thick, congested milk more easily. If the child is sleeping or breastfeeding proves too painful for the mother, the milk has to be expressed from the congested breast by hand. This process will cause her pain initially, but within just a few minutes the woman will notice a clear improvement and a relief from the pain. This is always accompanied with a lessening of tension in the inflamed breast. It often suffices to hand express the old, yellow, viscid milk which has collected just once. Sometimes, however, the procedure has to be repeated a second or third time on the days that follow. In most cases of mastitis, the body temperature goes down about half an hour after this treatment. Sometimes, however, it climbs to a very high level again before normalizing completely the following morning. In any case, the patient should stay in bed for a full additional day after the fever has disappeared. I urgently advise the mother to keep a watchful eye on both breasts and especially to protect them well from cold in the weeks that follow. For strange though it may seem, there are many cases in which the infection wanders from one breast to the other.

In the case of a breast infection it is moreover important to drink plenty of fluids so that the milk production does not decrease on account of the fever. The latter is a form of natural immunological defence which not only costs a lot of energy but also requires a lot of fluid. Moist body compresses or ablutions do the feverish patient good. Here the midwife is called upon to bring her nursing skills to bear and to teach the family a few "tricks". It is sad to see how much of this knowledge has been lost to families. We learn all kinds of things about mathematics and physics, but not the proper administration of a moist pack or an ablution – methods which contribute greatly to making a sick person feel better. When the patient begins to feel better, she is on her way back to health.

Mastitis is a serious illness and not always so easily overcome. Ask for help in good time, as soon as you notice congestion of the breast, to keep it from developing into a painful, febrile breast infection. In my antenatal classes, I always told the participants: "If you feel pain, discover redness or the breast feels very taut, pick up the phone in one hand and spread quark onto your breast with the other." The only decision there is to make is whether or not you want to continue breastfeeding. Then notify your midwife accordingly. Where necessary, she will engage the help of a doctor and the two will agree on the best method of treatment."

ⓢ Homoeopathic Treatment

As always, phenomena such as a wandering breast infection provide excellent pointers for finding the correct homoeopathic remedy. Conditions of this kind are described in homoeopathy; in this case the right choice would be *Lac caninum*. But there are also other substances to be considered, for example: *Aconitum, Belladonna, Bryonia, Chamomilla, Gelsemium, Lachesis, Phytolacca, Pyrogenium, Silicea*. I would like to describe a striking Belladonna mastitis "picture" in order to show how important it is to observe the condition carefully and study the repertories meticulously …

… Mrs. G. called to tell me that her temperature was above normal and one breast was red and painful. As described above, I began by assessing the condition of the breast and then undertook to express the milk by hand. She could not bear having her breast touched, said she would much rather stay in bed in her darkened bedroom and asked whether I knew of any homoeopathic remedy which could provide relief to her taut, overheated breast. I initially thought of giving her Bryonia and Phytolacca since it had often proven helpful to start out by administering these two remedies. This did not correspond to classical homoeopathic procedure, but, like my homoeopathy teacher himself, I knew from experience that these two substances were nearly always the correct treatment for mastitis. But suddenly I paused and reconsidered: This was not the typical infection, accompanied by a lumpy, painful breast. The redness of the breast looked different. The mother allowed me to open the curtains in the

bedroom for a minute and now I clearly saw that a red stripe had formed between the areola and the base of the breast. Upon close inspection, the symptoms now became distinct: a flushed face, sensitivity towards light, the desire for rest and the aversion to being touched. I referred to my book and, in the pharmacological picture for Belladonna, read the following: inflamed breast with reddening like the spokes of a wheel. That corresponded precisely to the woman's condition! I administered Belladonna C30, dissolved in a glass of water and stirred well. Half an hour later, Mrs. G. consented to having the milk pressed out of her congested breast. As always, after she had finished breastfeeding I spread quark on the affected area. When I rang her up later that day, the fever was already going down and the pain had disappeared entirely by the following day. The only symptom that remained for a few days longer was a certain sensitivity of the breast to being touched. This is completely normal, because, as elsewhere in the body, it takes a little while for a breast infection to heal completely.

With my knowledge of the healing powers of homoeopathic remedies, I am no longer afraid of breast infections. I can only confirm that, even for a midwife specialized in postnatal care, this method of healing is well worth the effort of learning.

⑤ Aroma Therapy and Breast Compresses

The administration of homoeopathic medication can be accompanied by spreading quark onto the painful, reddened area and leaving them there until they dry out. Either spread the quark directly onto the breast and cover them with a small towel or cloth, or wrap them in a large gauze pad by spreading them onto the pad and then folding it. A small, moist, cool cotton cloth soaked in essential oils or *Retterspitz External* represents a good substitute for a quark compress. Before applying the quark compress, you can gently rub *Stillöl/Nursing Oil 𝒟®* or *Rosengeranie-Lavendel-Massageöl/Rose-Geranium-Lavender Massage Oil 𝒟®* onto the breast. Never use plastic baggies or other plastic-coated materials on the breast, because they will block the escape of moisture. A small towel, woollen nursing pad or wool scarf are all good alternatives. When applying moisture in the form of curds or oil, make sure that the whole business isn't too wet and that the cold water doesn't reach the kidneys. Obviously, with a moist quark compress on your breast, you will have to stay in bed and not be up and around the house.

Even after a general improvement of the woman's condition, the curd treatment should be continued for at least one more day.

Another helpful measure is the application of *white cabbage leaves*. They have the same detoxifying effect as quark. Toxins form in the body on account of the fever; they put a strain on the organism and should therefore be excreted as quickly as possible. In this case it is best to support the process of excretion by way of the skin. To this end, the outer leaves are removed from the head of cabbage, then rolled with a rolling pin or bottle until they are soft and pliable and laid on the breast. As in the case of quark, a fresh leaf must be used for each new application. In the place of quark or cabbage leaves you can also apply Luvos *Healing Earth* to the breast, after having prepared it according to the instructions in the package. It doesn't matter what you use; ultimately the choice will be decided by what you happen to have in the house or can obtain quickly. When I was still making house calls, I had an arrangement with the manager of a nearby petrol station that he would always have "quark" (milk curds) on hand so that I could send the fathers out even at night and didn't have to keep raiding my own refrigerator.

Special Circumstances in Connection with the Child

Twins and Problem Children

Breastfeeding twins is essentially the same as breastfeeding a "oneling". Naturally, the mother is faced with the question: together or separately? There is no right or wrong answer; perhaps you can try both and decide which method you prefer. I have attended to many a mother of twins who mastered all of this like a "pro", simply by relying on her own instinct. With the help of your midwife, you are sure to find the right route to take. The fact that many twins grow up being partially breastfed and partially bottle-fed can often be attributed to the fact that the father or Grandma want to take a load off the mother, particularly with regard to feeding. But nappy-changing, washing the baby, cleaning house and cooking are also important duties!

As much as I would like to discuss everyday life with problem children, it would exceed the scope of this book. My chief concern is to enlighten my readers about natural methods of providing help when everything is proceeding normally. If your baby was born prematurely, ill, or in some way different, confide in a midwife. She will be as capable of helping you breastfeed your twins as of advising the mother of a baby with a cleft palate. Maybe there is an interest group of like-minded parents near where you live, who can likewise provide you with answers to your questions.

There are many situations in which it is not possible to breastfeed fully on account of the emotional or physical strain. Particularly if your child has to remain in the hospital, you will feel it is almost more than you can handle to pump the milk, go to the hospital every day, give your older children the proper care, tend to the household, etc. We occasionally hear of women who are afraid to call a midwife because they don't have their children at home yet. Gather your courage and make contact with a midwife! If you don't know of any, you can obtain addresses from the hospital, the doctor, the chemist's or your health plan team. I discover again and again that precisely these women do not receive any support or information for the simple reason that they don't know whom to turn to and are already at the limits of what they can manage. Actually, though, this difficult phase can, with all certainty, be relieved with a few good tips and pointers. It is especially important that you receive support and advice on breastfeeding, because sick and premature babies are even more dependent on the immunoglobulin in the mother's milk. Even if at first you don't succeed in breastfeeding fully, the baby should at least get the benefit of the milk you have. Be assured that even that "little bit" is better than nothing. When the day comes on which you are permitted to take your child home with you, I would once again like to advise you to ask a midwife to pay you a house call, because for you the day of discharge from the hospital is a day of being left alone with and having to take over full responsibility for your child. In that situation, you will undoubtedly be grateful for some pointers on caring for and breastfeeding your baby. With a lot of time and patience, you will soon be able to breastfeed your now healthy or meanwhile bigger "problem" child after all. Even if you still have to supplement the breast milk with infant formula, it's not the end of the world. As mentioned above: a bit of breast milk is always better than none at all. I have attended to many mothers who managed to breastfeed fully within a week. Naturally, it is important that you are prepared for what is more or less a delayed postnatal phase, i.e. that your husband has leave from work or one of the baby's grandmas can help you in the house.

Supplementing the Breast Milk

Bottle-Feeding

I am frequently asked if it is harmful to feed the baby a commercially prepared formula or home-concocted milk mixture from the bottle once a day. It goes without saying that, when the child is already several months old and the mother realizes that she simply no longer produces enough milk, she can supplement its diet with infant formula. Sometimes I have the impression that these days – in which breastfeeding has become more popular again – many mothers have a guilty conscience when they have to admit to themselves that they are no longer capable of breastfeeding their baby fully. But no woman should have to feel guilty for this reason. In these cases, I frequently tell women that it is preferable to supplement with infant formula – maybe a single bottle a day really will suffice – if it will help preserve harmony in the family, or if the mother is close to a nervous breakdown. It doesn't do the family any good if the baby is on a one-hundred-percent breast-milk diet but the mother is a nervous wreck as a result. A happy medium is always better than a forced, extremely stony path. As the mother, you yourself must decide what form of nutrition you feel most content and happy with for your child. Neither the baby nor your husband nor the rest of the family will be grateful to you for "sacrificing" yourself at the cost of your health. On the contrary, you'll constantly be reminded: "Yes, but this is the way you wanted it; now you'll just have to cope." Breastfeeding costs the woman enormous energy and can rarely be carried out at length without leading to a loss of strength. For this reason I would very much like to recommend my tonic "Aufbaumittel-

Stadelmann", a homoeopathic compound in powder form with which you can replenish your reserves of energy.

Solid Foods

Supplementation of the baby's diet with foods such as fruit, vegetables and solids is something which should be decided on an individual basis. When the mother begins to notice how the breastfeeding is consuming her energy and the child watches her eat with its mouth drooling, it is time to change to solids or at least supplement the breast milk with them. This generally occurs between the third and sixth months.

Be aware, however, that the baby's sense of taste is not yet as well-developed and diverse as yours or the product line of a baby food company. Here it can once again be helpful to seek contact with a breastfeeding group or mothers with more experience in these matters, or make an appointment with your midwife. These days you would think the nutrition of a small child was something extremely problematic and complicated, to read some of the brochures that are published on the subject. Use your common sense and rely on your maternal instinct. Even today, a baby really can still grow on grated apple, mashed banana, enhanced as time goes on by mashed cooked carrots, cauliflower and potatoes. Take the baby's limited sense of taste into account and increase the range of foods only very gradually.

Essentially, your baby can live on a diet consisting exclusively of breast milk until the end of the sixth month, as is recommended. But you don't have to follow this rule to a T. In particular, it is not advisable to stop breastfeeding from one day to the next, or even to reduce it by fifty percent. Rather, it should be a gradual transition, which begins in approximately the sixth month. It is around this time that the baby will express the desire to start eating and be capable of putting something into its mouth. That "something" doesn't have to be a toy, but can be something edible. It may take until your child is seven or eight months old to send out this signal. Be patient and react to your child's needs. Information brochures and advice from professionals can be helpful, but don't have to be considered an absolute must.

Breast Milk and Contaminants

A problem which affects everyone living today is that of pollutants. Particularly women who breastfeed will find themselves confronted with this issue. The first thing you should know is that the degree of contaminants in breast milk has been decreasing steadily for several years. But even if the levels of such substances as dioxins and PCBs have gone down markedly, thanks to new investigation methods a large number of other pollutants can now be detected – if only in minute quantities. An increasing proportion of synthetic aromas are likewise found in breast milk. The industry, and we as consumers, are therefore called upon to refrain from using all kinds of artificial substances in food, cosmetics, textiles and detergents – for the sake of our children and the coming generations.

In a sense, human breast milk is an indicator of the present state of environmental pollution. Even with this drawback, however, it is still the best nutrition we can offer our children. Due to its ideal composition and the protection it provides against illnesses, it is the most agreeable as well as the most healthful nutrition for the baby. Incidentally, it would be erroneous to think that infant formula offers a way out of the dilemma, because the contaminants are likewise detected in the commercially manufactured formulae.

The World Health Organization and the German national breastfeeding commission recommend breastfeeding for six months. If the breast milk is supplemented with solids, this period can be extended without causing the child any harm. If, however, you as a mother are uncertain in this respect, or think you may be or have been exposed to some particular pollutant, you can get in touch with your local public health office and request an analysis of your milk. In Germany, the analysis for dioxin contamination is only free of charge in justified cases because the accompanying tests are extremely expensive and have to be paid for by the state.

In order to avoid further increasing the level of contaminants in the breast milk, it is particularly important not to lose a weight unnecessarily during the breastfeeding period. Fasting or diets leading to quick weight loss and taking you below your initial pre-pregnancy weight level would cause your body to excrete toxins long stored in the fat tissue by way of the breast milk.

Weaning

At some point between the third month and the first or second year of the baby's life, you will have to inform yourself on the topic of weaning. Many children determine that point in time themselves and refuse the breast from one day to the next. Naturally, this is the ideal situation.

In many cases, the mother's desire to wean her child soon influences her milk production and the child. The milk quantity decreases from week to week, the baby takes pleasure in drinking from a bottle in the evening and eats more and more solid food.

Until the end of the first year it can be sensible to accustom the baby to formula gradually in the course of about two to three weeks, reducing the number of breast milk meals in the process. In some circumstances, this can be very difficult, particularly if the child has never drunk from a bottle before. In that case it will be better to wait and not wean the child until it is willing to eat solid food with a spoon. Incidentally, a child can grow up without ever having a bottle. But do allow your child some means of satisfying its sucking instinct for as long as possible. Sucking relaxes and contents it; it brings about a release of the "happiness hormone" and helps the child to fall asleep when it is tired, but also to cope with situations in which it is wrought up or distressed.

Babies can learn to drink fluids (tea and water) from a cup at a very early age. If it is still too small for that, however, you may have to employ a few tricks to get it accustomed to the rubber teat. Either you pump your own breast milk and feed it to the child in a bottle, or your place the rubber nipple over your own nipple so that the child can become accustomed to the new sensation. In this case, however, you should puncture a couple of extra holes in the teat because otherwise the child will become impatient, being used to drinking its fill from several milk ducts at once.

The more convinced you are about what you are doing, and the more time you leave yourself, the more smoothly the weaning process will go.

Perhaps, however, your child has become so accustomed to drinking from the breast that it refuses to accept any substitute. In my experience, this happens quite frequently with older children. Often there is only one solution. You take a holiday or go away for the weekend and your partner takes over on caring for and feeding the child. This is true "withdrawal treatment" but sometimes the only chance for success. It is only when the mother can no longer be seen nor heard nor – especially – smelled (she is sure to smell of breast milk) will the baby accept a substitute. But if you think to yourself, "No, I can't be that brutal and leave my screaming baby with my husband, the poor child!" then continue breastfeeding! I suspect that maybe you don't really want to stop breastfeeding yet.

On the other hand, there are children who suddenly favour the bottle over the breast. For the mother this is often linked with frustration and lots of tears. But console yourself with the thought that your child is so stable and independent that it no longer needs the intimacy of the breastfeeding relationship. This is not the first time your child will surprise you with a decision it has hatched in its own little head. Parting is painful in these moments, but is soon replaced by pride in the child's independence and maturity.

Often women are compelled to wean their babies because they urgently require a certain medication. I can only advise you to inform yourself carefully; this weaning advice is often given hastily and indiscriminately. There are excellent books in German about taking medications during pregnancy and the breastfeeding period (*Arzneimittel in der Schwangerschaft und Stillzeit* by Kleinebrecht and Windorfer; *Arzneiverordnung in Schwangerschaft und Stillzeit* by Schaefer and Spielmann) which I always refer to in these situations. There may well be comparable books in English. Another possibility is to ask the chemist or directly at the pharmaceutical company that makes the medication. Chemists can advise women and cooperate with the doctor to find an alternative medication. These procedures cost some time and effort, but our children should not be robbed of the best possible nutrition on account of thoughtlessness or false information.

Recommendations for Weaning

Reduce the amount of fluid you drink to a minimum. Avoid all diuretics such as beer, wheat beer, apple wine and sparkling wine. The best fluid for weaning is sage leaf tea, drunk in sips. If you are not receiving homoeopathic treatment, you can add a bit of peppermint to the sage. You can also drink and eat lemons in all variations.

Wear a rather tight, well-fitting bra and apply cold compresses to your breast as often as possible when you are at home. The old-fashioned tight breast wrap with a wide cotton bandage is just as effective a means as ever of stopping lactation. The bandage has to be so tight that the woman feels as if she is inside skin-tight "armour".

Homoeopathic Treatment

With the homoeopathic remedy *Phytolacca,* administered in a D2 or D3 potency in one-to-two-hour intervals, the mammary glands will no longer be able to secrete milk. As soon as your breasts remain soft, increase the intervals between doses until, after three or four days you only take five globuli three times a day. After a week, you must stop taking the remedy. *Lac caninum* or *Pulsatilla* may also be good choices. What matters most, as is so often the case, is the correct potency. Consult your midwife; even at this stage, she is still the right person to go to, and she will know which remedy is the right one for you. All three of those mentioned here, for example, should only be taken if truly indicated and not without sufficient knowledge.

Aroma Therapy

The *Original 𝒟*® Aroma Blend Salbei-Zypressen-Öl/Sage-Cypress Oil 𝒟®*, applied by means of a cold or quark compress, will undoubtedly be just as effective (see the passage on measures for reducing the milk quantity, p. 397 f.).

Regardless of when and how the intimate – but sometimes perhaps also burdensome – breastfeeding period comes to a close, it will always be connected with a bit of nostalgia. You may have longed for the freedom of not having to breastfeed, but soon you will realize: it was a beautiful, unforgettable and irrecoverable period, this "breastfeeding business". Don't plague yourself with thoughts about whether you weaned too soon or too late; just be happy about every drop of inestimably valuable breast milk you were able to give your child. Now the breastfeeding period is over, and it is undoubtedly good to have taken this step of letting go – letting your child go into a different world of nutrition. Sooner or later, every child must sever its ties with the mother's breast. No matter what the other people around you think, what is important is that you and your child agree on when the time has come for this separation.

THE LATE POSTNATAL PERIOD

Once the birth wounds have healed in the course of the first ten days, the above-described hormonal adjustments of the late postnatal period begin, a process lasting about eight weeks altogether. During this phase, the relationship between the newborn and the family becomes firmly established and the two begin to get to know one another. The initial euphoria is over and everyday life begins. As discussed in the introduction to the chapter on the postnatal period, the mother's inner balance is still unsettled. She may think everything has healed when she gets up from her bed about a week after birth. But she will soon become aware of her inner disarray.

She is no longer pregnant, no longer "freshly delivered", but she is also not the woman she was before getting pregnant. She usually feels unstable, inwardly topsy-turvy and in search of her self. Her pelvic floor aches in the evening and her back pains worsen in the course of the weeks; she often develops tension in the shoulders.

The pelvic floor is not yet firm enough to bear the weight of the body for hours on end. The feeling of pressure serves as a reminder that she has to start doing pelvic exercises regularly and conscientiously.

The tension in the back muscles is caused by an improper breastfeeding position and carrying the baby around to calm it down. After all, these muscles have not yet recuperated from the strains of pregnancy. The abdominal muscles are often still so soft and weak that the dorsal muscles are solely responsible for the body's stability. The uterus puts additional strain on the sacrum because the uterine ligaments are still slack and weak. As a result, the uterus often falls into a position of retroflexion.

The general instability and an unfavourable breastfeeding position lead to muscle tension in the upper body, perceivable as pain in the neck and shoulders.

All of these discomforts can be avoided if the mother is conscious of her condition and begins doing postnatal gymnastics on a regular basis about eight weeks after birth. The need to do exercises is what prompts many a women to make their way back to the midwife's practice and enjoy the atmosphere among other women in approximately the same situation.

Everyday Family Life/Being a Housewife

See to it that you have some help and support throughout the late postnatal period. If your girlfriend or the baby's Grandma offers to help, accept the offer gratefully: "Oh, that would be wonderful; I haven't managed to do the ironing and the windows desperately need cleaning!" Don't be afraid to ask for and accept assistance. Or if Grandma calls and says: "We'd like to come and see you and the baby again", you can – with a clear conscience – answer: "We'd love to have you – and we'd appreciate it no end if you could bring cake and dinner along for all of us." The grandmother will be glad to comply, because that way she won't feel so useless. Maybe it will even help her to come to terms with her new role as a grandmother. I could write an entire book just about complaining grandmothers. They are often sad that they're not allowed to help because "the young women of today want to do everything themselves." Really?

Your professional life is over for the time being, you're no longer receiving so much attention from your friends and relatives, your partner has to go back to work: In this phase, many women feel they can't cope, can't get enough sleep, and are afraid they can't meet the challenges of motherhood. For women who have given birth to their first child, an entirely new phase of life begins; for mothers with older children, family life undergoes some reshuffling. In the latter case, the mother has to come to terms with jealousy on the part of the baby's older sibling(s). Everyday life is discombobulated, the way it is in the weeks after you move house. On the outside, the mother is beaming, but inwardly everything is in disarray and needs to be reorganized. The mother and father have to adapt their relationship to the new situation. The man doesn't know when, where or how to approach the woman with regard to intimacy. "Is she ready for lovemaking yet or do I have to leave her alone for the time being?" is a standard question a man will ask, while the woman waits to be embraced, needs someone to lean on and lots of affection, but worries that he'll misunderstand and want to go "all the way". It takes the woman quite a long time to want "everything" again – physical love and sexuality – often because of a fear of pain or unfamiliar sensations. One man described this situation very aptly:

… *"We had to get to know one another all over again, like in the first phase of our relationship. Except that, back then, we were worried about our parents walking in on us. Now, every time we got started, the baby would cry. It was pretty darned nerve-racking during the first few weeks after the birth. Either I was unsure about asking, or my wife felt like it when I was exhausted, or our baby kicked up a fuss. But now it's more beautiful than ever. Our love has taken on entirely new aspects and is satisfying to a degree we never knew before."*

I attach great importance to making it clear to the family that it really does take at least eight weeks until a woman can bear a full load. My old midwife once said to me: "As long as it takes the child to grow [in the womb], that's how long it takes for the mother to recover. Where I come from, they used to say it takes nine months for the womb, the abdomen and the breasts to return to their old form." I didn't know what she was talking about back then; my own life was so fast-paced. Today I often recall her words. A mother's environment is not very likely to understand this gradual transformation. But I am quite confident that if women start insisting that the postnatal period be recognized as a phase in its own right, this process will become more tangible for everyone involved. The late postnatal period will bring far fewer depressions with it if you allow yourself the rest you need. Every young mother should have the right to a regular afternoon nap. Learn to relax for half an hour or an hour; the mountain of housework won't be any smaller afterwards but you'll be able to take care of it much more quickly if you have gathered fresh energy. I know that many people literally have to learn how to take an afternoon nap, but believe me, it's not that difficult. You simply have to give yourself permission. And maybe it would do the family good if everyone else followed suit.

It will boost your self-confidence to take an afternoon off and go out and buy yourself something, maybe a new blouse. In my opinion, clothing plays a big role in the late postnatal period. In many cases, it takes as long as thirty weeks until the old trousers and skirts fit again. Getting your day started in the morning after a strenuous night can be all the more frustrating when you look in the mirror and find bleary eyes, unkempt hair and jeans a size or two too small staring back at you. After a visit to the hairdresser's you'll like yourself better again – not just optically –; a new pair of trousers will help you to accept your soft, round tummy. Children not only love their mummy's soft bosom, but also her tummy. Whoever said that a mother has to be as slender as a beanpole? That was merely invented by advertising. Incidentally, many men also find soft women very cuddly. So be proud of your motherly curves.

I highly recommend that you join some kind of mother-baby group where you can get together with other mothers on a regular basis. After all, in professional life there are also team meetings in every department. When your partner comes home from work, don't tell him about all the things you didn't get around to, but report to him about the multifarious professional responsibilities you had to fulfil as a mother: those of the baby nurse, the kindergarten teacher, the cook, the cleaning lady, the general practitioner, the teacher and the psychologist. The everyday life of a mother encompasses all of these occupations. Don't be surprised if initially you have the feeling that "I just sat around at home all day" when you look back on your day or talk about it with others. Another important aspect is that you exhibit a constant willingness to learn in the years of motherhood. The bigger your children get, the sooner you should be in the habit of asking yourself what new challenges they will present you with on a given day. Learn not to doubt yourself and your child-raising methods constantly, but do question and examine them regularly, with a view to what you can do to improve them. Above all, you should get into the habit of looking at the problems that come up daily from the child's perspective. Things that were right for the first child will be different when the second child reaches that stage, and the third child will show you entirely new possibilities. Accept "just being home" as a new profession in which the foremost task is to face new challenges every day. You will be able to overcome them effortlessly if you approach them in a relaxed manner and, if possible, talk about your experiences with women who have raised or are raising more than one child. Be spontaneous and flexible and embark on an adventure. But don't forget to reward yourself every day – maybe you're not the only mother or the only househusband whose first act when the children are asleep is to reach for the chocolate. Give yourself regular treats, for example a regular massage, and in your partner relationship, get into the habit of praising one another every evening. And if in the midst of motherhood – which is strongly influenced by hormone fluctuations –

you find yourself having a "down", remember that only she who loves herself is loved by others.

Symptoms Accompanying the Late Postnatal Period

Bleeding

Again and again, a woman's body will show her the "red card", in other words (to stick to sports jargon) "send her off the field". The uterus tells her unequivocally that the internal wounds have not healed entirely yet. Physical or emotional strain will cause mucous membranes on the uterine wall to break off and be flushed out by means of bleeding.

You don't have to panic if you suddenly experience bright red, menstrual-type bleeding three weeks following childbirth. Take care of yourself in the manner recommended for the early postnatal period and be aware that the bleeding may have come about in connection with increased lactation.

You can relieve your symptoms with the same natural methods used in the early postnatal period, but if the bleeding continues, by all means consult a doctor.

First Menstruation

If such bleeding occurs six to twelve weeks after birth, it may simply be your first postnatal menstruation. Even mothers who breastfeed can start having their period regularly quite early on. This first menstrual bleeding will be quite heavy and often accompanied by severe pain in the small of the back and the lower abdomen. Cancel all dates and appointments and "call in sick" at home as well. If you take it easy, this first menstruation won't be so bad. Most women are disappointed that the menstruation-free phase is already over. At the same time, they're happy about the return of their period, because a regular cycle can bring about a harmonization of the hormone system. It is equally normal and natural not to begin menstruating until after you have stopped breastfeeding. But be careful! Breastfeeding is by no means a trustworthy method of contraception. As long as you breastfeed at four-hour intervals, the effect is supposedly as reliable as a coil. But don't forget: it is not at all uncommon for a woman wearing a coil to get pregnant! (On the topic of breastfeeding and menstruation, read the passage on p. ■.)

Pains in the Small of the Back

Many women complain of pain in the sacrum. The causes have been discussed above. Change your breastfeeding position or the height of the changing table if necessary. There are several reasons why it is better to carry your baby in a baby sling than in your arms; for one thing, it's easier on your back. Even if you have difficulties at first, be persistent and practice regularly. You will learn to tie the baby sling perfectly and entirely forget that you ever had problems with it. There is no substitute for this intimate connection with your child, and what's more, it's extremely practical. You'll see – your partner will enjoy it just as much as you do. Perhaps the midwife or breastfeeding group leader can help you and pass on a few tips and tricks.

Pains in the small of the back can, however, also be a sign of ovulation or the beginning of the first menstrual bleeding.

⑤ Homoeopathic Treatment

Homoeopathy – which, incidentally, can be used very effectively in combination with aroma therapy – has repeatedly proven helpful in coping with these discomforts. The following time-tested remedies are the most likely to be the right choice in this context: *Arnica, Hypericum, Rhododendron, Rhus toxicodendron, Kalium carbonicum* and *Sepia.*

⑤ Aroma Therapy

Kreuzbein-Massageöl/Lower Back Massage Oil 𝒟® will provide you relief and give your partner an excuse to spoil you with a massage. Many women continue to use this pleasant-smelling body oil even after the late postnatal period is over. Another helpful *Original 𝒟® Aroma Blend* for these symptoms is *Körperöl kräftigend/Body Oil Strengthening 𝒟®*, which – incidentally – fathers also enjoy as a back massage oil.

Debility

"Tell me, is this normal? My hair is falling out! If this goes on, I'll be bald soon." That is one of the questions most frequently asked by women during the late postnatal period. My answer: "In addition to the sweating and forgetfulness, the mother also sheds hair. And it's not the baby's fault, as many fathers seem to think."

In the weeks following childbirth, young mothers notice that they are constantly breaking out in a sweat, similar to the hot flashes of menopause. This is caused by hormonal fluctuations and is a natural means of protection for our bodies since it ensures that we stay home more often than we used to. This condition is certain to pass at the end of the late postnatal period, only returning for one or two days before your first menstruation.

The degree of hair loss during the late postnatal period varies from one woman to the next. Some mothers won't notice anything at all; others will keep a worried eye on their "receding hairline". But doesn't motherhood have something very mysterious about it? Soon beautiful, completely new hair will begin to sprout on all sides. Incidentally, some women's hair structure changes permanently. Thin hair becomes thick and full, straight hair becomes curly and vice versa.

During the late postnatal period, many women's partners lack an understanding for how forgetful their wives are. After being so considerate during pregnancy, during childbirth, during the early postnatal period, the partner simply refuses to adapt to this relatively harmless weakness. But it really does happen; you will notice that you forget the simplest things. Don't worry about this condition inordinately; just make yourself a shopping list; that will spare you endless discussions as to why this or that is missing in the house. This forgetfulness, by the way, is a "side effect" of the breast-feeding hormone, prolactin. What it signifies is that the mother should devote herself primarily to breastfeeding and nothing else. If she forgets an appointment, it will probably be of advantage to the baby. A breastfeeding mother has the feeling she is thinking with her bosom instead of her head; she hears her baby crying from miles away, but she lets something boil over on the stove. If she doesn't keep setting herself a timer, she's lost. Forgetfulness, however, can also be a sign of anaemia. If it really takes on "senile" dimensions, it may be worthwhile to have your blood tested for iron deficiency.

Most of the problems experienced by breastfeeding mothers are caused by exhaustion. Unfortunately, women rarely talk about this condition so clearly because they themselves find it difficult to believe that these "couple of pounds of baby" can be so strenuous. Formerly they held their own for entire days at their jobs and now this little bit of housework and infant care is suddenly so tiring? To make matters worse, many women start going back to work for a few hours a week even before they have stopped breastfeeding. What's more, people of today have apparently forgotten that women used to breastfeed their children, but they weren't responsible for all of the rest of the work that needs doing. There was often a grandmother, a great-aunt or other women around, often living in the same house or on the same farm. Where this was not the case, a subsequent birth often meant the woman's death because she had become so weak.

When breastfeeding mothers come to us with their problems, we midwives therefore often know the cause: They feel drained, they're exhausted, and they complain about the accompanying discomforts. Often they haven't managed to make up for the loss of blood during labour and are accordingly suffering from a double sapping of their energy. In addition to blood loss and lactation – as much as one litre/one quart per day –, they are also drained by the loss of fluid brought about by the nocturnal perspiration attacks. I myself remember the months following the births of my own children only too well. Hormonal fluctuations and the loss of energy often detracted from my feelings of happiness and gratefulness for the healthy, happy child. Many women confirm that they feel completely spent, literally as though the baby had sucked out all of their life energy.

Herbal Medicine

One of the most helpful tea blends for this period is *Frauentee nach I. Stadelmann/ Women's Tea after I. Stadelmann*, containing lady's mantle, St.-John's wort, lemon balm, chaste tree and yarrow. This blend provides support to the female hormone system and helps stabilize a woman's nerves and emotions for the burdens she is bearing.

Incidentally, *blackthorn juice* is a beverage with very good strengthening and lactation-promoting qualities and therefore makes an excellent present for any woman in the postnatal period.

⑤ Aroma Therapy

The *Original D® Aroma Blend Wochenbettbauchmassageöl/Childbed Abdominal Massage Oil D®* is sure to provide optimal support. Maybe it will even become your new favourite body oil. Particularly the yarrow it contains helps prevent you from falling into a postnatal depression. The yarrow appears to me to be the most appropriate essential oil for the postnatal phase and will work wonders in helping the mother find her inner balance again. I created my *Körperöl festigend/Firming-Up Body Oil D®* especially for women suffering from depression in addition to general exhaustion. The essential oils verbena, jasmine, clary sage, myrtle, rose geranium, yarrow, vetiver and cypress work to strengthen and stabilize the hormone system.

The most suitable oils for the aroma lamp are those I mentioned in connection with the early postnatal period. I can highly recommend grapefruit as a fresh scent that is guaranteed to cheer you up and get you smiling again, help you rediscover motherhood – and maybe even experience it as a wonderful adventure.

⑤ Homoeopathic Treatment

Years ago, during one of my own postnatal experiences, I was desperately in search of an appropriate homoeopathic remedy which would restore my depleted energy, raise my iron level and stop my hair from falling out. My homoeopathist prescribed me a tonic which was a fairly good help but, in my opinion, contained too much Vitamin A and D. So I sat down myself to look for the most suitable homoeopathic substance. I soon discovered, however, that there were a great many pharmacological pictures which corresponded with the situation of the exhausted mother in the postnatal period. So I took my request to the Bahnhof-Apotheke in Kempten, and together the pharmacist and I concocted a homoeopathic compound which we called *"Aufbaumittel Stadelmann"* and which has since helped many a person in a state of depleted energy: pregnant women, women in the postnatal period, breastfeeding women and people recovering from serious illnesses. In the meantime it is often even prescribed by doctors. May all classical homoeopathists forgive me, but the success of this powder speaks for itself (composition, see p. 441). It can either be taken as needed or regularly twice to three times a day in doses of one teaspoon at a time, dissolved on the tongue. Many midwives confirm my experience and, incidentally, also use the powder for women whose strength ebbs during labour or when the dilation phase is very tedious and energy-consuming. During a home birth, the powder can take the place of an infusion. It has also proven extremely effective in cases of iron deficiency or circulatory problems during pregnancy. Due to its lactose basis and the glucose D1 the powder contains, the homoeopathic iron is immediately absorbed by the body. The tonic has been taken by many women as a means of avoiding conventional iron supplements, and they report that their iron level rises rapidly as a result. And fellow midwives have told me that they have prescribed a pinch of the powder to icteric newborns who don't suckle well and thus managed to cope with the problems without the child's having to be admitted to the hospital. I highly recommend keeping a bottle of this powder in the house and administering it whenever a member of the family is at the end of his or her energy rope. It will help activate the body's natural self-help mechanisms.

Sexuality after Childbirth/Contraception

Frequently the midwife or the parents themselves will bring up the topic of sexuality during one of the last house calls, a topic which goes hand in hand with the question of contraception.

Sexuality

What both partners should know is that, during the breastfeeding period, the lactation hormone prolactin can decrease the woman's sexual desire and cause the vagina to dry out. A lack of sexual desire is therefore not a sign that the woman has a sexual aversion to the man. The woman's organism simply has another priority for the time being, so to speak: to care for the baby, before she concentrates on something else again. It should not be forgotten that the foremost purpose of sexual intercourse is to preserve the species, and that task has just been successfully fulfilled.

Women who do not contract any injuries during childbirth are often sexually active again far sooner than those who do. Often they already ask the midwife within a few weeks after birth whether there is any reason to refrain from sexuality. These couples enjoy the experience of the birth and their affection for one another on all levels and with all pleasure quite soon.

There are widely differing statements concerning the woman's ability to experience an orgasm after childbirth. A lot is written on the subject and many claims are made, but the topic nevertheless remains a taboo. It is entirely possible that, following a traumatic birth, a woman needs more time before she can turn her attention to physical love again. But the rumour that a woman can no longer have an orgasm after giving birth is nothing but nonsense! On the contrary, I have attended to many a couple who reported that it was only after the birth of their children that they experienced truly fulfilling sexuality.

If for some reason the birth of the new child was a difficult one to come to terms with, it is important that the couple learn to talk to one another about this delicate subject, perhaps with the help of the midwife or a counsellor or therapist. This aspect is unfortunately often placed at the bottom of the priority list, because the newborn initially demands the parents' attention "twenty-four/seven". In the course of the weeks and months that follow, however, it will be important for the partner relationship to consist not only of an emotional connection but also comprise the physical aspect again, because good sexuality is a decisive factor in a relationship. We midwives unfortunately often witness situations in which the couple simply accepts the fact that everything has been different since the birth of the child. The woman devotes herself to motherhood – and finds fulfilment there – and soon returns to her job, thus taking on an enormous double burden; the man spends more time than ever on sports. Sooner or later the breastfeeding period ends; life gets back to normal and the lack of sexual satisfaction is expressed in the form of increasing tension, lack of harmony and bad moods. Both partners suffer from the absence of the "happiness hormones": as is the case during childbirth, sexual intercourse activates sex hormones and leads to an indescribable feeling of happiness, a regular endorphin "trip". The feeling of floating on Cloud Nine, a bit closer to heaven, helps the parents cope with the normal problems of everyday life – to say nothing about the fact that these hormones contribute decisively to one's overall emotional and physical well-being and stabilize the immune system. Even a child who has developed into the family's sunshine can never replace this endorphin high.

Domestic harmony is thus not solely dependent on whether or not the newborn sleeps through the night, the kindergarten child is obedient and willing to learn, the school child does well in school, etc. but on the relationship between the parents. If their sex life is unhappy or has ceased to exist, the parents sub-consciously place increasingly high expectations on the children and the relationship automatically becomes more and more crisis-ridden. What is more, an enormous unconscious burden is placed on the backs of the children. In our society, sexuality is a constant topic in the media, but in reality it is still much too taboo a topic between young parents.

These problems may be brought up for discussion by the midwife leading a post-natal exercise class, or by the participants themselves. It would be a shame, however, if they then merely talked *about* and not *to* the men. Now and then there is a couple who pluck up the courage to broach the subject with the midwife and ask for her help in finding a solution. We midwives are an excellent choice in these situations, because during the intense phases of pregnancy, childbirth, the postnatal period and breastfeeding we have gotten to know the parents extremely well and gained insight into their relationship. Naturally, a midwife is seldom trained in couples counselling, but she has all of the experience of her profession and her own partnership to draw from. If the midwife advises the couple to get counselling, her words are more likely to be heeded than if they are voiced by someone the parents don't know. It took me several years to realize that the gynaecologist, for example, is not necessarily the right person to turn to, because his focus is directed primarily towards the physical conditions for sexuality. He will tend to say something like: "Everything has healed and there is no further obstacle to resuming your sexual relationship; I assume you have already discussed contraception with your husband." Often doctors simply don't have the time, and women can't explain their sexual problems to them on their way from the internal examination to the changing room.

The holistically minded midwife often finds a means of helping the couple in the naturopathic treasure chest. A homoeopathic remedy, Bach flowers, an essential oil blend and the advice to go and see a skilled craniosacral therapist have often helped to solve this sensitive topic to the point where it wasn't a topic at all anymore and the young family's happiness was restored.

Family planning associations, for example the German "Pro Familia", also offer help with problems related to sexuality and generally have offices in all of a country's large cities.

If you are a couple who really need time and sensitivity to come to terms with the birth experience, I would like to encourage you to be patient with yourselves and leave yourselves all the time in the world. Things will never be the way they were, because now you are parents, but your sexuality can become more beautiful and more open than ever! Maybe you can leave the child in the hands of a competent and trusted babysitter and treat yourselves to a wellness day which will help you to encounter one another as a twosome: with a pleasant relaxation massage, an energy-boosting sunbath, a romantic candlelight dinner and a massage oil with aphrodisiacal qualities on your night table.

Sooner or later you will sense a desire to have another child, whether only on the mental level or on the physical level as well. Give yourselves and another child the opportunity to experience birth again. Perhaps you will find, like countless other couples, that the second birth will reconcile you with the first! The birth of a second child can help you to attain closure and make peace with the subject of childbirth. Third children are then often the result of true physical desire – and being tired of using contraception. In many relationships one of the partners realizes that children really are the true point in life and their conception should not be the result of rational planning. My view is confirmed again and again: the first child is the product of two hearts in love, the second a rational decision, the third a result of physical desire.

New Challenges in Conjunction with Sexuality

Among the many different reasons for the fact that sexuality becomes a critical topic during the breastfeeding period are the injuries contracted during childbirth, which are still "sensitive to the touch" on the emotional as well as the physical level, and are associated with strange, new feelings. It is not only the woman, but also often the man who has problems after a birth which has ended with surgical measures or an episiotomy and doesn't know how to come to terms with them. There is not only the wound and the scars on the perineum, vagina and/or labia and the emotional uncertainty, but also physical obstacles: the dryness of the vaginal milieu and the lactating breasts. Under these new conditions, physical union can become a challenge for both parties. The "missionary position" should be used with great care during the first three months, because it exposes the perineal scar to considerable pressure which can cause the woman pain. The couple are called upon to be imaginative in the lovemaking context, just as they were during the phase of getting to know one another and again during pregnancy. They can think up new ways of showing affection and new lovemaking positions and shouldn't forget that *Dammmassageöl/Perineum Massage Oil D®* not only made the genital tissue supple for childbirth but is also a suitable and effective means of making the scars in that zone less sensitive. There is hardly a human being on earth who doesn't like to be caressed! If you have some *Geburtsöl/Childbirth Oil D®* left over, it is also appropriate for application to the vagina. When the bottle has been used up, many couples like to switch to *Massageöl blumig/Massage Oil Flowery D®* or *Massageöl Frisch/Massage Oil Fresh D®* . Please be advised, however, that fatty plant oils make condoms porous – i.e. their safety as a means of contraception can no longer be guaranteed.

For some couples, the presence of the newborn in the parents' bed turns into a major obstacle. One woman remarked to me: "I don't know what my husband's problem is. While I was pregnant, the baby witnessed what we were doing from inside the womb, and now from the outside?!" If the family is already larger, there is the light sleep of the "big" kids to contend with, who are suddenly found standing in the doorway saying: "When you guys are finished, I just wanted to tell you that …" And, naturally, it should not be forgotten that some days are so strenuous – after all many a night's sleep is cut short with a newborn in the house – that now the woman, now the man falls asleep the minute his or her head hits the pillow.

Contraception

And when the moment finally arrives that every obstacle has been overcome, the children are taken care of, the evening was romantic, the leftover *Geburtsöl/Childbirth Oil D®* has already been poured into a little bowl for use during a sensitive foreplay massage, the woman is melting with desire, suddenly it occurs to the couple: "Wait a minute, what if I'm already capable of conceiving again?"

Contraception is a topic which sometimes goes unresolved for months and robs the parents of the pleasure of sexuality. The two of them have gotten accustomed to the woman's milk-producing bosom – the baby is likely to be suckling at it pleasurably at this very moment – can live with the whole family sharing the parents' bed because the living-room sofa turned out to be too uncomfortable, have taken care of the problem of dryness by massaging each other with oil, and gotten rid of inhibitions about physical contact because he learned to tell her: "I love to look at you; the scar doesn't bother me at all" and she was able to confirm that she can enjoy the massages and the phase of tuning in to one another the way she used to and a wonderful feeling of sensitivity has returned to her pelvis. And nevertheless, perhaps she won't be able to have her accustomed orgasm the first few times because the couple hasn't had time to talk about the issue of contraception. This is understandable: she's worried the condom might not be entirely reliable, and anyway, oil can't be used in conjunction with a condom or vice versa because the plant oils can disintegrate the rubber, but without oil intercourse might hurt because of the dry state of the vagina. She can't take the pill because she's breastfeeding, and she doesn't want to take gestagen because she's so tired of taking pills. Neither partner likes the coil as a means of contraception because it actually only prevents the ovum from embedding itself in the lining of the uterus, but not conception. Or she has already had a coil but had it removed because she menstruated so heavily and she just couldn't get used to the feeling of having a foreign body inside her. What remains are the so-called barrier methods – the diaphragm, cervical cap and LEA contraceptivum, all of which may be strange and unfamiliar. What now? There's the contraception computer Ladycomp, but it's quite expensive. Parents who have already had several children may consider sterilization. But the mother went through the pregnancies and the births and thinks now it's time her husband did his share, but he's afraid to take such an irrevocable step. Really no more children, ever again?

A solution can only be found together. Leave yourselves time; perhaps talk to your midwife about it again. You may find that you come to the same conclusion as the man who said: "Oh, let's just forget it for the time being; when she's done breastfeeding we'll just take our chances until another baby comes. After all, my wife is the happiest when she's pregnant or breastfeeding!"

Perhaps the best route, therefore, is for the man to be patient. Thanks to this new child, the partner relationship will revolve around other things for the time being anyway. What is important, though, is that he regularly communicates to her that he likes and appreciates her. Every loving word, every little gesture, an affectionate hug, a gentle caress gives rise to moments of happiness – and with them, the so-called "happiness hormones".

Remember, moreover, that sexuality may be an important part of every relationship, but it's not everything! When your hearts are happy, your pelvises will follow suit and you can be very sure that a phase of the most fulfilling hours of lovemaking – complete with orgasms – will come. I have heard many women say: "You know, natural contraception is the best form, because it makes me stay in tune with my body, and even my husband knows exactly when I'm capable of conceiving or not. We lived with the contraception computer for ages, and it showed us red (the sign of fertility) again and again, but the feeling of bliss and desire were so great that we ended up just ignoring that machine!" Incidentally, I would also like to take this opportunity to refute the widespread belief that women who have had several children are frigid because their vaginas are stretched out. That is simply not true! On the contrary, many home birth parents (not one of those women had an episiotomy) have reported that the most beautiful sex they experienced was after their children had all been born.

The Adventure of Parenthood

Having reported so extensively on the physical discomforts and emotional strains a woman is subjected to during the postnatal period, last but certainly not least, I would like to point out that the experience of motherhood is a wonderful one in the life of a woman. I have no doubt that nature introduces the elevating feeling of motherhood only to those women who have the good fortune of being able to go through this experience.

For you as the mother and father, every new day in your life with your child will bring new surprises. Enjoy every day anew, with an awareness that this happiness is a great gift. It can be over so soon: nobody knows how long the child will be permitted to remain with you. Some people live only very briefly; no-one signs a contract with eternity when they are born. However great the strain, effort and pain – physical as well as emotional –, however sleepless the nights, as your children grow, you will learn what it means to have them: it means not to be alone. But also remember that you will only accompany your child for one stretch along the path of its life. The day will come when you have to let go.

"The wings to freedom grow in letting go."

Try to make this guideline your own; perhaps it will help you when, one day, the children grow up, leave home and live their own lives. You as parents can look back on a meaningful, fulfilled life. The experience of the child's first conscious hand games, its first laugh in an otherwise very exhausting night, will reward you for all the effort. Its first steps, its first "Mama" and "Dada", the happy gurgling when "Dada" walks through the door will erase the strains of the day at work in a flash.

Life without children would be empty and tedious. I wish you strength and staying power so that you can consciously experience your child's growth in many hours of calm and relaxation.

BASIC PRINCIPLES OF HERBAL MEDICINE

History

Herbal medicine is as old as mankind itself. Its history dates back to the very earliest sources. In Chinese medicine, there is knowledge of the author of a pharmacological study of plants dating from the period around 3700 bc. In India, herbal medicine was described more than 1,500 years ago in the *Book of Ayurveda*. The herbal-medicinal knowledge of the Mediterranean regions was first recorded by the Greek physician Dioscorides in his work *De Materia Medica* of the first century AD. The thread of herbal medicine (also referred to as phytotherapy) thus runs throughout history; knowledge of it has come down to us from the Egyptians, the Romans, the Jews and the Teutons.

Among the most well-known German-language medical works are the twelfth-century AD writings of the abbess Hildegard von Bingen which are presently being rediscovered with a great deal of enthusiasm. In fact, medieval convents and monasteries played a significant role in this context since, thanks to the herbal books written there, that period's knowledge of the healing powers of plants is available to us today.

The identification of the substances contained in plants and research on their effects have become recognized sciences. After technology was introduced to medicine, however, herbal medicine led a shadowy existence for many decades, although it is – and always has been – one of the fundamental elements of scientific medicine. With the aid of chemical analysis methods as well as pharmacological and toxological studies, it has been possible to identify, isolate and improve on substances which today are still the core element of many medicines, for example acetylsalicylic acid, which is obtained from the salicin found in the bark of certain willows.

In 1978, along with homoeopathy, herbal medicine was granted the status of a special form of therapy under German law.

Production of Plants for Herbal Medicine

The plants are frequently cultivated in special gardens where they receive meticulous care and are harvested under the appropriate conditions.

Plants (or parts thereof) obtainable from pharmacies are referred to in herbal medicine as drugs; they must be of high quality and correspond to the presently valid pharmacopoeias with regard to identity, purity and active ingredient content. They must moreover be tested for toxic residue.

The active ingredients are extracted from the leaves, fruits, seeds, bark and roots of the plants in the optimal manner.

The Use of Medicinal Plants

Medicinal plants are used in medicine successfully every day in the form of tea, tincture, extract creams and lotions, etc. Active ingredients extracted from plants can also be included among the ingredients of standardized medicinal products.

Due to their active ingredients, phyto-pharmaceuticals (pharmaceutical products made from plants) can be classified as prescription or non-prescription drugs; in Germany a distinction is also made between non-prescription drugs which must be sold in a pharmacy and those which can also be sold elsewhere. At the same time, however, the same substances, if contained in herbal tea, can legally be classified as food.

To serve as *tea*, the plants or their parts are carefully dried and crushed. Where possible, they should be obtained from areas which have been tested for toxins. Only a small spectrum of active ingredients is present in tea.

Tincture is generally an alcoholic extract with a ratio of 1:5 to 1:10. The alcohol content and the form of extraction are selected in such a way as to obtain the broadest possible active ingredient spectrum.

Tincture offers a number of advantages over tea, since it contains not only the water-soluble substances but also those soluble in fat and alcohol.

A *plant extract* is the concentrated tincture or the dry extract of plant parts.

The Effects of Medicinal Plants

Medicinal plants can heal illnesses, help to prevent them and relieve the discomforts they cause. Support in the healing process can be attained by means of internal and external applications.

Compresses are used primarily with tinctures and – as described further on in the section on aroma therapy – always be applied in accordance with the basic phytotherapeutic principle, for example hot compresses to stimulate circulation and cold in cases of inflammations and injuries characterized by heat.

The use of medicinal herbs is sensible when the potentials and limitations of their application are observed closely.

Medicinal Plants in Midwifery

Medicinal plants are used traditionally in the context of midwifery. Reports on experience with medicinal plants clearly show that their effects in the treatment of pregnant and birthing women and women in the postnatal period are not to be underestimated – as is perhaps evidenced most clearly by Verbena officinalis as well as the spices cinnamon, cloves and ginger. During pregnancy, they can bring about inordinately strong uterine contractions; during birth, on the other hand, they can be used in the place of medicinal induction methods. Recent observations show that women should be cautious with the intake of poppy seeds, which can cause bleeding.

The Application and Dosage of Herbal Tea Blends

Unless otherwise specified, all herbal teas discussed in this book are blended as follows:

• equal parts of all ingredients

Preparation of tea for the expectant or postpartum mother:

• one heaping teaspoon to one cup (125 ml/4.5 fl. oz.) of water

Preparation of tea for the newborn
• ½ teaspoon to one cup of water

Tea should not be taken in great quantities or for prolonged periods. Generally its administration for several weeks and a maximum of three months suffices. Exceptions to this rule can be made during pregnancy and the breastfeeding period. Here again, however, it is important to observe the recommendations as to when the intake of an herbal tea blend can or should be discontinued.

Preparation

Pour boiling water over the dried herbs and allow them to steep for ten minutes. For this purpose, a large tea net can be used, or the tea poured through a sieve once it has steeped.

Tea blends in teabags are not recommended because the herbs in them are too finely cut/ground and, moreover, the packaging of each teabag separately to protect the aroma causes a lot of waste. Teabag blends are often supplemented with essential oils in microcapsules since the oils naturally present in the herbs are lost due to the fine cutting. Instant tea generally consists of spray-dried glucose syrup or glucose granulate supplemented with dry extracts and essential oils. The readymade granulate blends contain approximately ten percent dry extract, corresponding to about fifty percent fresh herbs.

Seeds such as caraway, fennel and anise should be freshly crushed (not ground but gently crushed, just to the point where the outer shell is opened) so that the effects of the essential oils can develop. The crushed seeds only keep for about three weeks in an airtight container. Fennel tea, for example, will only serve to counteract wind if it is prepared with freshly crushed seeds as opposed to teabags.

Dosage

To avoid undesirable side effects, the maximum amount per day – specified in the sections of this book wherever relevant – should not be exceeded. The proportion of water can, however, be increased.

For infants, a few teaspoons a day generally suffice.

The tea should be drunk in sips at a lukewarm to warm temperature (not cold).

Storage Life of Herbal Tea

Once prepared, the tea should be drunk within twelve hours, after which the danger of microbial contamination is too great. Tea which is left standing for several hours moreover tends to take on a bitter taste.

Storage Life of Dried Herbs

Dried herbs can be kept for half a year to a year at the very most. After that they take on a musty taste.

Application of Tinctures

In general, the instructions enclosed in the packaging should be observed for the application of herbal tinctures. The latter should never be administered to open wounds in undiluted form.

Interaction with Other Forms of Treatment

Herbal applications often complement homoeopathic or aromatherapy treatment well. Other alternative healing methods, for their part, do not impair the effects of herbal extracts.

During treatment with homoeopathic remedies, peppermint tea should be avoided. Many homoeopathists also advise against the intake of chamomile tea during homoeopathic treatment.

Contraindications during Pregnancy

Pregnant women should avoid the intake of senna leaves and frangula bark. They have the effect of strongly stimulating the intestines and can lead to a disturbance of the electrolyte balance and, at worst, induce premature contractions.

Important for the Use of Chamomile

Particularly in the case of newborns, parents frequently make the mistake of applying a chamomile infusion to the child's eyes to treat conjunctivitis (pinkeye).

Chamomile should never be used on or near the eyes; the appropriate medicinal plant for this purpose is euphrasy, also called eyebright! An infusion must always be free of particles which can get caught beneath the lower eyelid and further irritate the infected eye/s.

Important for the Use of Stinging Nettle

It is frequently claimed that stinging nettle should not be used to treat oedema on account of its "beta-sitosterol" content, which supposedly promotes oedema. Beta-sitosterols are present only in the roots of the plant and are moreover not water-soluble.

BASIC PRINCIPLES OF HOMOEOPATHY

Classical homoeopathy was founded by Samuel Hahnemann (1755–1845). A pharmacist, chemist and physician, he was considered a leading scientist in his day.

The Simile Rule and the Pharmacological Picture

Samuel Hahnemann is above all famous for his simile rule:

Similia similibus curentur –
Like cures like.

This principle can be explained easily with the aid of an example:
A healthy person eats a belladonna (deadly nightshade) berry and suffers from the symptoms of poisoning which can also be experienced by an ill person who has not consumed belladonna: high fever, red head, delirium, sweating, hypersensitivity to the sun, thirst without the urge to drink a lot, etc.
Ill persons suffering from these symptoms will be helped by belladonna.

Hahnemann experimented with the mother tinctures of plants and determined that they had substantial side effects and in extreme cases could even cause death. He began diluting and potentiating the tinctures by succussing (vigorously shaking) the diluted remedy. What he discovered was that:

- In healthy persons the symptoms occurred only in a very weak form.
- In ill persons, the substance helped to cure the illness.

Hahnemann recorded the *pharmacological pictures* – the symptoms occurring in healthy persons on whom the substance was tested. The catalogue of pharmacological pictures is still being expanded today, since homoeopathy is a limitless form of empirical medicine.

The pharmacological pictures consist of so-called *guiding symptoms* and *modalities* such as:

- improvement or worsening of the symptoms
- the effects of cold and heat, activity and rest
- change of symptoms depending on time of day, season, side of body, intake of food, thirst, skin reactions, perspiration.

In homoeopathy, no diagnoses are drawn up and treated, but rather the patient is viewed as a whole.
In other words, homoeopathy is a holistic therapy which takes the patient into consideration from head to toe and with all physical and emotional symptoms. Like all naturopathically oriented holistic therapies, homoeopathy regards:

- an illness as a weakening of the vital forces
- healing as a strengthening of the vital forces.

Through the simile rule, the substance gains access to the body's blocked/ weakened forces and the mechanisms of order and defence and promotes the healing process.

Homoeopathy represents a form of active support for the body's natural healing mechanisms.

The aim is not to repress or dispel the symptoms or to counteract the illness. Homoeopathy is also referred to as a form of stimulation therapy because it stimulates the body's self-help mechanisms and harmonizes and balances body and soul.

It can also not be considered a preventive form of treatment since it should only be used when the vital forces are disturbed, i.e. an illness has developed. Pregnancy, childbirth and a postnatal process which proceed normally thus require no medication but represent entirely normal conditions in the life of a woman.

The Effects of Homoeopathic Remedies

The effects of homoeopathic remedies are governed by *Hering's Law*, which states: When the pathological process develops from the upper to the lower parts of the body and from the deepest part of the organism to the external parts, for example:

- the pregnant woman still has a feeling of nausea but no longer suffers from it
- the birthing woman is capable of performing the labour of birth again
- the feverish child calms down, its fear dissipates
- in cases of restlessness, sleep comes
- fear is replaced by a sense of confidence
- the congested nose starts running,

then the illness is taking the desired course and will be cured. In other words, if a fever is followed by a skin rash, it is a good sign. The rash should not be repressed, but permitted to take its course. The skin is the outermost layer of the body and a major excretion organ. If, however, a rash is followed by an asthma attack, the illness is taking the wrong course; the condition is worsening and should be treated (or further treated with a change in the choice of remedies) as quickly as possible.

The Production of Homoeopathic Remedies/Potentiation Techniques

In keeping with the book of homoeopathic substances, the remedies are made of plants, animals, minerals, metals and pathogens.

The potentiation of the substances is still carried out according to a method established by Hahnemann. Solid substances are ground, then mixed with a dilution substance such as lactose or alcohol at a ratio of 1:99 and potentiated by a precisely described method of pulverization in the case of lactose and succussion in the case of alcohol. By these means, the C1 potency is produced. One part of the resulting substance is then mixed with ninety-nine parts of the dilution substance to obtain the C2 potency, one part of which is mixed, in turn, with ninety-nine parts of the dilution substance to obtain C3. The process is repeated to dilutions as high as C200 and more.

In Germany, homoeopathic remedies are often produced in D potencies. To this end, one part of the initial substance is added to nine parts of the dilution substance. This first potentiation is referred to as D1, which, mixed with nine parts of the dilution substance and succussed, produces D2 and so on.

Forms of Medication and Storage Life

The remedies are available in various forms: in liquid form in water-alcohol blends referred to as *dilutions (dil.)*, in powder form as a product of pulverization on a lactose basis, referred to as *triturations (trit.)*, in pressed form as *tablets (tabl.)* and in *globuli/pills (glob.)*, tiny sucrose globuli coated with remedies in liquid form and then dried. A number of homoeopathic remedies are also available in ampules for injection.

German law rules that homoeopathic remedies can be stored for seven years, but this ruling does not correspond to the actual storage life. Many homoeopathists are of the opinion that the remedies will virtually keep forever as long as they are not exposed to X-rays or other forms of radiation. If a remedy is not effective despite confident reportorization, it should be replaced.

The Dosage of Homoeopathic Remedies

Homoeopathic remedies are apportioned in different ways by different homoeopathic therapists. For pregnant women and children, the therapist usually prescribes the most suitable substance in the form of globuli, of which two to five constitute one *dose*. The globuli are to be placed beneath the tongue or in the inside of the cheek and left to dissolve. Alternatively, five drops or one tablet are administered.

The choice of *potencies* is likewise variable. A selection must be made between high and low potencies. Your homoeopath will choose the appropriate remedy in the appropriate potency for you. The easiest way to determine the potency is by trying to ascertain whether the symptom is a purely physical one or whether mental/emotional symptoms are more in the foreground. In the case of physical discomfort it has proven best to prescribe low potencies and, conversely, if the problems are on an emotional level it is better to work with high potencies. In acute phases, either the low potency can be frequently administered, or the patient can be given a single dose of the high potency. In cases of high potencies, it is particularly important to recognize the simile correctly in order not to confuse the acute picture. For if a patient takes the wrong remedy, he or she will develop the symptoms associated with that remedy in addition to the symptoms he/she already has. This would make further homoeopathic treatment all the more difficult. Moreover, out of ignorance, pregnant women are sometimes treated with high potencies and then have no-one to turn to when they undergo a so-called "initial aggravation" of their symptoms. In many cases, the woman will now turn to allopathic measures after all, though she actually wanted to avoid them in the interest of her child's safety. Homoeopathy must be taken seriously and applied holistically, and not be sold as harmless globuli doses. Particularly pregnant women and small children react very sensitively and well to homoeopathy. For that reason, brief treatment with low potencies or a single administration of a C30 or C200 potency usually suffices.

When choosing the potency, the rule of thumb is:
the more physical the symptoms, the lower the potency
the more mental/emotional the problem, the higher the potency.
When deciding on the frequency of the administration:
the more acute the problem, the higher the potency and the more frequent its administration.

In the case of *low potencies*, i.e. under C30, the following simple dosage plan has proven effective:
The remedy is taken as often as the potency degree can be multiplied to obtain twenty-four. In other words a D/C6 dose can be taken four times in twenty-four hours, a D/C12 twice. It is recommended that pregnant women and infants be prescribed one dose fewer per day because, on account of their increased sensitivity, the healing process sets in effectively and quickly.
In the case of *high potencies*, a single dose normally suffices. If necessary, the remedy can be diluted once again in a glass of water and drunk in sips. In acute situations this procedure can be repeated. If no improvement comes about, it is necessary to check the symptoms and modalities again with all precision and consider whether perhaps a different remedy must be administered.

The intake of the remedy is to be ceased as soon as an improvement has come about. Homoeopathic remedies are often taken for too long a time – again, due to ignorance – essentially leading to the same problem that occurs when the wrong remedy is chosen: if the patient is already healed of the symptom(s) and continues to take the remedy, the effect will be to bring about those symptoms he/she just got rid of. Then it is often erroneously assumed that the homoeopathy wasn't effective.
Here I would like to point out once again that, during pregnancy, childbirth and the postnatal period, you (assuming you are a layperson with regard to homoeopathy) should never undertake any experiments with this method of treatment, and certainly never proceed on the assumption that the more you take, the better the effect. Instead, I urgently advise you to consult a health provider with training and experience in homoeopathy. And I would like to recommend to all midwives that they take the time to study the pharmacological pictures and not to learn homoeopathy exclusively from books but to attend seminars on the subject.

Homoeopathic Complexes
Contrary to the simile rule mentioned previously, various mutually enhancing remedies can be administered together in the form of a so-called complex. Well-known companies such as Weleda, Wala, Heel and Cefak manufacture such complexes, which have proven very effective.
A time-tested complex for women in the postnatel period and persons whose

strength and energy has been sapped by physical or emotional problems is my tonic "Aufbaupulver Stadelmann", available from the Bahnhof-Apotheke in Kempten, Germany. It contains the following triturations: Calcium carbonicum D3 (4g), Calcium phosphoricum D3 (6g), China D6 (2g), Ferrum metallicum D6 (10g), Ferrum phosphoricum D6 (5g), Magnesium carbonicum D6 (7,5g), Magnesium phosphoricum D6 (7,5g), Silicea D4 (6g), Stannum D6 (2g), Zincum metallicum D6 (2g) and Glucose D1 (128g). Your pharmacy may be able to obtain the "Aufbaumittel Stadelmann" for you, but be sure to compare the prices first; you may save money by ordering it directly.

Interaction with Other Medicines

In the area of phytopharmacy there are plant extracts, essential oils and other healing substances which have a strong effect and can impede the healing function of a homoeopathic remedy. For this reason, the following advice should be heeded when undergoing homoeopathic treatment:

Do not use genuine peppermint in any form, even in toothpaste, chewing gum or similar products.

Many homoeopaths are furthermore of the opinion that the consumption of coffee reduces the effect of homoeopathic remedies or even destroys it altogether. Every homoeopathic therapist will have to rely on his/her own experience on this point, although it is probably sensible to avoid such strong stimulants during homoeopathic treatment. Many homoeopathists also recommend avoiding vinegar and chamomile tea

but, here again, different people have had different experiences and it is not possible to formulate a general rule. If the simile has been chosen well, the body itself will have a sense of what does it good and send the appropriate signals – which, after all, is the aim of homoeopathic treatment.

Essential Oils and Homoeopathic Remedies

Many people are of the opinion that no essential oils can be administered during homoeopathic treatment. This point urgently requires clarification, because in obstetrics both therapies have been used simultaneously for years – successfully. Naturally, certain strong oils such as camphor, peppermint and eucalyptus should be avoided in conjunction with homoeopathy.

All other aroma-therapy essences can be used without concern during homoeopathic treatment.

Homoeopathy in Midwifery

Throughout midwifery care in the hospital as well as at home, homoeopathy has become a popular – and effective – method of helping pregnant and birthing women to undergo natural childbirth and of helping children to enter the world without the burden of allopathic medicine's many undesirable side effects.

These days if a pregnant woman wants the birth of her child to be supported homoeopathically, she is likely to be able to find a hospital in her area in which there are midwives with training in homoeopathy. Self-employed midwives who work in antenatal and postnatal care often have substantial knowledge of this healing method.

Homoeopathy should not, however, be regarded as the only effective and satisfactory medicine in the obstetrics context. In other words, it should be thought of as an effective form of care for mother and child in the areas in which it can help, and be used in conjunction with other methods which can help in other areas. If the maternal pelvis is too narrow, there are no homoeopathic remedy which can widen it. Homoeopathic and other natural healing methods should be used in such a way that childbirth becomes achievable and medicines with undesirable side effects can be avoided.

BASIC PRINCIPLES OF AROMA THERAPY

History

Essential oils were used as long ago as 3000 BC in Mesopotamia, where flowers and herbs were distilled in order to extract hydrolytes. The ancient Egyptians are also known to have used essential oils for mummifying bodies, and for healing and cosmetic purposes. In the Middle Ages, the Arabs rediscovered distillation and developed it further. Having gone through another period of neglect, aroma therapy enjoyed a revival in Western countries towards the end of the 1980s, and in more recent years it has established itself on an increasingly broad basis.

Essential Oils

Essential oils are the odoriferous substances of plants which attract insects for pollination and prevent animals from eating the plants. A plant's scent molecules protect it from extreme heat or cold. Some plants even produce essential oils with an antibiotic effect. Plants also communicate with one another via their scents.

One and the same plant may diversify the scents it produces, depending on the time of day or the season, and it can store scent molecules in its different parts in varying amounts and combinations. It is extremely important that some flowers, such as roses and jasmine, are picked at the right time of day in order to obtain as much aroma as possible before the warmth of the sun makes the plant release it into the atmosphere.

Essential oils can be found in almost all colours of the spectrum – from pale yellow through green and blue to dark brown – and their consistency ranges from watery to resinous. Fragrant substances evaporate easily and are highly flammable.

Extraction Methods

There are several methods of extracting essential oil from plants: steam distillation, cold pressing, extraction, effleurage (in exceptional cases only), and a new and expensive method of extraction using supercritical carbon dioxide.

Ingredients

Essential oils are living substances and, depending on where they are produced, their ingredients are subject to variations attributable to climate, local method of harvesting and distillation. Furthermore, the therapeutic effect of an oil cannot be measured just by demonstrating the presence of a few important main ingredients; it is necessary to consider the whole range and interaction of all the active components present in the complex mixture.

The individual substances have an extensive range of actions; their effects may be antiseptic, sedative, antiviral, hypotensive, stimulating, uplifting, antifungal, spasmolytic, expectorant, anti-inflammatory, antidepressant, immunostabilizing, diuretic, analgesic, hormonal, and they can even cause severe skin irritation, abortion or neurological damage.

How Essential Oils "Work"

Essential oils and aroma blends act on our olfactory system and are absorbed by the skin or mucous membranes. It is a recognized fact that the sense of smell is the first of the senses to develop while the embryo is in the uterus and that the embryo is capable of perceiving smells in the womb within just a few weeks of conception. The sense of smell is extremely keen between birth and the age of twelve weeks, after which it becomes weaker up until age three and then builds up again to reach its peak in a person's mid thirties; it then declines by approximately thirty percent towards old age.

By acting on our limbic system and on the mechanism for responding to stimuli, essential oils can have an effect on our bodies, create a feeling of well-being and enhance the healing process. Scent molecules are transported within minutes via the bloodstream into the blood, metabolized and then excreted within a few hours. When administering aroma therapy, it is therefore important to work only with naturally pure substances. Whether essential oils enter the human body through inhalation, the skin or, less commonly, by ingestion, the mechanism for identifying them always functions by way of the sense of smell. This must be borne in mind with every therapy.

The pharmaceutical aspect is often neglected. Precisely because fragrant essences are highly concentrated and contain a large number of different active ingredients, the proven healing properties of essential oils should not be underestimated. Therapies with fragrant oils, bath agents and ointments should therefore only be administered by persons with a basic grounding in aroma therapy or, better still, expert knowledge of the field.

Quality and Purity

Only pure essential oils have healing properties! Because poor quality or adulterated products are available on the world's markets, quality must always take priority over quantity when carrying out aroma therapy.

The following detailed information on the label will help you when purchasing products:

- English and Latin plant names
- Country of origin
- Type of cultivation: controlled organic cultivation)/Demeter = Demeter cultivation/collected from natural environment/conventional cultivation
- Details on part of plant processed
- Extraction method: steam distillation/CO_2-distillation/cold pressing/effleurage/alcohol extraction/hexane distillation (= absolute)
- Batch number: enables the user to trace the origin of the oil from the supplier's bottling date right back to the farm of harvest
- Expiry date or bottling date
- Warnings regarding possible dangers of accidental ingestion

Quality Control

It is not sufficient to test essential oils and mixtures of essential oils for therapeutic use simply by smelling them, and it is not possible to use physical tests to examine with certainty whether oils have been contaminated, falsified or tampered with. Chemical analysis is therefore the only method which can verify all of the ingredients. When testing the quality of essential oils, it is certainly true to say: trust in a product is all very well, but close inspection is better.

Pharmacopoeia Quality
Any chemist can easily obtain the few essential oils listed in the *European Pharmacopoeia* (Ph. Eur.). Since the quality of these oils complies with legal requirements, they are approved for the manufacture of therapeutic blends. If a chemist chooses to use these monographed oils and requests the official inspection certificates from the manufacturer, he saves himself the trouble of having to carry out his own costly investigations. However, this small collection of just fifteen monographed DAB- or Ph.-Eur.-approved oils is not sufficient for in-depth aroma therapy. What is more, it is not possible to carry out holistic treatment with these oils because details of their cultivation and production methods are not taken into account and there is accordingly no guarantee that they are of the best quality.

Nature-Identical Essential Oils
However authentic they may smell, synthetic fragrances contain very few significant therapeutic ingredients and are therefore of little or no use at all. Aroma therapists describe these oils as dead substances since they are not extracted from plants. Again and again, allergies have been linked with nature-identical and synthetic fragrances.

Storage and Shelf Life
All essential oils should be stored in dark bottles at room temperature between approximately 18°C and 20°C/ 65°F and 68°F. After use, the bottles must be sealed again immediately to prevent the essential oil from evaporating. The quality of the oil could change as soon as the oxygen content in the bottle increases. Not only oxygen, but also light can cause chemical processes to occur in the oils which can lead to changes in their quality and efficacy. Please take note of the "use-by" date printed on the label.
Bear in mind that essential oils must be kept out of the reach of children!

Applications and Dosage
These nine golden rules will help you to carry out aroma therapy in a holistic manner and to ascertain the correct proportion of the oil you have selected.
With regard to the person being treated, the rules are:
> *the younger – the more sparing*
> *the lighter – the less*
> *the more sensitive – the less*
> *the older – the more frequent*

With regard to the person's condition, the rules are:
> *the greater the pain – the more oil*
> *the more chronic the symptoms – the longer the treatment*

With regard to the amount of essential oil, the rules are:
> *the fresher the scent – the more*
> *the more precious the fragrance – the more sparing*
> *the heavier the oil – the less*

Treatment is continued for as long as a

fragrance is pleasing to the nose and the body responds positively. If it fails to please, or if the body no longer has the need for it, the therapy is discontinued – intuition tells us quite clearly whether a specific treatment should be carried out more frequently or not.

Essential Oils in Midwifery

Since a feeling of well-being is conducive to relaxation, raises the pain threshold and has a positive effect on the vegetative nervous system, it stands to reason that there are many uses for soothing oils in midwifery. Drugs should be used as little as possible during pregnancy and childbirth to prevent undue strain on the baby and, above all, to convey the message to the mother that she herself is capable of giving birth. This is exactly what aroma therapy can achieve in pregnancy and childbirth. Mothers also enjoy pleasantly fragrant baths and massage oils to aid recovery and wound-healing in the postpartum period.

Aroma Lamps

Several factors, such as the quality of the lamp, the size of the room and the number of people in it, all influence how effective essential oils are when used in an aroma lamp. If the lamp is to be used for therapeutic purposes, then it should be borne in mind that the essential oil will affect all persons present. Aroma lamps made of various materials are available; the heat source is provided by either a candle or a light bulb. Make sure that there is sufficient space between the heat source and the water

bowl and that the water bowl is the correct size. It is also important to ensure that the oil lamp bowl is cleaned regularly.

The aroma lamp casing should be designed in such a way that there is no risk of fire. For safety reasons, naked candles may not be used in clinical areas under any circumstances. Although electric aroma lamps are more expensive, they are more durable and also more economical because the temperature always remains constant.

Duration of use: It suffices to have a lamp burning for about one hour, during which time the aroma molecules can evaporate and fill the room.

It is best to refrain from refilling the lamp with essential oils for the next eight hours.

Dosage: A smaller number of drops is required for creating general well-being than for treating cases of physical discomfort.

In a room measuring approximately 25 m²/82 sq. ft. with a ceiling 2.50 m/ 8 ft. 3 in. high, for example, three to four drops of the *Original D®* *Aroma Blend Entbindungsduft/Childbirth Aroma* are sufficient to create a sensual aroma for a few pleasant hours, or for childbirth.

Just one single drop of pure essential rose oil, or five drops of rose oil diluted in 10% jojoba wax, are sufficient to create a wonderful rose fragrance in the room. For a common cold, ten drops of *Erkältungsöl wärmend/Common-Cold Warmth Oil D®* are needed for a room of the same size. However, if there are any young children or pregnant women in the room, the dose of essential oil must be cut in half. If a room is to be made fragrant and has very small children in it – i.e. between one and three years of age – then just a quarter of the usual dose is used.

It is important always to start with a small number of drops because another one or two drops can easily be added if the room is not fragrant enough.

Body Oils

Fragrant oils must always be combined with an emulsifier, such as a fatty plant oil, in order to take effect via the skin. The higher the unsaturated fat content of the basis oil and the warmer the skin, the more quickly absorption takes place. The essential oil usually takes effect in the body within a few minutes. As a general rule, essential oils together with their fatty basis oil are fully absorbed by the skin within approximately one hour, and after about ninety minutes they have been completely metabolized.

Duration of use: A sick person's current metabolic condition must be taken into consideration; usually, two treatments per day are sufficient. However, if the person is suffering from pain lasting over a period of hours and the metabolic rate is raised, as when suffering from labour pains or gastro-enteritis, more regular treatments via the skin will be both desirable and necessary.

Dosage: The following rough guidelines should be followed when making up one's own compositions of essential oils in fatty basis oils:

Body oil should contain a maximum dose of one percent essential oil, i.e. a maximum of 0.5 ml essential oil may be added to 50 ml of fatty plant oil; this is between seven and fifteen drops, depending on the essential oil.

Massage oil may contain up to ten percent essential oil which is the equivalent to a maximum of 5 ml, or between 30 and 150 drops, of essential oil per 50ml. In most cases, five percent essential oil is sufficient.

Therapeutic oil, e.g. for the treatment of pain, may contain as much as thirty percent essential oil. This means that 3 ml, or between 30 and 90 drops, may be added to 7 ml of plant oil. This highly alcoholic blend may only be used for a short period, or preferably for just one treatment.

The following rule of thumb applies to aroma therapy just as it does to all areas of natural medicine:

Less is more!

Baths

Bathing in essential oils is a very pleasant and effective form of aroma therapy. It has the advantage that the essential oil can take effect through the entire surface area of the skin. It is important to note that essential oils should never be added undiluted to the bath water but must be mixed with a suitable, pure vegetable emulsifier such as honey, dairy cream, neutral soap, whey or salt.

Dosage: Between three and fifteen drops are added to a bathtub full of water. It is also important to consider whether the purpose of the bath is purely sensual or to treat tension or pain, and whether it is for an adult, a pregnant woman or a child.

Pregnant women and children should be given no more than half, babies and toddlers just one third of the amount specified above!

Washes

Sick patients in particular benefit from washing with essential oils if they are bedridden or only able to get up for brief periods. The gentle stimulation of the skin helps to strengthen the immune system, revive the circulation and bring the vegetative nervous system into harmony. This is a good way of treating circulatory problems, fatigue or exhaustion and insomnia.

Dosage: The chosen essential oil must be mixed with an emulsifier before being added to the water for washing. One to two drops of essential oil are usually sufficient. When washing sick children, one drop is enough, for adults five drops of essential oil is the maximum to be used.

The quickest way to release essential oils or blends thereof in water is with a small amount of soap. The oils can also be combined with a teaspoon of vinegar; this has a particularly pleasant effect on patients suffering from fever because it accelerates evaporation and at the same time boosts the skin's protective acidity.

Wraps and Compresses

Make sure that you always have the necessary equipment on hand. Ursula Uhlemayr's "Wickel & Co." dressing kits are a practical way of always having everything at the ready. They are available at the Bahnhof-Apotheke Kempten, and similar kits can also be found in health food shops or obtained from health-product mail-order companies.

Additives such as onions, potatoes, lemons, healing earth, quark and essential oils make wraps (also known as "packs") and compresses more effective. These Kneipp applications help to strengthen the body's defence system, enhance cardiovascular functions and stimulate the body's detoxification mechanism. Do not leave children unattended and observe them for allergic reactions. Remove the wrap if there are signs of discomfort. Wraps can be reapplied depending either on the symptoms of the ailment or on the decision of the patient, who can usually tell whether he/she feels any benefit.

Temperature: The wrap may be cold or warm, depending on the needs of the patient. In cases with acute symptoms, such as inflammation or fever, it is usually preferable to apply a cooling wrap to extract heat. Moist warm wraps are far more effective than dry warm applications. They improve circulation and are used to relieve cramps and tension. Wraps made with ingredients from the kitchen should be applied at room temperature at least or, preferably, at body temperature.

Dosage: Because the wrap has several layers, the essential oil cannot easily evaporate outwards and works through the skin with a sustained, long-lasting effect. Pure essential oils must always be mixed with an emulsifier; for wet wraps salt water is best (1 teaspoon of salt to 1 litre/quart of water). Depending on the age and sensitivity of the patient, use between one and seven drops of oil, or, alternatively, massage the affected area with the appropriate *Original D® Aroma Blend* oil and then apply the wrap.

Curd cheese/quark is an excellent cure for inflammatory conditions such as mastitis and phlebitis. Make a sufficient amount to cover the body surface with a ratio of one tablespoon of quark to one or two drops of essential oil or the corresponding amount of an *Original D® Aroma Blend*. The quark is then spread onto a cotton or linen cloth or made into a wrap and applied to the affected area.

Duration: Depending on how comfortable the patient feels, an exposure time of between half an hour and a maximum of one hour is usually sufficient.

Compresses and Wound Dressings

For the treatment of wounds, the appropriate essential oil or *Original D® Aroma Blend* should be sprinkled onto a moistened, sterile wound dressing.

Duration: In cases where symptoms and pain are acute, the dressing may be applied repeatedly at short intervals of approximately one hour; if treatment is to be carried out over a longer period the dressing may be renewed twice daily. When treating wounds, it is always essential to seek expert advice or consult a doctor.

In the clinical area, any suitable essential oil can be worked into the usual wound irrigations, dressings or creams. *Rose-Teebaum-Essenz/Rose-Tea-Tree Essence D®* can also be sprinkled onto air-permeable dressings and compresses at short intervals to begin with and then twice daily. No more than one to five drops of essential oil should be used, depending on the size of the wound.

Please note that fresh oils in their pure form, such as lavender extra and tea-tree oil, are suitable only for short-term use, i.e. one to two days. If they are to be used over a long period, all oils, including the two already mentioned above, must be mixed with a fatty oil or worked into creams from the second, or at the latest, the third day of treatment, because even these skin-friendly oils will eventually cause irritation. As soon as new skin has formed over the wound, the healing process can be helped along with a fatty plant oil such as St John's Wort oil.

Fatty Plant Oils

Cold-pressed oils extracted from the seeds and fruits of olive, almond, hazel, walnut, jojoba and macadamia plants or from rose hip, black caraway, wheat and evening primrose are gentle to the skin and have healing properties. The same applies to macerates such as aloe-vera oil and arnica, marigold, and St. John's Wort oil.

Quality, Storage and Shelf Life

High quality fatty plant oils are available on the market. Oils gained from the first cold pressing are the only ones to be used for therapy and body care because they are high in unsaturated fatty acids. Fat soluble essential oils are easily absorbed when mixed with fatty oils and penetrate into the deeper layers of the skin. From there, they are taken up by the smallest capillaries and thus enter the blood stream. This process varies according to the area of skin involved and also depends on body temperature. The warmer and more delicate the skin, the more relaxed the muscles are and the more quickly the blood flows, so that the active ingredients of the fatty and essential oils quickly reach the person's circulation and are metabolized more rapidly.

Basis oils which are particularly high in monounsaturated and polyunsaturated fatty acids are very good for the skin; some of them even aid epithelialisation and regeneration and are especially useful for treating wounds. If cold-pressed plant oils are used, the skin remains permeable and is nourished, thus helping skin problems to improve.

It is important to ensure that, to the extent possible, the basis/carrier oils used are extracted from plants grown according to controlled organic methods. This is the only way to guarantee that oil used for massage and skin care is residue-free; otherwise, highly toxic substances such as pesticides, insecticides or heavy metals bind easily with fatty substances and can enter the human body through the skin.

Basis oils have high levels of unsaturated fatty acids and therefore only keep for a limited length of time. These acids, also known as essential fatty acids, react to oxygen, causing the oil to become rancid. The more nourishing the oil, or the richer it is in unsaturated fatty acids, the shorter its shelf life will be. As a general rule you should check every fatty plant oil to see whether it is rancid, even if it supposed to keep for another six months. The shelf life of the individual plant oils always depends on the storage method.

The way in which a plant oil is stored determines how long it can be used once it has been opened.

As soon as the bottle is in regular use it should be smelt before each application to check whether the fatty oil smells unpleasant, decomposed or rancid.

Fatty plant oils which have become rancid should no longer be administered, whether externally or internally. The change is caused mainly by oxygenation, as a result of which free radicals accumulate, which are harmful to health.

In order to prevent changes from occurring prematurely, plant oils should be stored in dark bottles in a cool dry place. Direct light facilitates the oxidation process and should therefore be avoided. The amount needed for use should be taken from a larger storage bottle, or the oils should be bought in small quantities.

Refined Plant Oils

Although these are described as plant oils, they are extracted mechanically. Having been bleached, deodorized and supplemented with solvents, colourings and vitamins, these so-called "user-friendly", tasteless, artificially scented, long-lasting oils are introduced onto the market. Refined fatty oils do not contain any unsaturated fatty acids because the latter are destroyed in the refining process.

Paraffin Oils – Vaseline

I strongly wish to draw your attention to the fact that these are poor quality oils. These cheap oils, manufactured from petroleum, can be described as dead oils. Paraffin oils are present in vast quantities in products sold by the baby industry but it is almost impossible to absorb them through the skin, let alone make use of them, and so they are simply stored in the body. Vaseline, the "dry matter" gained from this crude oil product, blocks the pores and, at best, acts as a water-barrier or protects against freezing in winter.

Interaction with Other Medicinal Products and Contraindications

The strongest contraindication to using an essential oil or blend is that one's own nose has an aversion to it. If the oil smells unpleasant – even if there are no other indications that it should not be used – to be on the safe side, it is nevertheless best not to use it.

In the following section, specific oils and their areas of use are explained. Because these oils are only present in small amounts in the *Original D® Aroma Blends*, their effects are less problematic and, what is more, when the oils themselves are purchased, special care is taken to ensure that they contain the smallest possible quantities of the ingredients which may cause complications. *Original D® Aroma Blends* contain no preservatives or chemical additives and you can therefore be sure that they are of the best untreated natural quality.

Pregnancy

Camphor, eucalyptus and peppermint oils may not be used during pregnancy because they may cause premature contractions. The following oils are particularly unsuitable for pregnant women: basil, verbena, ginger, cardamom, clove, oregano, cypress and cinnamon, since they likewise stimulate contractions. Lavandin, rosemary, ravintsara,

hyssop and thyme thymol oils all have a hypertensive effect and should only be used after consulting a midwife or doctor with aromatherapy experience. If the blood pressure is too low, it is best to avoid lavender extra, marjoram, clary sage, nard and ylang ylang.

Infants and Young Children

Scents should not in fact be used at all near infants, since they may irritate the nose and inhibit bonding. It is therefore best to use essential oils on babies for therapeutic purposes only; for example, in order to stimulate digestion, the essential oils of cumin, fennel, aniseed and coriander can be added to massage oils if necessary.

Above all, oils with extremely fresh and stimulating aromas, such as eucalyptus, peppermint, rosemary, sage and lemon, should not be used on small children. Strong-smelling substances such as camphor and menthol are generally associated with the risk of respiratory arrest and glottal oedema.

For this reason, these substances should never be applied directly onto or near an infant's nose. These active ingredients, which are mainly found in eucalyptus and peppermint oil, are not used at all in the Original D® *Aroma Blends for Children*.

Oils Unsuitable for Sunbathing and in Cases of Allergy

When using body oil containing citrus oils, French verbena, lemon balm, angelica root or yarrow, it is best not to expose the skin to the sun for four hours following application because these oils can increase the skin's sensitivity to light and cause so-called light spots and pigment disorders. These spots may reappear as soon as the area of skin is exposed to the sun again, a phenomenon which can continue for a few months or, in some cases, for the rest of the affected person's life. The same applies to fatty St.-John's-Wort oil. Some substances, however, have not yet been sufficiently researched in this respect and many of the warnings relating to herbal medicine have simply been adopted, although this does not necessarily mean that they actually apply to the particular essential oils. I know for a fact that many of my fragrant blends do not cause any problems, even though they contain ingredients which, according to the textbooks, aggravate the skin. As always, it is the dosage which turns a substance into a poison.

Photosensitizing oils can also cause skin irritation in persons with allergies. All people with sensitive skin should therefore observe the following: first, carry out a skin test by applying the essential oil mixed with a little fatty oil to the crook of the arm and let it take effect for about ten minutes or longer. If it causes itching or blistering, refrain from using this oil. The same applies for any aroma blend.

Oils Unsuitable for Persons Suffering from Epilepsy or Asthma

Persons suffering from chronic diseases should be cautious with all substances. For them in particular, it is absolutely necessary to smell the bottle of essential oil first. When doing this, epileptics and asthmatics should ensure that they hold the bottle at an appropriate dis-

tance from the nose. On no account must they use rosemary, camphor, sage or hyssop. Fennel and aniseed oils may be used with caution, if their content have been checked beforehand, as is the case with the *Original D*® *Aroma Blends*.

Counteractive Measures

If, in spite of the precautions taken, skin reactions do occur, the therapy must be discontinued immediately. The next measure is to wash well with soap and take a purgative to speed up metabolism and excretion. A cup of strong coffee helps the metabolic process.

If essential oil has made its way into the eyes, they must be rinsed profusely under running water. It is then essential to seek medical advice.

Homoeopathy and Aroma Therapy

The extent to which these two forms of therapy exclude or complement one another is frequently discussed. It is an undisputed fact that camphor should not be used directly in combination with any homoeopathic medicine. The same applies to all essential oils similar to camphor, such as eucalyptus and all types of mint.

Apart from these exceptions, the two fields of medicine combine well with each other.

Creating Blends

If individual prescriptions are made up by a chemist, it is sufficient to check the basic ingredients according to the laws governing the operation of pharmacies in the country in question. If blends are manufactured in advance, certain conditions must be met before they are put into use. In Germany, for example, these conditions are laid down in the AMG (= Arzneimittelgesetz/German Drug Law) for medications, in the respective regulations for cosmetics and in the LMBG (= Lebensmittel-, Bedarfsgegenstände- und Futtermittelgesetz/Foodstuffs, Consumer Goods and Animal Feed Law) for aroma oils not intended for direct use on humans. It is not only necessary to carry out the relevant investigations, but also to examine all documents relating to approval and registration, such as toxicological certificates, etc. Failure to attend to these matters at the outset could result in inspections being carried out by pharmaceutical advisory bodies, visits from the government inspection agency, or, at a later date, liability issues.

Therapists who make their own blends for patients bear full liability for the whole range of risks – from intolerance to reflex respiratory arrest – because no insurance company will cover for the unauthorized manufacture of drugs (formulae used for therapy are automatically classified as drugs).

This applies as a basic rule for all categories, irrespective of whether they are aroma oils or teas.

Original *D*® Aroma Blends

The fragrance of each blend will always depend on the quality of the individual oils and the particular manufacturing companies, and it will alter with each year's new harvest.

For that reason, I deliberately do not give any details of measurements, because I have often heard of treatments supposedly failing, or skin irritation occurring, if blends have been prepared by a different chemist or with essences from other firms. So many plagiarists have made bad copies of my *Original D*® *Aroma Blends*, presumably in order to lower costs, by using fewer drops of oil or by using poorer quality essential oils. As a result, the fragrance is different and, not surprisingly, the effect is altered. I hope that you will understand my decision not to publicize the formulae for my blends in order to protect you and my blends from plagiarists whose interests are presumably purely market-oriented.

Be very wary of blends made by other manufacturers and chemists, because in most countries they are legally permitted to work with oils which only have to meet minimum requirements rather than be of the best quality. Emphasize that you require oils which are one hundred percent pure and make sure that they are of the best quality. The regular laboratory tests carried out during storage and production at the Bahnhof-Apotheke Kempten prove that it is worth one's while to be rigorously cautious.

The quality stamp on bottles of *Original D*® *Aroma Blends* is your guarantee that they contain oils of the highest quality. The aroma blends are produced under my supervision at the Bahnhof-Apotheke Kempten. I value this teamwork with the Bahnhof-Apotheke very highly and would like to ask all the chemists and companies who make requests, sometimes very forcefully, for details on my formulae, to respect this. There is only one chemist with whom I am able to carry out this intensive and well-researched work.

We select the essential oils together on the basis of our own analytical laboratory procedures. As an example, the amount of α-thujone (a type of ketone) found in samples from suppliers can vary by between four and forty-eight percent in genuine sage oil or, by contrast, by between just zero and four percent in lavender oil. When purchasing, we choose the most suitable oil for our blends by looking for the best possible combination of all the active ingredients and the fragrance.

I would like to take this opportunity to express my thanks to the pharmacist, Mr Wolz. On numerous occasions I have come to realize that the success of such excellent, straightforward teamwork between midwife and pharmacist cannot just be taken for granted.

Our dedication to working for the Forum Essenzia e.V. is another way in which we try to further the cause of essential oils and to pass on our knowledge and experience in order to promote the use of aromas.

A MIDWIFE'S CARE FOR MOTHER AND CHILD

Facts about the Work of the Midwife

Pregnancy

During your pregnancy, the midwife plays an important role as your specialist advisor and you should make sure that you contact her at an early stage. You may see her in her practice, she can make a home visit or you can phone her for advice.

The midwife has the following responsibilities:

- to offer personal advice with regard to
  - healthy living
  - medical examinations which need to be carried out
  - sexuality and partnership
  - preparing for your baby
  - social benefits available to expectant mothers
- to give advice on pregnancy-related complaints
- to carry out antenatal check-ups
- to hold antenatal classes.

Childbirth

The midwife is an independent practitioner responsible for the management of any normal labour and birth, whether it is a

- home birth: responsibility for labour, birth and postpartum period at home
- independent birthing centre birth: responsibility for birth in the independent birth centre and for the postpartum period at home
- out-patient delivery: responsibility for birth in hospital and postpartum period at home
- hospital birth: responsibility for birth and the initial postpartum period in hospital.

The midwife will use her specialist knowledge to support and accompany you through all stages of pregnancy, childbirth and the postpartum period. She will observe, examine and keep records on your condition and that of your child. The midwife will help you to start breastfeeding and she will carry out the first check-ups on your baby.

The Postnatal Period

In Germany every mother has the right to daily visits from a midwife for the first ten days following the birth of her baby. This right remains valid even after she has been discharged from hospital. If complications arise, visits may continue until the end of the postnatal period or until breastfeeding has finished. Therefore, if you wish, you can be cared for by a midwife in your own home.

Postnatal care includes:

- observation of the baby's development
- help and advice on the healing and care of the umbilical cord, problems with wind, latching onto the nipple and neonatal jaundice
- taking blood samples to test for metabolic disorders
- observation of the postpartum moth-

er's progress and of involution of the uterus (return to normal size and position)

- help in dealing with breast engorgement, cracked and sore nipples, retention of the lochia, digestive and other problems
- active help with breastfeeding
- practical guidance on infant care
- information on bottle feeding, the prevention of allergies, routine check-ups and family planning.

Midwives offer courses on postnatal exercises, pelvic floor exercises and baby massage.

They also offer support and advice to parents in difficult situations, for example if their child is sick or stillborn, or has died after birth.

What parents ought to know:
- The midwife is an expert practitioner.
- The midwife works in accordance with the legal guidelines relating to midwifery in the country in question.
- The midwife seeks medical help if there are any deviations from the normal course of events.
- In Germany, midwifery costs are covered by the health insurance system.
- Find out about midwifery services in the country where you live. For up to date information, consult the internet pages of the respective midwives' associations (see below).

Information is also available in Germany from all
- regional midwives' associations

- health authorities
- family educational institutions, or ask your own doctor for information.

Helpful Addresses for the German-Speaking Countries (see Internet for addresses of midwives' associations in English-speaking countries)

Bund Deutscher Hebammen e.V.
Postfach 17 24
76006 Karlsruhe
Tel.: +49 (0)721 / 98 18 90
Fax: +49 (0)721 / 981 89 20
E-Mail: info@bdh.de
www.bdh.de

Bund freiberuflicher Hebammen Deutschlands e.V.
Kasseler Str. 1a
60486 Frankfurt
Tel.: +49 (0)69 / 79 53 49 71
Fax: +49 (0)69 / 79 53 49 72
E-Mail: geschaeftsstelle@bfhd.de
www.bfhd.de

Schweizerischer Hebammenverband
Rosenweg 25 C, Postfach
3000 Bern 23
Tel.: +49 (0)31 / 332 63 40
Fax: +49 (0)31 / 332 76 19
E-Mail: info@hebamme.ch
www.hebamme.ch

Österreichisches Hebammengremium
Postfach 4 38
1061 Wien
Tel./Fax: +43 (0)1 / 597 14 04
E-Mail: oehg@hebammen.at
www.hebammen.at

Further helpful addresses:

Arbeitsgemeinschaft Gestose Frauen
e.V.
This organization provides information
on Pre-eclampsia and its treatment.
Kapellener Str. 67a
47661 Issum
Tel.: +49 (0)2835 / 26 28
Fax: +49 (0)2835 / 29 45
E-Mail: info@gestose-frauen.de
www.gestose-frauen.de

Bundeszentrale für gesundheitliche
Aufklärung (BZgA)
Offers a highly informative and recom-
mendable brochure on the subject of
antenatal diagnostics
51101 Köln
Tel.: +49 (0)221 / 89 92-0
Fax: +49 (0)221 / 89 92-300
E-Mail: order@bzga.de
Download: http://www.bzga.de/bzga_
stat/pdf/13625100.pdf

FORUM ESSENZIA e.V.
Non-profit association for the promo-
tion and protection of aroma therapy
and aroma care, aroma culture
Kotterner Straße 81
87435 Kempten
Tel.: +49 89 7145391
E-Mail.: info@forum-essenzia.org
www.forum-essenzia.org

Initiative REGENBOGEN
»Glücklose Schwangerschaft« e.V.
A contact group for parents who have
lost a child before, during or after
childbirth
c/o Renate Dreier
Westring 100
33378 Rheda-Wiedenbrück
Tel.: +49 (0)5242 / 352 97
E-Mail: HGST@initiative-regenbogen.
de
www.initiative-regenbogen.de

Gesellschaft für Qualität in der außerklinischen Geburtshilfe (QUAG) e.V.
Federation of German midwives' associations for the documentation and
quality management of extraclinical
births
c/o Anke Wiemer
Elisabethenstr. 1
63579 Freigericht
Tel./Fax: +49 (0)6055 / 5781
E-Mail: geschaeftsstelle@quag.de
www.quag.de

Verwaiste Eltern in Deutschland e.V.
Help for mothers, fathers, siblings,
grandparents in mourning and persons
accompanying them
c/o Christine Fleck-Bohaumilitzky
Eichenstr. 14
85232 Bergkirchen-Lauterbach
Tel./Fax: +49 (0)8135 / 87 06
E-Mail: kontakt@veid.de
www.veid.de

Zentralverband der Ärzte für Natur-
heilverfahren und Regulationsmedizin
(ZÄN) e.V.
The oldest and largest physicians' asso-
ciation for natural healing methods
Am Promenadenplatz 1
72250 Freudenstadt
Tel.: +49 (0) 74 41 / 9 18 58-0
Fax: +49 (0) 74 41 / 9 18 58-22
E-Mail: info@zaen.org
www.zaen.org

SUPPLIER REFERENCES

Wickel & Co.®

The wraps and compresses recommended in the book can be obtained from the Bahnhof-Apotheke Kempten (address see below) in ready-to-use sets in various sizes for children and adults. These sets are manufactured from high-quality, natural textiles by Ursula Uhlemayr in the Allgäuer Werkstätte.

Natural Textiles

Natural baby and children's clothing, nappies and related products, crib/bassinette textiles, breastfeeding cushions and animal skins are available from

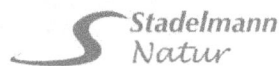

Stadelmann Natur

Stadelmann Natur
An der Schmiede 1
87487 Wiggensbach
+49 8370 209069
www.stadelmann-natur.de

Essential Oils and Aroma Blends
Original D® Aroma Blends

The aroma therapy products described in the book are manufactured with the assistance of the author in the
Bahnhof-Apotheke Kempten
Bahnhofstr. 12
87435 Kempten
+49 831 5 22 66 11
info@bahnhof-apotheke.de
www.bahnhof-apotheke.de
The *Original D® Aroma Blends* and essential oils of other firms (Primavera, farfalla, Wadi) can be ordered directly from those firms and obtained in all German pharmacies.

In Switzerland, the *Original D® Aroma Blends* can be obtained from
Farfalla Essential AG
Florastr. 18
CH-8610 Uster
Tel. 0 44 - 905 99 00
www.farfalla.ch

Primavera®-Aromaprodukte can also be ordered directly from
Primavera Life GmbH
Naturparadies 1
D-87466 Oy-Mittelberg
Tel. 08366-8988-0
Fax 08366-8988-4099
info@primaveralife.com
http://www.primaveralife.com

Further Products for Pregnancy, Breastfeeding and the Postnatal Period.

In addition to the *Original D® Aroma Blends* the following products mentioned in the book are likewise available from Bahnhof-Apotheke Kempten:

- "Aufbaumittel Stadelmann"
- homoeopathic remedies
- original tea blends by Ingeborg Stadelmann
- natural silk maternity pads
- wool/silk breast pads
- hygiene articles
- silk dolls
- amber necklaces with/without teething stone
- orrisroot
- practical guides/literature

The Author

Ingeborg Stadelmann (b. 1956), independent midwife and mother of three children, is co-founder of the midwives' practice "Erdenlicht" in Kempten and was active in midwifery care at home for many years. Her primary concern in the practice of her profession is the holistic care of pregnant women and mothers. To this end, aside from classical homeopathy, Ingeborg Stadelmann made comprehensive and successful use of the methods of aroma therapy.

For several years, the author has been exclusively involved with the supplementary training of midwives and nurses (including those specializing in elderly care) as well as with adult education. She holds lectures and seminars on the subjects of natural obstetrics, herbal medicine, homeopathy and aroma therapy throughout the German-speaking areas.

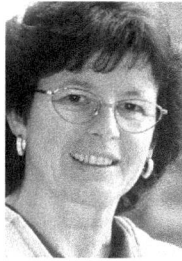

In 2004, Ingeborg Stadelmann was awarded the Diamond Brooch of Honour by the Bayerischer Hebammenverband (Bavarian Midwives' Association). In 1999 she received the "Goldener Apfel" from the women's association Kempt'ner Frauenliste for her services as a midwife and initiator of the "Erdenlicht" independent birthing centre.

Her most recent projects include the aroma and medicinal plant garden on the Burghalde in Kempten (Allgaeu, Germany), which she initiated jointly with the pharmacist Dietmar Wolz. The garden was opened in July 2005.

More information on Ingeborg Stadelmann can be found at www.stadelmann-verlag.de

ACKNOWLEDGEMENTS FOR THE FIRST EDITION

Here I would like to extend my thanks to all the persons who assisted me in the "birth" of this book - first and foremost all the children who were born into my hands. Through them, I had the opportunity to gather experience and knowledge. I would like to thank all parents who allowed me to accompany them during the births of their children. I would like to let the mothers know that I not only shared their labour pains and all of their feelings with them, but also experienced great strength in the countless hours I spent attending to births. The power and energy produced by birthing women gave me the staying power I needed for this book. During the book's nine-month pregnancy, the weeks of its birth and the subsequent afterpains of the initial proofreading, I felt strongly connected to the women I attended to during that phase. It really did take me nine months and six weeks to write the manuscript and prepare the book form printing.

The act of passing the manuscript on to the copy editor and the publisher was like placing my confidence in the midwife and concluding the postnatal period. I even had to undergo a postnatal "down" with my book and come to the realization that I would have to raise the "child" myself. For a number of well-known publishing companies, the book was too comprehensive and too "user-unfriendly". I was told I would have to wait until 1995/96. That was too long; it was not how I had envisioned things. After friends helped me find a copy editor and a book designer, there was no longer any obstacle to publishing the book myself. Now, exactly a year after its birth, the book will appear in print. My heartfelt thanks go to you, dear Klaus, for your editing work and the nocturnal hours you devoted to my book. Dear Julia, thank you for your untiring efforts in the production of the book. Torill, I am particularly happy to have made your acquaintance. I am very happy that your Norwegian perspective is eternalized in my book. I would bet anything that your little secret helped you in the creation of these artworks.

I am especially indebted to all those who had to do without me during the period in which the book was coming into being, above all my family, the pregnant women who were disappointed not to find me at "Erdenlicht" as expected or as usual.

My fellow midwives were a huge support; they stood by me with lots of perseverance and took over on my midwifery duties without a word of complaint. Thank you, dear Brigitte and dear Elisa; you were indispensable helpers.

Gisela became a friend and great help to me, indefatigably and attentively correcting my many spelling, typing and grammar errors in the manuscript to the very end. The comments supplied by Vera were an important aid for the first trial reading.

In the process of creating this book, the collaboration with you, Dietmar, was – as always – proved to be a pleasant, happy and irreplaceable help. I am highly indebted to you for putting your extensive knowledge at my service and answering my questions with constant patience.

I would furthermore like to mention Dr. Friedrich Graf, who – with his confirmations and seminars – not only gave me knowledge about homoeopathy but also the courage to stick it through in homebirths. ("Maybe one day you will come to appreciate the aroma essences too, Friedrich – the feminine counterpart to your masculine homoeopathy.")

Thanks to all the women who encouraged me to write this book.

And my heartfelt appreciation to my dear colleague Frauke for the critical corrections of the second edition, the production of which went smoothly despite a certain amount of excitement that accompanied it.

Thank you, Joachim, for your assistance.

Ermengerst 1995

ACKNOWLEDGEMENTS FOR THE NEW EDITION

I would hereby like to express my thanks to all the persons who contributed to this newly revised and designed edition of my book. My sincere thanks go to all who wrote to me, communicating their suggestions and requests. And I am especially grateful to you, dear Marina, for putting my letters and words in order in your reliably consistent manner. God bless you, my dear "Erdenlicht" colleagues, for telling me your thoughts on the new edition, and especially you, Gabi, for your critical reading of the manuscript. I cannot even conceive of writing and publishing a book without your help, Johanna, and I thank you for your sincere friendship. Torill, I thank you as well; with you it was a fast and uncomplicated decision as to how the design could be improved.

The collaboration with the Kosel printing press was as good as ever, even if Joachim wasn't there for the revision. But you, Martin, put a lot of effort into acquainting yourself with the subject.

My special thanks go as well to the people who taught, encouraged and accompanied me on my naturopathic path. Without teachers there would be no students, and without diligent hands there would be no high-quality natural products. Thank you, Friedrich, for your enormous knowledge, which you have now made available to us midwives in books you likewise publish yourself. It gives me great pleasure that we not only went the same route in founding publishing houses, but – especially – that you refer to my *Original $\mathcal{D}^{\circledR}$ Aroma Blends* in your books and grant them the place they deserve alongside homoeopathy. Maybe one day we will find the time to take a closer look at the similarities between aroma and homoeopathic medicine. I would furthermore like to acknowledge Ute Leube and Gian Furrer and their teams. Your information from the world of essential oils is just as important as the exchange of views and experience with all the experts at the association Forum Essenzia. United we are strong, and it is my great hope that, through our efforts, essential oils will continue to be available in genuine quality for many generations, despite the political difficulties. But it is you, Dietmar, to whom I am indebted for the fact that these oils are available in optimal, ready-to-use form – and all of your perfectly trained and knowledgeable employees. It takes many little parts to form something complete and whole!

Finally, I owe my heartfelt thanks to my children, who are already investing their efforts into continuing the alliance already begun and feeding it with new energy. As always, I would also like to thank my family for the sacrifices they made while I was writing the manuscript and taking such affectionate care of me in my office. Thank you, Konrad, for making it possible for me to devote myself to my "hobby" – writing – even during holidays, and for tolerating my passion – the work in the pharmacy with Dietmar – without a word of objection.

Ermengerst 2005

BIBLIOGRAPHY

Obstetrics/Midwifery

Aas, Kjell: Das allergische Kind. Thieme, Stuttgart 1981

Balaskas Janet: Aktive Geburt. Kösel, München 1993

Balaskas, Janet: Natürliche Schwangerschaft. Mosaik, München 1990

Berg, Dietrich: Schwangerschaftsberatung und Perinatalogie. Thieme, Stuttgart 1972

Body Shop Team: Mamatoto. Verlagsgesellschaft, Köln 1992

Geist, Christine (Hrsg.): Hebammenkunde. de Gruyter, Berlin 1995.

Davis, Elizabeth: Das Hebammen-Handbuch. Kösel, München 1992

Fedor-Freybergh, Peter G.: Pränatale und perinatale Psychologie und Medizin. Saphir, Älvsjö 1987

Goeschen, Klaus: Kardiotokographie-Praxis. Thieme, Stuttgart 1980

Grospietsch, Gerhard: Erkrankungen in der Schwangerschaft. Wissenschaftliche Verlags-Gesellschaft, Stuttgart 2000

Hertl, Michael: Kinderheilkunde und Kinderkrankenpflege für Schwestern. Thieme, Stuttgart 1979

Kitzinger, Sheila: Geburt ist Frauensache. Kösel, München 1993

Kitzinger, Sheila: Natürliche Geburt. Kösel, München 1991

Kitzinger, Sheila: Schwangerschaft und Geburt. Kösel, München 1982

Kleinebrecht, Jürgen/Fränz, Jürgen/Windorfer, Adolf: Arzneimittel in der Schwangerschaft und Stillzeit. Wissenschaftliche Verlags-Gesellschaft, Stuttgart 1986

Leboyer, Frédérick: Geburt ohne Gewalt. Kösel, München 1991

Leboyer, Frédérick: Fest der Geburt. Kösel, München 1985

Leboyer, Frédérick: Die Kunst zu atmen. Kösel, München 1983

Leboyer, Frédérick: Sanfte Hände. Kösel, München 1983

Lippens, Frauke: Geburtsvorbereitung. Staude, Hannover 1992

Lothrop, Hanni: Das Stillbuch. Kösel, München 1993

Lothrop, Hanni: Gute Hoffnung Jähes Ende. Kösel, München 1992

Mändle, Christine/Opitz-Kreuter, Sonja/Wehling, Andrea: Das Hebammenbuch. Schattauer, Stuttgart 1995

Martius, Gerhard: Hebammenlehrbuch. Thieme, Stuttgart 1990

Martius, Gerhard: Lehrbuch der Geburtshilfe. Thieme, Stuttgart 1974

Martius, Gerhard: Geburtshilfliche Operationen. Thieme, Stuttgart 1971

Odent, Michel: Erfahrungen mit der sanften Geburt. Kösel, München 1986

Odent, Michel: Die sanfte Geburt. Kösel, München 1979

Ploil, Oja: Frauen brauchen Hebammen. Aleanor, Nürnberg 1991

Pschyrembel Klinisches Wörterbuch. 259. Aufl. de Gruyter, Berlin 2002

Pschyrembel, Willibald/Dudenhausen, Joachim W: Praktische Geburtshilfe. de Gruyter, Berlin 1991

Schindele, Eva: Gläserne Gebärmutter. Fischer, Frankfurt 1990

Schneider, Ernst: Nutze die Heilkraft unserer Nahrung. Saatkorn, Hamburg 1978

Sichtermann, Barbara: Leben mit einem Ungeborenen. Fischer, Frankfurt 1991

Thews, Gerhard/Mutschler, Ernst/Vaupel,

Peter: Anatomie, Physiologie, Pathophysiologie des Menschen. Wissenschaftliche Verlags-Gesellschaft, Stuttgart 1999.

Herbal Medicine

Eberwein, Eva/Vogel, Günther: Arzneipflanzen in der Phytotherapie. Kompendium gemäß Monographien der Kommission E. Kooperation Phytopharmaka, Bonn 1990.

Fischer, Susanne: Blätter von Bäumen. Hugendubel, München 1991

Fischer, Susanne: Medizin der Erde. Hugendubel, München 1991

Gehrmann, Beatrice: Arzneidrogenprofile für die Kitteltasche. Deutscher Apotheker-Verlag, Stuttgart 2000

Madaus, Gerhard: Lehrbuch der biologischen Heilmittel. Band 1–11. Mediamed, Ravensburg 1990

Pahlow, Mannfried: Das große Buch der Heilpflanzen. Gräfe und Unzer, München 1993

Uhlemayr, Ursula: Wickel & Co. Urs-Verlag, Burgberg 2003

Van Wyk, Ben-Erik/Wink, Coralie/Wink, Michael. Handbuch der Arzneipflanzen. Wissenschaftliche Verlags-Gesellschaft, Stuttgart 2004

Weiss, Rudolf Fritz: Lehrbuch der Phytotherapie. Hippokrates, Stuttgart 1985

Wichtl, Max (Hrsg.): Teedrogen und Phytopharmaka. Wissenschaftliche Verlags-Gesellschaft, Stuttgart 2002

Willfort, Richard: Gesundheit durch Heilkräuter. Tranner, Linz 1959

Homoeopathy

Boericke, William: Homöopathische Mittel und ihre Wirkungen. Verlag Grundlagen und Praxis, Leer 1986

Braun, Artur: Methodik der Homöopathie. Sonntag, Stuttgart 1992

Charette, Gilbert: Homöopathische Arzneimittellehre. Hippokrates, Stuttgart 1985

Coulter, Catherine: Portraits homöopathischer Arzneimittel. Haug, Heidelberg 1988

Eichelberger, Otto (Hrsg.): Kent-Praktikum. Haug, Heidelberg 1984

Friedrich, Edeltraud/Friedrich, Peter: Charaktere homöopathischer Arzneimittel. Traupe, Höhenkirchen 2004

Graf, Friedrich: Homöopathie und die Gesunderhaltung unserer Kinder und Jugendlichen, Sprangsrade Verlag, Sprangsrade 2003

Graf, Friedrich: Homöopathie in der Geburtshilfe, Sprangsrade Verlag, Sprangsrade 2001

Graf, Friedrich: Ganzheitliches Wohlbefinden. Homöopathie für Frauen. Herder, Freiburg 1994

Graf, Friedrich: Homöopathie für Hebammen und Geburtshelfer. Teil 1 mit 7. Staude, Hannover 1990

Hahnemann, Samuel: Organon der Heilkunst. Haug, Heidelberg 1986

Imhäuser, Hedwig: Homöopathie in der Kinderheilkunde. Haug, Heidelberg 1987

Kent, James T.: Arzneimittelbilder. Haug, Heidelberg 1990

Kent, James T.: Repertorium I, II, III. Haug, Heidelberg 1989

Köhler, Gerhard: Lehrbuch der Homöopathie. Band 1 u. 2. Hippokrates, Stuttgart 1988

Schlüren, Erwin: Homöopathische Frauenheilkunde und Geburtshilfe. Haug, Heidelberg 1987

Stadelmann, Ingeborg: Homöopathische Haus- und Reiseapotheke. Stadelmann Verlag, Ermengerst 2004

Vermeulen, Frans: Kindertypen in der

Homöopathie. Sonntag, Regensburg 1988

Vithoulkas, George: Die wissenschaftliche Homöopathie. Burgdorf, Göttingen 1986

Wiesenauer, Markus: Gynäkologisch-geburtshilfliche Praxis. Hippokrates, Stuttgart 1987

Yingling, W. A.: Handbuch der Geburtshilfe. O-Verlag, Berg 1985

Aroma Therapy

Carle, Reinhold: Ätherische Öle. Wissenschaftliche Verlags-Gesellschaft, Stuttgart 1993.

Gildemeister, Eduard/Hoffmann, Friedrich: Die ätherischen Öle. Akademie-Verlag, Berlin 1968.

Franchomme, Pierre/Jollois, Roger/Pénoël, Daniel: L'aromathérapie exactement. Ed. Roger Jollois, Limoges 1990.

Stadelmann, Ingeborg: Bewährte Aromamischungen. Mit ätherischen Ölen leben, gebären, sterben. Stadelmann Verlag, Ermengerst 2003

Stadelmann, Ingeborg: Aromatherapie von der Schwangerschaft bis zur Stillzeit. Stadelmann Verlag, Ermengerst 2005

Zimmermann, Eliane: Aromatherapie für Pflege- und Heilberufe. Sonntag, Stuttgart 2002

Index

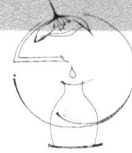

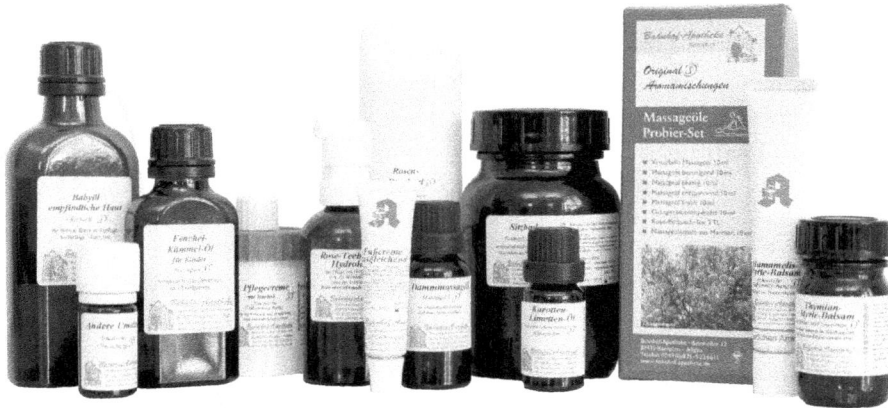

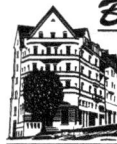

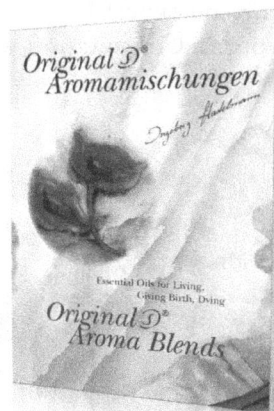